General Anesthesia: New Evidence and New Challenges

General Anesthesia: New Evidence and New Challenges

Editor: Mercy Rogers

MURPHY & MOORE
www.murphy-moorepublishing.com

www.murphy-moorepublishing.com

MURPHY & MOORE

Cataloging-in-Publication Data

General anesthesia : new evidence and new challenges / edited by Mercy Rogers.
p. cm.
Includes bibliographical references and index.
ISBN 978-1-63987-795-9
1. Anesthesia. 2. Anesthetics. I. Rogers, Mercy.
RD81 .G46 2023
617.96--dc23

Murphy & Moore Publishing
1 Rockefeller Plaza,
New York City,
NY 10020, USA

ISBN 978-1-63987-795-9

Contents

Preface

Anesthesia is a state that is characterized by a temporary loss of sensation and awareness. It facilitates the execution of painful medical procedures that can cause severe distress and pain to the patient. Anesthesia is classified into three categories, namely, general anesthesia, sedation and local anesthesia. General anesthesia involves putting the patient into a medically induced coma. It can be administered either intravenously or can be inhaled by the patient. The types and degree of anesthesia vary depending upon the medical procedure to be performed. These drugs have a variety of effects on the body such as loss of consciousness, loss of reflexes on the autonomic nervous system, and amnesia. This book aims to shed light on some of the unexplored aspects of general anesthesia and the challenges in its administration. From theories to research to practical applications, studies related to all contemporary topics of relevance to this type of anesthesia have been included herein. This book is appropriate for students seeking detailed information in this area of medicine as well as for experts.

The information contained in this book is the result of intensive hard work done by researchers in this field. All due efforts have been made to make this book serve as a complete guiding source for students and researchers. The topics in this book have been comprehensively explained to help readers understand the growing trends in the field.

I would like to thank the entire group of writers who made sincere efforts in this book and my family who supported me in my efforts of working on this book. I take this opportunity to thank all those who have been a guiding force throughout my life.

Editor

Comparison of the effect of sevoflurane or propofol anesthesia on the regional cerebral oxygen saturation in patients undergoing carotid endarterectomy

Sanghee Park[1], Keunbae Yook[1], Kyung Yeon Yoo[1], Jeong Il Choi[1], Hong-Beom Bae[1], Youngwook You[1], Baoyuan Jin[1,2] and Seongtae Jeong[1,2*]

Abstract

Background: The monitoring of regional cerebral oxygen saturation (SrO_2) using near-infrared spectroscopy is useful method to detect cerebral ischemia during. Sevoflurane and propofol decrease cerebral metabolic rate ($CMRO_2$) in a similar manner, but the effects on the cerebral blood flow (CBF) are different. We hypothesized that the effects of sevoflurane and propofol on SrO_2 were different in patients with deficits of CBF. This study compared the effect of sevoflurane and propofol on SrO_2 of patients undergoing cerebral endarterectomy (CEA).

Method: Patients undergoing CEA were randomly assigned to the sevoflurane or propofol group ($n = 74$). The experiment was preceded in 2 stages based on carotid artery clamping. The first stage was from induction of anaesthesia to immediately before clamping of the carotid artery, and the second stage was until the end of the operation after clamping of the carotid artery. Oxygen saturation (SrO_2, SpO_2), haemodynamic variables (blood pressure, heart rate), respiratory parameters (end-tidal carbon dioxide tension, inspired oxygen tension), concentration of anesthetics, and anesthesia depth (bispectral index score) were recorded.

Results: During stage 1 period (before carotid artery clamping), the mean value of the relative changes in SrO_2 was higher ($P = 0.033$) and the maximal decrease in SrO_2 was lower in the sevoflurane group compared with the propofol group ($P = 0.019$) in the contralateral (normal) site. However, there is no difference in ipsilateral site (affected site). SrO_2 decreased after carotid artery clamping and increased after declamping, but the difference was not significant between two groups. Changes in mean arterial blood pressure was lower in sevoflurane group than propofol group after the carotid artery declamping ($P = 0.048$).

Conclusion: Propofol-remifentanil anesthesia was comparable with sevoflurane-remifentanil anesthesia in an aspect of preserving the SrO_2 in patients undergoing carotid endarterectomy.

Keywords: Carotid endarterectomy, Regional cerebral oxygen saturation, Near-infrared spectroscopy, Propofol, Sevoflurane

* Correspondence: anesjst@jnu.ac.kr
[1]Department of Anesthesiology and Pain Medicine, Chonnam National University Medical School and Hospital, 42 Jebong-ro, Dong-gu, Gwangju 61469, South Korea
[2]The Brain Korea 21 Project Center for Biomedical Human Resources, Chonnam National University, Gwangju, South Korea

Background

Carotid endarterectomy (CEA) is a useful surgical treatment for reducing the cerebral infarct risk in patients with carotid artery stenosis [1]. Ischaemic brain injury is one of the most severe complications of CEA, caused by cerebral hypoperfusion during temporary carotid artery clamping [2]. Cerebral hyperperfusion syndrome is also a critical, rare complication [3]. Monitoring of cerebral blood flow is essential to prevent these complications; however, continuous monitoring throughout the entire period of CEA is not easy [4].

Monitoring of the regional cerebral oxygen saturation (SrO_2) using near-infrared spectroscopy (NIRS) is a non-invasive method to observe the oxygen balance of the brain. SrO_2 determined by arterial oxygen saturation, cerebral blood flow (CBF), haemoglobin and cerebral metabolic rate ($CMRO_2$) reflect the balance of oxygen supply and demand of brain tissue [5]. Previous studies indicated that it is possible to detect the changes in CBF and predict the occurrence of cerebral ischaemia by monitoring of SrO_2 [5–8]. Furthermore, monitoring of SrO_2 using NIRS is suggested to be a useful method to detect brain ischaemia during CEA [7].

Sevoflurane and propofol are common agents used to maintain general anaesthesia in CEA. Both agents decrease the $CMRO_2$ in a similar manner, but the effects on the CBF are different. CBF changes in parallel to the $CMRO_2$—a decrease in $CMRO_2$ is accompanied by a decrease in CBF, and vice versa. However, sevoflurane per se has a vasodilatory effect and increases the CBF at concentrations > 1 MAC (minimal alveolar concentration). Thus, CBF is abundant compared with $CMRO_2$ [9, 10]. Meanwhile, propofol has no vasodilatory effect; it decreases the CBF as $CMRO_2$ is reduced. [9] Moreover, the reduction of CBF exceeds that of $CMRO_2$ by propofol, resulting in a decrease in the CBF/$CMRO_2$ ratio [11, 12]. There have been several reports that the brain oxygen balance is well maintained in sevoflurane anaesthesia compared with that induced by propofol [13–15].

Recent studies measuring cerebral oxygen saturation using NIRS showed higher oxygen saturation in sevoflurane anaesthesia than that induced by propofol [16, 17], suggesting that sevoflurane is better than propofol to maintain the cerebral oxygen balance. However, in these studies, the patients had neither cerebral vascular disease nor deficit of CBF, and the CBF was preserved with both agents from the viewpoint of clinical safety.

In the present study, we hypothesized that the effects of sevoflurane and propofol on SrO_2 in patients undergoing CEA with deficits of CBF, were different compared to those without any CBF deficits. The primary outcome of the study was the comparison of the effects of sevoflurane and propofol on SrO_2 in patients undergoing CEA with deficits of CBF. Secondary outcome was the occurrence of any neurologic or hemodynamic deterioration.

Methods

This prospective randomized controlled trial was approved by the institutional ethics committee of our institution (CNUH-2015-159) and registered in the ClinicalTrials.gov (NCT02609087). After receiving the written informed consent, 74 patients (age, 19–80 years) scheduled to undergo CEA under general anaesthesia were randomly allocated into the sevoflurane group or propofol group by a pre-assembled list generated at random using Excel program. The exclusion criteria were patients with American Society of Anesthesiologists (ASA) physical status ≥4 with low cardiac function, anemia, end-stage renal disease, patients who were low oxygen saturation with pulmonary disease, both carotid artery stenosis, and other neurological disease not related to carotid artery disease. This study was conducted in accordance with the Consolidated Standards of Reporting Trials (CONSORT) 2010 statement [18].

General management

Patients were given triazolam (Halcion®; Pfizer Korea, Seoul, Korea) for anxiolysis 1 h before arriving in the operating room. After arrival in the operating room, 5-lead electrocardiography, pulse oximetry, and non-invasive automatic blood pressure cuff and end-tidal capnography were implemented for basic monitoring. To assess the depth of anaesthesia, BIS® A-2000™ (Aspect Medical Systems, Natick, MA, USA) was attached to the forehead, and an INVOS®5100B cerebral oximeter using NIRS (Somanetics, Troy, MI, USA) was applied for monitoring of SrO_2. The two probes were placed at the forehead just above the bispectral index score (BIS) probe facing the medial margin of the other. For continuous blood pressure monitoring (Deltran; Utah Medical Products, Midvale, UT, USA) and to obtain samples for arterial blood gas analysis, a 20-gauge catheter was placed in the radial artery after local anaesthetic infiltration. TOF-watch®SX (Organon Ireland Ltd., Swords, Co. Dublin, Ireland) was used to measure the acceleration of the adductor pollicis muscle as a means of monitoring proper muscle relaxation.

In the sevoflurane group, general anaesthesia was induced by infusion of remifentanil (Ultiva®; GlaxoSmithKline Manufacturing; San Polo di Torrile, Italy) using a target-controlled infusion (TCI) pump (Orchestra Base Primea®; Fresinius, Brezins, France) at a target concentration of 3 ng/dL with bolus injection of 1.5 mg/kg of propofol (1% Anepol®; Hana Pharmaceutical Co., Seoul, South Korea). After confirmation of the loss of consciousness by testing the eyelid reflex, 0.6 mg/kg of rocuronium bromide (Esmeron®; MSD, Kenilworth, NJ, USA) was given for muscle relaxation. A facemask and manual ventilation were applied until adequate sedation (BIS < 60) and muscle relaxation (TOF count 0) were achieved. Endotracheal intubation was then performed. General anaesthesia was maintained with 50% O_2 at 3 L/min with sevoflurane (Sevofran®; Hana Pharmaceutical Co.), with adjustment of the sevoflurane concentration to maintain a BIS value of 40–50. In the propofol group, anaesthesia induction and maintenance were performed by continuous infusion and changing the concentration of propofol (Fresofol MCT®; Fresinius Kabi, Granz, Austria) with remifentanil at a concentration of 3 ng/dL using a TCI pump. After endotracheal intubation, controlled ventilation was established at a tidal volume of 7 mL/kg and rate of 12/min with $FiO_2 = 0.5$, and end-tidal carbon dioxide ($ETCO_2$) was maintained between 35 and 40 mmHg by respiratory rate control.

If mean arterial blood pressure (MAP) decreased by < 55 mmHg or was ≥25% of the baseline value, or the systolic arterial pressure dropped below 90 mmHg [19], 100 μg of phenylephrine was injected for correction. Dopamine was infused when hypotension was sustained despite proper anaesthetic depth or if an inotropic agent was required after vessel clamping. If the operator requested, 12.5–25 mg of diluted indocyanine green (Indocyanine Green®; Dongin-Dang Pharmaceuticals; Seoul, Korea) was added. At the end of the operation, total infused fluid volume, blood loss, urine output, anaesthesia time, operation time, and vessel clamping time were assessed.

Cerebral oxygen saturation and haemodynamics record

This study was divided into two stages. The first stage was from induction of anaesthesia to immediately before carotid artery clamping, and the second stage was from carotid artery clamping to the end of surgery. Before induction of anaesthesia, the basal levels of blood pressure, heart rate, oxygen saturation, BIS, and SrO_2 in room air were recorded. When haemodynamic stability was established with mechanical ventilation ($FiO_2 = 0.5$) after induction of anaesthesia, blood pressure, heart rate (HR), oxygen saturation, BIS and SrO_2 were recorded (post-induction baseline). At 1-min intervals, blood pressure, HR, oxygen saturation, BIS, SrO_2, ET_{CO2}, anaesthetic concentrations, type and dosage of inotropic agent were assessed after skin incision for 10 min. These values were then recorded every 5 min before carotid artery clamping. After clamping and declamping of the carotid artery, the values were recorded every 1 min for 10 min, including maximal decrease after carotid artery clamping and maximal increase after declamping of SrO_2. The recording interval was then returned to 5 min.

Statistical analysis

Previous studies in patients free of cerebrovascular disease showed maximal decreases in SrO_2 of 9.6% ± 7.7% in the sevoflurane group and 4.2% ± 7.0% in the propofol group. Student's *t*-test (2-tail) was performed using the G-power program to calculate the sample size showing the difference of maximal decrease between the two groups (effect size = 0.7338623) and 34 patients per group were required to achieve adequate power ($P = 0.05$; $\beta = 0.8$) to detect a difference. Considering possible dropout, 37 patients were enrolled per group. Patients' characteristics and intraoperative variables were analysed using Student's *t*-test or Pearson's chi-square test. Changes in SrO_2 were analysed using Student's t-test. Continuous variables, including SrO_2, BIS, blood pressure and heart rate, were analysed by repeated measures analysis of variance (ANOVA) with time as a within-subject repeated measure and the group as a between-subject variable. Statistical analysis was performed using the IBM SPSS Statistics version 20 statistical package (IBM, Chicago, IL, USA). All data are expressed as means ± standard deviation. In all analyses, $P < 0.05$ was taken to indicate statistical significance.

Results

Among the 74 patients initially included in the study, 2 patients (1 in the sevoflurane group and 1 in the propofol group) with low SrO_2 (pre-induction basal value < 50%) and 2 patients in the propofol group that showed sustained hypotension or arrhythmia intraoperatively were excluded (Fig. 1). Patients' characteristics including gender, weight, and height, were similar in both groups. There were no significant differences in intraoperative total fluid administration, blood loss, or urine output between the groups (Table 1). There were no significant differences in preoperative values of SrO_2, arterial blood pressure, peripheral arterial oxygen saturation, or heart rate between the groups (Table 2). The mean concentrations of intraoperative anaesthetic agents were 1.36 ± 0.19 Vol% for sevoflurane and 2.53 ± 0.37 μg/mL for propofol. The mean remifentanil concentrations were 2.16 ± 0.62 ng/mL in the sevoflurane group and 2.87 ± 1.0 ng/mL in the propofol group; the difference was not significant.

Changes from the pre-induction period until carotid artery clamping

SrO_2 increased significantly in both groups after induction of anaesthesia compared with baseline ($P < 0.001$ in the sevoflurane group and $P = 0.012$ in the propofol group). However, there was no difference in the change in SrO_2 between the groups (Fig. 2a). The mean value of the relative change in SrO_2 was higher ($P = 0.033$) and the maximal decrease in SrO_2 was lower in the sevoflurane group compared with the propofol group ($P = 0.019$) in the contralateral site. However, there is no difference in ipsilateral site (affected site) (Table 3). MAP, HR and BIS were similar from induction until 30 min after skin incision, and there were no differences between the groups (Fig. 2).

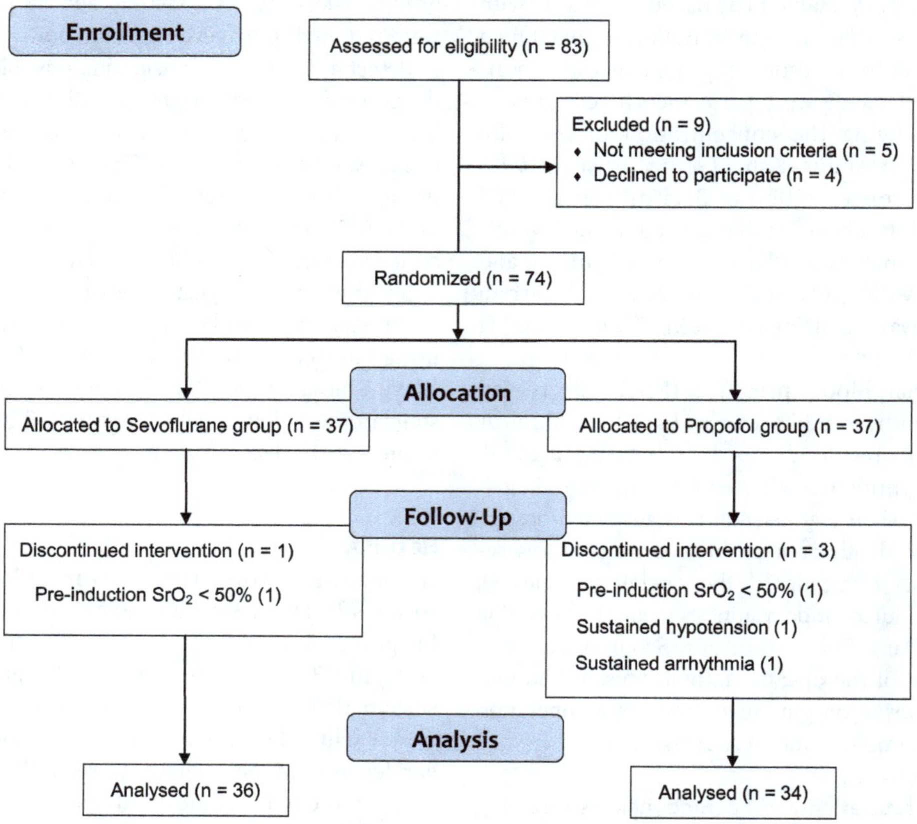

Fig. 1 CONSORT flowchart showing the flow of patients through the trial

Table 1 Patients Characteristics and Intraoperative Variables

	Sevoflurane ($n = 36$)	Propofol ($n = 34$)	P value
Sex (Male/Female)	31/5	27/6	0.562
Age (yrs)	69 ± 8	67 ± 7	0.212
Height (cm)	163 ± 7	164 ± 7	0.322
Weight (kg)	64 ± 10	66 ± 10	0.513
Hemoglobin (g/dL)	12 ± 1	13 ± 1	0.273
Underlying diseases			
Hypertension	30	24	0.413
DM	13	15	0.389
Total anesthesia time	181 ± 29	174 ± 26	0.914
Total operation time	161 ± 19	158 ± 17	0.806
Artery clamping time	39 ± 8	38 ± 10	0.401
Fluid administered (mL)			
Crystalloid	1412 ± 377	1618 ± 441	0.069
Colloid	338 ± 218	256 ± 237	0.201
Bleeding (mL)	90 ± 42	116 ± 72	0.159
Urine (mL)	577 ± 279	762 ± 400	0.109

Values are mean ± SD or numbers

Changes from cardioid artery clamping until the end of surgery

SrO_2 decreased significantly after carotid artery clamping in both groups ($P < 0.001$), but there was no difference between the two groups (7.6% ± 4.8% in the sevoflurane group vs. 7.6% ± 5.3% in the propofol group, $P = 0.857$) (Fig. 3a). After carotid artery declamping, SrO_2 increased significantly, but there was no difference between the two groups (10.0% ± 11.3% in the sevoflurane group vs. 11.8% ± 10.2% in the propofol group, $P = 0.473$) (Fig. 3a). The change in MAP was significantly lower in the sevoflurane group than the propofol group after declamping of the carotid artery ($P = 0.048$) (Fig. 3b). There was no difference in heart rate and BIS score between groups (Fig. 3c and d).

SrO_2 decreased by > 20% of baseline during surgery in one patient in the sevoflurane group and in five patients in the propofol group, but the differences between groups were not statistically significant ($P = 0.06$). The SrO_2 of five patients (three in the sevoflurane group and two in the propofol group) fell below 50%. In the pre- and post-carotid artery periods, SrO_2 decreased by > 20% in two patients. Mild stroke occurred in two patients at postoperative follow-up (one in the propofol group and one in the sevoflurane group), and the SrO_2

Table 2 Baseline hemodynamic and oximetry values

	Sevoflurane ($n = 36$)	Propofol ($n = 34$)	P value
SrO_2 (%)-Ipsilateral	64.2 ± 5.7	66.0 ± 5.9	0.074
SrO_2 (%)-Contralateral	64.1 ± 7.6	67.4 ± 9.2	0.096
SpO_2 (%)	97 ± 2	97 ± 2	0.407
Mean arterial pressure (mmHg)	103 ± 16	110 ± 20	0.092
Heart rate (beats/min)	66 ± 12	70 ± 17	0.222

Values are mean ± SD. SrO_2 = regional cerebral oxygen saturation; SpO_2 = peripheral arterial oxygen saturation

decreases in each patient were assessed: 18% of basal level and 26% of pre-clamping period in a patient in the propofol group; 11% of basal level and 18% of pre-clamping level in a patient in the sevoflurane group. SrO_2 increased sharply, > 20% of basal level, after reperfusion in one patient in the sevoflurane group; however, no neurological disorders were found.

Continuous infusion of dopamine was required for maintenance of MAP in the majority of patients, and there were no differences in dopamine dosage or vasopressor requirements.

Discussion

Regional cerebral oximetry using NIRS is a non-invasive method to evaluate the balance between cerebral oxygen supply and cerebral tissue oxygen demand [20]. SrO_2 indicates the percentage of oxygenated and deoxygenated haemoglobin detected by near-infrared irradiation at two

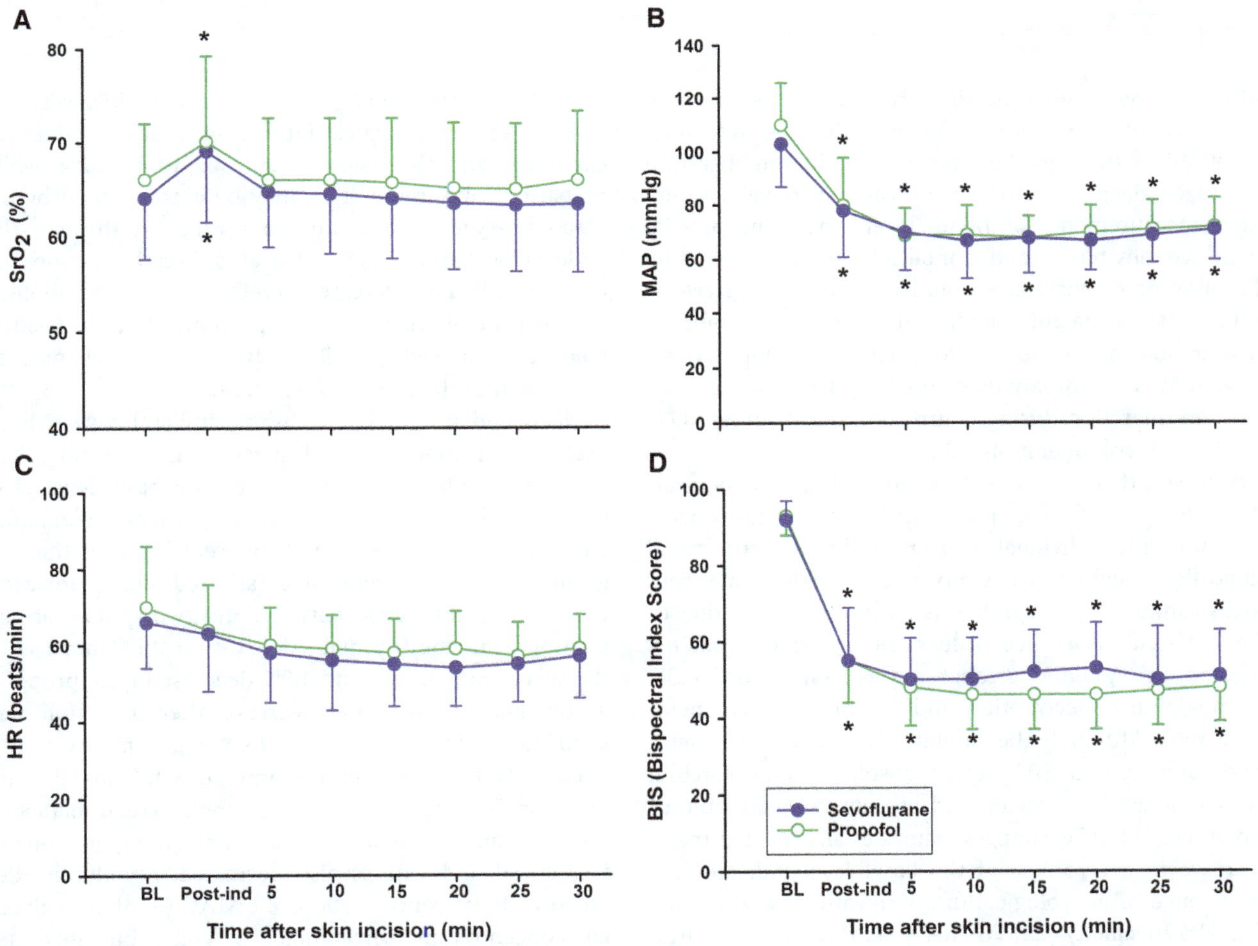

Fig. 2 Changes from the pre-induction period until carotid artery clamping. Changes in (**a**) regional cerebral oxygen saturation (SrO_2), (**b**) mean arterial pressure (MAP), (**c**) heart rate (HR), and (**d**) Bispectral index score (BIS) before carotid artery clamping. BL = baseline before anesthesia induction; Post-ind = post-induction. Groups: Sevoflurane = anesthesia with sevoflurane and remifentanil; Propofol = anesthesia with propofol and remifentanil. Data are expressed as mean ± standard deviation. *$P < 0.05$ vs Baseline in each group

Table 3 SrO_2 Values in before arterial clamping

	Sevoflurane ($n = 36$)	Propofol ($n = 34$)	P-value
Ipsilateral			
Mean SrO_2 (%)	63.9 ± 6.6	65.3 ± 6.4	0.452
Minimum SrO_2 (%)	61.8 ± 6.6	63.1 ± 7.1	0.407
Mean value of relative changes in SrO_2			
compare to baseline (%)	1.3 ± 8.0	− 1.6 ± 8.0	0.237
Relative maximum decrease in SrO_2 (%)			
compare to baseline	3.3 ± 8.8	4.8 ± 9.7	0.504
compare to post-induction	9.9 ± 6.2	8.1 ± 6.2	0.250
Contralateral			
Mean SrO_2 (%)	67.1 ± 7.5	67.3 ± 6.9	0.452
Minimum SrO_2 (%)	66.3 ± 8.0	66.3 ± 7.1	0.992
Mean value of relative changes in SrO_2			
compare to baseline (%)	9.1 ± 20	−1.9 ± 22	0.033
Relative maximum decrease in SrO_2 (%)			
compare to baseline	−3.9 ± 10.1	0.7 ± 10.5	0.019
compare to post-induction	4.4 ± 3.7	6.6 ± 5.1	0.038

Values are mean ± SD. SrO_2 = regional cerebral oxygen saturation

different wavelengths passing through the skull. The near-infrared irradiation used for NIRS shows high penetrability through the scalp and skull, and therefore can reach deep brain tissue for cerebral oxygen saturation measurements of tissue layers including arterial blood, venous blood, and frontal lobe tissue supplied by the anterior cerebral artery and middle cerebral artery. NIRS is a convenient, rapid, non-invasive and continuous method that is superior to other monitoring devices; as such, it is commonly used to monitor cerebral ischaemia and infarction during neuro- or cardiac surgery [21] and in high-risk operations [22].

However, there are limitations for NIRS, such as localised reflection of oxygen saturation only in focal areas and large interindividual differences due to extracranial blood flow including the scalp. The numerical data from NIRS cannot be interpreted as simple numbers due to the different reference values in individual patents affected by systemic arterial oxygen saturation, CBF, haemoglobin concentration and cerebral oxygen metabolic rate. Although the limitations restrict the assessment of recorded SrO_2 as an absolute value, cerebral ischaemia can be detected and prevented by continuous monitoring of SrO_2 changes. Samra et al. reported that a decrease in $SrO_2 > 20\%$ of the basal level indicates the occurrence of neurological disorder with 80% sensitivity and 82% specificity [23]. Michel et al. reported that NIRS can recognise cerebral ischaemia during carotid artery clamping in CEA patients with 80% sensitivity and 94% specificity, and it is 6.5 min faster than the somatic-evoked potential [24].

In the present study, SrO_2 increased rapidly with induction and endotracheal intubation until carotid artery clamping, and then slowly returned to baseline while preparing for surgery. This may be accompanied by increased oxygen supply due to ventilation through the endotracheal tube ($FiO_2 = 0.5$) after breathing room air ($FiO_2 = 0.21$) and decreased cerebral oxygen metabolism due to general anaesthesia. A previous study in healthy volunteers showed a similar pattern of SrO_2 changes to those seen in the present study [25].

Mean and minimal SrO_2 were similar between both groups from induction and incision until carotid artery clamping. SrO_2 was influenced by the basal level ($P <$ 0.001), and average values of SrO_2 change compared with the basal level were not different between the two groups at the ipsilateral side (affected side). However, there was a difference between the two groups at the contralateral side (normal side), with a 9.1% increase in the sevoflurane group and 1.9% decrease in the propofol group, and the maximal decrease after induction was significantly different between the two groups.

The effects of sevoflurane and propofol on CBF are different. Both agents decrease cerebral oxygen metabolic rate by a similar amount and, as a result, oxygen demand is reduced and CBF is also decreased. Sevoflurane decreases CBF at concentrations < 1 MAC (minimum alveolar concentration; sevoflurane = 2 Vol%) but increases CBF at concentrations > 1 MAC [9, 26], which are thought to be due to the cerebral vasodilation effects of sevoflurane and cerebral autoregulation [27, 28]. Meanwhile, propofol decreases CBF in a dose-dependent manner [12, 29].

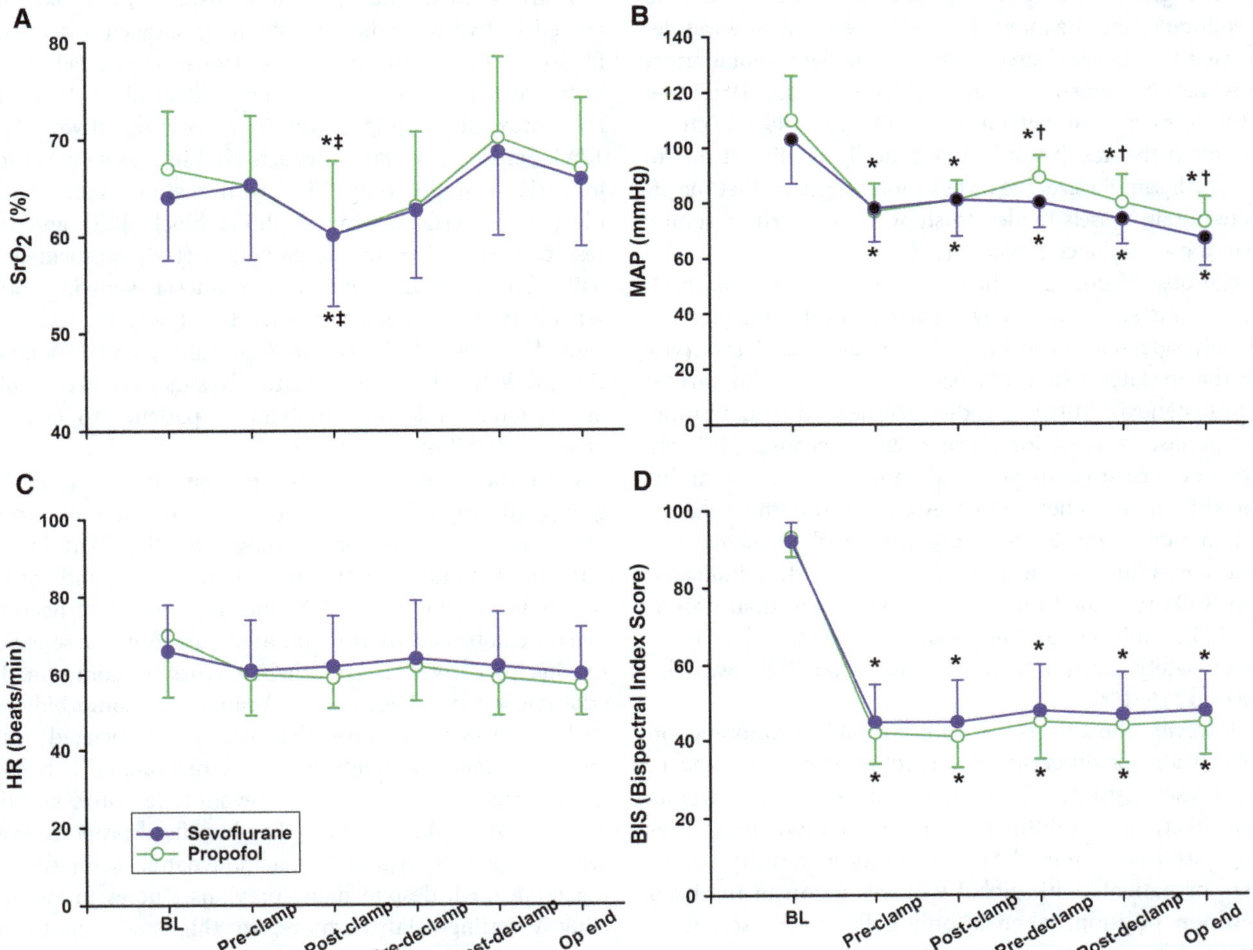

Fig. 3 Changes from carotid artery clamping until the end of surgery. Changes in (**a**) regional cerebral oxygen saturation (SrO_2), (**b**) mean arterial pressure (MAP), (**c**) heart rate (HR), and (**d**) Bispectral index score (BIS) from cardioid artery clamping until the end of surgery. BL = baseline before anesthesia induction; Pre-clamp = immediate before carotid artery clamping; Post-clamp = maximum decrease in SrO_2 after artery clamping; Pre-declamp = immediate before declamping the artery; post-declamp = maximum increase in SrO_2 after artery clamping; Op end = operation end. Groups: Sevoflurane = anesthesia with sevoflurane and remifentanil; Propofol = anesthesia with propofol and remifentanil. Data are expressed as mean ± standard deviation. *$P < 0.05$ vs Baseline, ‡$P < 0.05$ vs Pre-clamp in each group. †$P < 0.05$ vs Sevoflurane group

In the present study, sevoflurane was administered at a concentration < 1 MAC throughout the entire operation time, and the mean sevoflurane concentration was 1.36 vol%. This result suggests that the effect of sevoflurane on change in CBF may be reduced compared with the pre-induction period. However, SrO_2 was elevated compared with the baseline, which was thought to be due to increased oxygen supply and decreased cerebral oxygen metabolic rate. The mean value of the relative change in SrO_2 and maximal decrease were significantly higher in the sevoflurane group than the propofol group. This may have been because the decrease in CBF by propofol is more profound than that by sevoflurane, although the decrease in $CMRO_2$ was similar between the two agents.

Interestingly, the SrO_2 change only occurred on the contralateral but not the ipsilateral side, and there was no significant difference on the ipsilateral side in the peri-clamping period between the two groups. This was associated with differences in drug responses between ipsilateral and contralateral sides. Severe internal carotid artery stenosis induces blood–brain barrier injury and impairs the autoregulation to interrupt vasodilation or vasoconstriction on the ipsilateral side. McCulloch et al. reported stump pressure elevation of the clamped ipsilateral carotid artery after switching anaesthetic agent from sevoflurane to propofol in patients with CEA, and they assumed that this was caused by the vasodilation effect of sevoflurane and vasoconstriction effect of propofol [29]. Simultaneously, the middle CBF rate was decreased when anaesthetic agent was changed from sevoflurane to propofol (ipsilateral side, 53 ± 22 → 43 ± 17 cm/s, $n = 14$; contralateral side, 53 ± 19 cm/s → 37 ± 7 cm/s, $n = 7$). In another group, the agent was changed from propofol to sevoflurane, and the internal carotid artery pressure was decreased to a lesser degree when the middle cerebral artery flow rate remained constant (ipsilateral side, $51 \pm 22 \rightarrow 52 \pm 25$ cm/s; contralateral side, $43 \pm 15 \rightarrow 49 \pm 17$ cm/s). Although this result was not statistically significant due to the small sample size, the observation suggested that the affected brain vessels tended to show a lower drug response than those on the contralateral side.

The observation that the data difference between both agents was significant only on the contralateral (non-affected) side may have been due to decreased reactivity on the ipsilateral (affected) side in patients with carotid artery stenosis. Further studies are needed to determine the precise reasons for these results, because CBF rate was not measured in our study and SrO_2 can be influenced by many other factors. After carotid artery clamping in our study, SrO_2 changes showed no significant differences in both groups. Previous studies indicated that SrO_2 remained higher with sevoflurane than propofol [25], and sevoflurane was considered to secure a wider safety margin than propofol when CBF was decreased [16, 17].

However, the effects of propofol and sevoflurane on SrO_2 were not different after carotid artery clamping in the present study. These discrepancies in the results were likely due to differences in the methods used. Previous studies examined SrO_2 changes in healthy volunteers or patients with global CBF reduction in the head elevation position, whereas only collateral vessels were supplied because a large vessel was clamped and main CBF was blocked in the present study. During the vessel clamping period, SrO_2 was decreased by 7.5% compared with the pre-clamping period in both groups in the present study. These observations indicated that cerebral blood supply from the collateral artery could not satisfy the cerebral demand resulting in increased collateral blood flow to compensate for blockage of the main blood flow by clamping. This cerebral haemodynamic state offset the reactions of sevoflurane and propofol to CBF, or blunted the vessel reactivity to both agents.

Another consideration of our study is the effect of intraoperative shunt flow during clamping. Intraoperative carotid bypass (shunt) was not conducted in all patients in the present study. Although placement of carotid artery shunt can increase SrO_2 especially in symptomatic carotid disease patients [30], the optimal threshold of SrO_2 for selective shunting using NIRS have not been established [31]. Furthermore routine or selective shunting has no evidence for the better neurologic outcome comparing with no shunting [32]. As a result, haemodynamic control for prevention of stroke guided by evoked potential monitoring during clamping is used instead of shunting in our institution.

In the present study, postoperative mild stroke occurred in two patients, one of whom showed a decrease in $SrO_2 > 20\%$ of the basal level (sensitivity, 50%), while decreases of > 20% in SrO_2 occurred in six patients in the entire study population (positive predictive value, 17%). Sensitivity of 80% was achieved in a previous study in patients undergoing CEA with regional anaesthesia (deep or superficial cervical plexus block) [23], and the results were revised in a large cohort study performed in 549 patients with general anaesthesia showing 30% sensitivity, 98% specificity, and 37% positive predictive value [33]. Our study with 50% sensitivity and 17% positive predictive value in a relatively small cohort should be repeated in larger numbers of patients to achieve greater reliability.

With the exception of two patients in the propofol group, inotropic agents were used to maintain blood pressure within the normal range in other patients in our study population. Haemodynamic instability often occurs in patients with CEA, and impairment of haemodynamic autoregulation by blunted baroreceptor sensitivity due to carotid artery atherosclerosis is common. In addition, advanced age and medications for comorbidities, such as hypertension or diabetes, are associated with haemodynamic instability. Propofol maintained a higher mean arterial pressure than sevoflurane after carotid artery clamping in this study. The benefit of propofol over sevoflurane with regard to haemodynamic stability was not confirmed, despite many previous studies in various clinical settings. Furthermore, in this study, inotropic agents were necessary to maintain stable arterial blood pressure in both groups, and variation of mean arterial blood pressure tended to be uneven. Therefore, we cannot conclude that propofol is a better agent than sevoflurane for providing haemodynamic stability in patients with CEA, and further research is required.

Conclusions

Propofol-remifentanil anesthesia was comparable with sevoflurane-remifentanil anesthesia in an aspect of preserving the SrO_2 in patients undergoing carotid endarterectomy.

Abbreviations

BIS: Bispectral index score; CBF: Cerebral blood flow; CEA: Carotid endarterectomy; $CMRO_2$: Cerebral metabolic rate; HR: Herat rate; MAP: Mean arterial pressure; NIRS: Near-infrared spectroscopy; SrO_2: Regional cerebral oxygen saturation

Acknowledgements

None.

Author's contributions

SJ, KYY designed the study. SJ and SP drafted manuscript. SP and YWY performed study and obtained data. SJ and HBB performed statistical analysis. KY, JIC and BJ assisted literature search and data collection. JIC and HBB reviewed statistical analysis. All authors read and approved the final manuscript.

References

1. Silver FL, Mackey A, Clark WM, Brooks W, Timaran CH, Chiu D, Goldstein LB, Meschia JF, Ferguson RD, Moore WS, et al. Safety of stenting and endarterectomy by symptomatic status in the carotid revascularization endarterectomy versus stenting trial (CREST). Stroke. 2011;42(3):675–80.
2. Henderson RD, Eliasziw M, Fox AJ, Rothwell PM, Barnett HJ. Angiographically defined collateral circulation and risk of stroke in patients with severe carotid artery stenosis. North American symptomatic carotid endarterectomy trial (NASCET) group. Stroke. 2000;31(1):128–32.
3. Bouri S, Thapar A, Shalhoub J, Jayasooriya G, Fernando A, Franklin IJ, Davies AH. Hypertension and the post-carotid endarterectomy cerebral hyperperfusion syndrome. Eur J Vasc Endovasc Surg. 2011;41(2):229–37.
4. Pennekamp CW, Moll FL, de Borst GJ. The potential benefits and the role of cerebral monitoring in carotid endarterectomy. Curr Opin Anaesthesiol. 2011;24(6):693–7.
5. Casati A, Spreafico E, Putzu M, Fanelli G. New technology for noninvasive brain monitoring: continuous cerebral oximetry. Minerva Anestesiol. 2006; 72(7–8):605–25.
6. Bhatia R, Hampton T, Malde S, Kandala NB, Muammar M, Deasy N, Strong A. The application of near-infrared oximetry to cerebral monitoring during aneurysm embolization: a comparison with intraprocedural angiography. J Neurosurg Anesthesiol. 2007;19(2):97–104.
7. Moritz S, Kasprzak P, Arlt M, Taeger K, Metz C. Accuracy of cerebral monitoring in detecting cerebral ischemia during carotid endarterectomy: a comparison of transcranial Doppler sonography, near-infrared spectroscopy, stump pressure, and somatosensory evoked potentials. Anesthesiology. 2007;107(4):563–9.
8. Ogasawara K, Konno H, Yukawa H, Endo H, Inoue T, Ogawa A. Transcranial regional cerebral oxygen saturation monitoring during carotid endarterectomy as a predictor of postoperative hyperperfusion. Neurosurgery. 2003;53(2):309–14 discussion 314-305.
9. Kaisti KK, Metsahonkala L, Teras M, Oikonen V, Aalto S, Jaaskelainen S, Hinkka S, Scheinin H. Effects of surgical levels of propofol and sevoflurane anesthesia on cerebral blood flow in healthy subjects studied with positron emission tomography. Anesthesiology. 2002;96(6):1358–70.
10. Reinsfelt B, Westerlind A, Ricksten SE. The effects of sevoflurane on cerebral blood flow autoregulation and flow-metabolism coupling during cardiopulmonary bypass. Acta Anaesthesiol Scand. 2011;55(1):118–23.
11. Jansen GF, van Praagh BH, Kedaria MB, Odoom JA. Jugular bulb oxygen saturation during propofol and isoflurane/nitrous oxide anesthesia in patients undergoing brain tumor surgery. Anesth Analg. 1999;89(2):358–63.
12. Van Hemelrijck J, Fitch W, Mattheussen M, Van Aken H, Plets C, Lauwers T. Effect of propofol on cerebral circulation and autoregulation in the baboon. Anesth Analg. 1990;71(1):49–54.
13. Iwata M, Inoue S, Kawaguchi M, Takahama M, Tojo T, Taniguchi S, Furuya H. Jugular bulb venous oxygen saturation during one-lung ventilation under sevoflurane- or propofol-based anesthesia for lung surgery. J Cardiothorac Vasc Anesth. 2008;22(1):71–6.
14. Kaisti KK, Langsjo JW, Aalto S, Oikonen V, Sipila H, Teras M, Hinkka S, Metsahonkala L, Scheinin H. Effects of sevoflurane, propofol, and adjunct nitrous oxide on regional cerebral blood flow, oxygen consumption, and blood volume in humans. Anesthesiology. 2003;99(3):603–13.
15. Kawano Y, Kawaguchi M, Inoue S, Horiuchi T, Sakamoto T, Yoshitani K, Furuya H, Sakaki T. Jugular bulb oxygen saturation under propofol or sevoflurane/nitrous oxide anesthesia during deliberate mild hypothermia in neurosurgical patients. J Neurosurg Anesthesiol. 2004;16(1):6–10.
16. Jeong H, Jeong S, Lim HJ, Lee J, Yoo KY. Cerebral oxygen saturation measured by near-infrared spectroscopy and jugular venous bulb oxygen saturation during arthroscopic shoulder surgery in beach chair position under sevoflurane-nitrous oxide or propofol-remifentanil anesthesia. Anesthesiology. 2012;116(5):1047–56.
17. Kim SJ, Kwon JY, Cho AR, Kim HK, Kim TK. The effects of sevoflurane and propofol anesthesia on cerebral oxygenation in gynecological laparoscopic surgery. Korean J Anesthesiol. 2011;61(3):225–32.
18. Schulz KF, Altman DG, Moher D, Group C. CONSORT 2010 statement: updated guidelines for reporting parallel group randomised trials. BMC Med. 2010;8:18.
19. Brain Trauma F, American Association of Neurological S, Congress of Neurological S, Joint Section on N, Critical Care AC, Bratton SL, Chestnut RM, Ghajar J, FF MCH, Harris OA, et al. Guidelines for the management of severe traumatic brain injury. I. Blood pressure and oxygenation. J Neurotrauma. 2007;24(Suppl 1):S7–13.
20. Jobsis FF. Noninvasive, infrared monitoring of cerebral and myocardial oxygen sufficiency and circulatory parameters. Science. 1977;198(4323): 1264–7.
21. Goldman S, Sutter F, Ferdinand F, Trace C. Optimizing intraoperative cerebral oxygen delivery using noninvasive cerebral oximetry decreases the incidence of stroke for cardiac surgical patients. Heart Surg Forum. 2004; 7(5):E376–81.
22. Casati A, Fanelli G, Pietropaoli P, Proietti R, Tufano R, Montanini S, Collaborative Italian study group on Anaesthesia in elderly P, Danelli G, Nuzzi M, Mentegazzi F, et al. Monitoring cerebral oxygen saturation in elderly patients undergoing general abdominal surgery: a prospective cohort study. Eur J Anaesthesiol. 2007;24(1):59–65.
23. Samra SK, Dy EA, Welch K, Dorje P, Zelenock GB, Stanley JC. Evaluation of a cerebral oximeter as a monitor of cerebral ischemia during carotid endarterectomy. Anesthesiology. 2000;93(4):964–70.
24. Michel A, Weigand MA, Eckstein HH, Martin E, Bardenheuer HJ. Measurement of local oxygen parameters for detection of cerebral ischemia. The significance of cerebral near-infrared spectroscopy and transconjunctival oxygen partial pressure in carotid surgery. Anaesthesist. 2000;49(5):392–401.
25. Valencia L, Rodriguez-Perez A, Kuhlmorgen B, Santana RY. Does sevoflurane preserve regional cerebral oxygen saturation measured by near-infrared spectroscopy better than propofol? Ann Fr Anesth Reanim. 2014;33(4):e59–65.
26. Mielck F, Stephan H, Weyland A, Sonntag H. Effects of one minimum alveolar anesthetic concentration sevoflurane on cerebral metabolism, blood flow, and CO2 reactivity in cardiac patients. Anesth Analg. 1999;89(2): 364–9.
27. Ogawa Y, Iwasaki K, Shibata S, Kato J, Ogawa S, Oi Y. The effect of sevoflurane on dynamic cerebral blood flow autoregulation assessed by spectral and transfer function analysis. Anesth Analg. 2006;102(2):552–9.
28. Cho S, Fujigaki T, Uchiyama Y, Fukusaki M, Shibata O, Sumikawa K. Effects of sevoflurane with and without nitrous oxide on human cerebral circulation. Transcranial Doppler study. Anesthesiology. 1996;85(4):755–60.
29. McCulloch TJ, Thompson CL, Turner MJ. A randomized crossover comparison of the effects of propofol and sevoflurane on cerebral hemodynamics during carotid endarterectomy. Anesthesiology. 2007;106(1):56–64.
30. Cuadra SA, Zwerling JS, Feuerman M, Gasparis AP, Hines GL. Cerebral oximetry monitoring during carotid endarterectomy: effect of carotid clamping and shunting. Vasc Endovasc Surg. 2003;37(6):407–13.
31. Pennekamp C, Immink R, den Ruijter H, Kappelle L, Bots M, Buhre W, Moll F, de Borst G. Near-infrared spectroscopy to indicate selective shunt use during carotid endarterectomy. Eur J Vasc Endovasc Surg. 2013;46(4):397–403.
32. Chongruksut W, Vaniyapong T, Rerkasem K. Routine or selective carotid artery shunting for carotid endarterectomy (and different methods of monitoring in selective shunting). Cochrane Database Syst Rev. 2014;6: CD000190.
33. Mille T, Tachimiri ME, Klersy C, Ticozzelli G, Bellinzona G, Blangetti I, Pirrelli S, Lovotti M, Odero A. Near infrared spectroscopy monitoring during carotid endarterectomy: which threshold value is critical? Eur J Vasc Endovasc Surg. 2004;27(6):646–50.

2

Retrospective analysis of cases of intraoperative awareness in a large multi-hospital health system reported in the early postoperative period

Amanda S. Deis[1], Michael P. Schnetz[1], James W. Ibinson[2,3,4] and Keith M. Vogt[2,5,6*]

Abstract

Background: Awareness with recall under general anesthesia remains a rare but important issue that warrants further study.

Methods: We present a series of seven cases of awareness that were identified from provider-reported adverse event data from the electronic anesthesia records of 647,000 general anesthetics.

Results: The low number of identified cases suggests an under-reporting bias. Themes that emerge from this small series can serve as important reminders to anesthesia providers to ensure delivery of an adequate anesthetic for each patient. Commonalities between a majority of our identified anesthetic awareness cases include: obesity, use of total intravenous anesthesia, use of neuromuscular blockade, and either a lack of processed electroencephalogram (EEG) monitoring or documented high depth of consciousness index values. An interesting phenomenon was observed in one case, where adequately-dosed anesthesia was delivered without technical issue, processed EEG monitoring was employed, and the index value suggested an adequate depth of consciousness throughout the case.

Conclusions: Provider-reported adverse event data in the immediate post-operative period are likely insensitive for detecting cases of intraoperative awareness. Though causation cannot firmly be established from our data, themes identified in this series of cases of awareness with recall under general anesthesia provide important reminders for anesthesia providers to maintain vigilance in monitoring depth and dose of anesthesia, particularly with total intravenous anesthesia.

Keywords: Intraoperative awareness, General anesthesia, Depth of consciousness monitoring, Processed electroencephalogram

* Correspondence: vogtkm@upmc.edu
[2]Department of Anesthesiology & Perioperative Medicine, University of Pittsburgh School of Medicine, 3459 Fifth Avenue, UPMC Montefiore, Suite 467, Pittsburgh, PA 15213, USA
[5]Department of Bioengineering, Swanson School of Engineering, University of Pittsburgh, Pittsburgh, USA

Background

Accidental intraoperative awareness with recall (AWR) is the unanticipated explicit recollection of intraoperative events during anesthesia. Though important to understand and prevent, it is fortunately a rare event. In fact, the incidence estimates vary widely, likely due to methodology differences in identification of awareness events. Several randomized controlled trials with AWR as the primary endpoint have used structured interviews to detect awareness events and expert panel review to adjudicate possible cases of AWR [1–6]. Averaging across the data from these trials gives an incidence of 0.25% for definite AWR and an additional 0.32% of patients having possible AWR. This is corroborated by an incidence of 0.44% in a recent meta-analysis that included randomized trials focused on either anesthetic regimens or anesthetic depth monitors (but not necessarily specifically focused on AWR detection) [7].

Retrospectively identifying cases of AWR, when no structured patient interview has been conducted, is expected to have a lower sensitivity. This is illustrated by much lower calculated incidences of AWR within retrospective studies of varying methodology: 0.023% in a single-institution retrospective chart review [8] and 0.0051% in the United Kingdom's 5th National Audit Project [9]. Thus, retrospective anlayses have limited sensitivity, and may detect AWR events at rates 10–100 times lower than propsective trials. Surveying practicioners seems equally insensitive, with rates of 0.0043% [10] and 0.0065% [11] reported.

Despite this low prevalence, AWR is a clinically important phenomenon to understand and prevent. The Psych-SOS study completed post-traumatic stress disorder (PTSD) assessments of patients from three major awareness prevention trials and found a 43% incidence of PTSD in those who experienced AWR, compared to 16% in a matched cohort without AWR [12]. Though the longevity of PTSD has not been studied in a large cohort of AWR patients, symptoms can last for many years after the event [13, 14]. Even without a PTSD diagnosis, many AWR patients experience some negative symptoms such as sleep disturbance, anxiety, fear, panic, depression, and inability to work [15–17].

The purpose of this investigation was to identify cases of AWR at our institution by a retrospective review of routinely collected adverse event data. We expected to find many AWR cases, based on the very large number of anesthetic records available for review. However, the small number of cases identified precluded a formal analysis. Our results are presented as a truncated AWR case series, focused on general anesthetics. Commonalities between these cases are discussed to highlight some important considerations to maintain vigilance in AWR prevention.

Methods

Cases of AWR were collected from the Electronic Anesthesia Record (EAR) system of the University of Pittsburgh Medical Center. This is a large multi-hospital health system, with a mix of tertiary/academic centers and suburban hospitals that share a centralized EAR. The system-wide EAR was queried for all available electronic anesthesia records over the period 9/13/2010 to 1/12/2019. Patients with AWR were identified using quality improvement records attached to our EAR. In this system, providers voluntarily denote an adverse event flag (labelled "Intraoperative Recall") any time before the EAR chart is finalized, which is typically after patient discharge from Post-Anesthesia Care Unit (PACU). Following identification of those anesthetics that had the adverse event flag for "Intraoperative Recall", the patient charts were reviewed by the authors for data thought to be relevant to the awareness event. We limited the subsequent analysis to cases done under general anesthesia. Data abstracted included the surgery performed, anesthetics administered, patient characteristics, and the patient's past medical and surgical histories. Written documentation was searched for descriptions of the character of the experiences reported by the patients during the awareness event. All authors reviewed the documentation available for each case and made a determination by consensus of the likelihood of an AWR event (rated as Probable, Possible or inconclusive). Additionally, cases were classified using the Michigan Awareness Classification Instrument [18]. Case durations were calculated using the induction and emergence times documented on the EAR. In the UPMC system, the BIS monitor (Medtronic/Covidien, Mansfield, MA, USA) is the processed electroencephalographic (EEG) monitoring device typically available in most anesthetizing locations. Age-adjusted minimum alveolar concentration (aaMAC) was calculated for any volatile agents used, using previously-established formulas [19]. For the purposes of describing patient body habitus, we classified body-mass index (BMI) as normal-range (BMI = 18.5–30), obese (BMI = 30–40), and morbidly obese (BMI > 40).

Results

During the study period, 1,273,060 total anesthetic records were available for query. Only 10 cases were identified in which the "Intraoperative Recall" event flag was marked. Thus, the calculated incidence of AWR from this dataset, using this method of identification was only 0.00079%. Three of these cases were documented as sedation with monitored anesthesia care, and these were excluded from further analysis. The number of general anesthesia cases queried was 647,009, giving a calculated incidence of 1:92,429 (0.0011%) of AWR under general anesthesia in our EAR. We briefly describe the 7 identified cases of AWR during general anesthesia in a condensed case series below. A summary of key case details is provided in Table 1. To retain patient anonymity, no patient-specific information has been included.

Case 1 occurred in a male patient in his 30's with American Society of Anesthesiologists (ASA) physical status (PS) II presenting for elective spine surgery. This patient had a normal-range BMI. The patient was premedicated with 50 mg of fentanyl and 2 mg of midazolam. General anesthesia was induced with 130 mg of propofol, and muscle paralysis initiated with 50 mg of rocuronium. Intermittent boluses of rocuronium were used to maintain paralysis. Maintenance of anesthesia was with sevoflurane, and the lowest concentration during the majority of the 3.5 h-long case was 1.77% (aaMAC = 1.11). However, the concentration decreased to 0.9 to 1.1% (aaMAC = 0.57–0.69) in the approximately 10 min prior to turning the patient supine. This volatile anesthetic was augmented with a remifentanil infusion at 0.1 to 0.2 mcg/kg/min, and this infusion was discontinued approximately 10 min prior to turning supine. A total of 200 mcg of fentanyl was given in divided doses after extubation, approximately 20 min after discontinuation of the remifentanil infusion. Mean arterial pressures (MAP) was maintained in the range 80 mmHg to 120 mmHg, but this required a phenylephrine infusion at rates up to 0.5 mcg/kg/min plus intermittent boluses of ephedrine. His heart was in sinus rhythm, rates ranging 45 to 80 beats per minute (bpm). Processed EEG monitoring was not used.

Case 2 occurred in a morbidly obese male patient in his 70's, ASA-PS III, for elective head/neck surgery. He was premedicated with 50 mcg of fentanyl and 2 mg of midazolam. General anesthesia was induced with 200 mg of propofol and 100 mcg of fentanyl. Muscle paralysis was maintained with boluses of rocuronium. Maintenance of anesthesia was achieved with intermittent boluses of fentanyl and sevoflurane; the lowest end-tidal sevoflurane concentration was 1.45% (aaMAC = 0.98). Vitals were remarkable for atrial fibrillation, with heart rates between 60 to 95 bpm and no hypotension. Processed EEG monitoring was not used. Case duration was 2.5 h.

Case 3 occurred in an obese female patient in her 60's, ASA-PS III, for orthopedic surgery following a traumatic fracture. She was premedicated with 2 mg of midazolam. General anesthesia was induced with 180 mg of propofol, and 100 mg of lidocaine was given. Muscle paralysis initiated with 190 mg of succinylcholine and 30 mg of rocuronium. Maintenance of anesthesia was achieved

Table 1 Summary of key characteristics of identified AWR cases done under general anesthesia

Case #	Surgery Type	Age (decade)	Gender	ASA PS	Premedication	Patient risk factors for AWR	Maintenance anesthetics used	Notes	Classification of Recall
1	Spine	30s	M	2	midazolam & fentanyl	none	Sevoflurane, remifentanil	Early lowering of anesthetic agent and discontinuation of remifentanil infusion. BIS not used.	Possible; Class 2
2	Head & Neck	70s	M	3	midazolam	morbid obesity	Sevoflurane	BIS not used	Possible; Class 1
3	Orthopedic	60s	F	3	midazolam	obesity	Sevoflurane	Sevoflurane < 0.5 aaMAC for much of case, with BIS < 60	Probable; Class 5D
4	General	30s	F	3	none	morbid obesity	TIVA with propofol, dexmedetomidine, & ketamine	BIS > 65 during entire case	Possible; Class 2
5	General (abdominal)	50s	F	3	midazolam	none	TIVA with propofol, dexmedetomidine, & ketamine	BIS < 47 for entire case	Possible; Class 2
6	General	60s	F	2	midazolam	none	TIVA with dexmedetomidine and remifentanil, then propofol	BIS > 60 for much of case	inconclusive
7	Plastic	20s	F	2	midazolam	obesity	TIVA with propofol, & dexmedetomidine & ketamine	IV infiltration occurred. BIS not used	inconclusive

Classification of recall event is based on concordance of authors. Each case is classified as Probable, Possible, or inconclusive, for the likelihood of a true AWR event. Further, the perceptions described are described using the Michigan Awareness Classification Instrument [18], as described in the text with sevoflurane, and end-tidal concentrations ranged from 0.3 to 1.3% (aaMAC = 0.19–0.82) during the case. The BIS™ monitor was applied, and the highest BIS index value recorded was 54.8. Case duration was 2 h. Vital signs during the case were heart rates between 55 to 75 bpm and MAP ranging from 95 mmHg to 115 mmHg, with minimal support by intermittent phenylephrine and ephedrine.

Case 4 occurred in a morbidly obese female patient in her 30's, ASA-PS III. She presented for elective abdominal surgery and received no premedication. Anesthesia was induced with 200 mg of propofol, 16 mcg of dexmedetomidine, and 20 mg of ketamine. Muscle paralysis initiated with 160 mg of succinylcholine and 90 mg of rocuronium with intermittent boluses of rocuronium throughout the case to maintain paralysis. The patient had a history of difficult airway management but was uneventfully intubated with a Glidescope. Total intravenous anesthesia (TIVA) was maintained with three infusions: propofol ranging from 100 to 150 mcg/kg/min, with additional intermittent boluses; dexmedetomidine at 0.4 mcg/kg/hr; and ketamine at 0.2 mg/kg/hr. Processed EEG monitoring was utilized during the case, but not applied until 5 min after incision, which was about 30 min after induction. The BIS index ranged 65–75 in the first 30 min after application. At this time, a relief in hands-on providers occurred, and midazolam 2 mg was given. The highest recorded BIS index was 79.2, and this occurred during the middle portion of the case approximately 45 min after induction. The BIS index was > 65 for the majority of the surgical case. Vital signs were unremarkable with no support. Case duration was just over 2 h.

Case 5 occurred in a female patient in her 50's, ASA-PS III, with normal range BMI. She presented for general surgery. She was premedicated with midazolam 2 mg. Anesthesia was induced with 150 mg of propofol followed by rocuronium 30 mg to facilitate tracheal intubation. TIVA was maintained using a propofol infusion with a basal rate of 100 mcg/kg/min, with intermittent boluses, dexmedetomidine infusion at 0.2 mcg/kg/hr and ketamine infusion at 0.2 mg/kg/hr. The highest documented BIS index was 46.6. Vitals signs were remarkable only for mild bradycardia, with heart rates in the 50's pre-induction. She was normotensive throughout the two-hour case, with no support.

Case 6 occurred in a female patient in her 60's, with ASA-PS II and normal-range BMI, who underwent an elective plastic surgery. Prior anesthesia complications included postoperative nausea and vomiting. She was premedicated with midazolam 2 mg. General anesthesia was induced with 50 mg of propofol and 50 mcg of fentanyl. Paralysis was maintained with intermittent boluses of rocuronium. Maintenance of anesthesia employed remifentanil at 0.2 to 0.6 mcg/kg/min and dexmedetomidine between 0.2 to 0.7 mcg/kg/hr. Approximately 20 min after surgical incision (and 40 min after induction) a propofol infusion at 50 mcg/kg/min was started, and the dose was subsequently increased to 75 mcg/kg/min for the last hour of the case. Vitals were unremarkable, with minimal intermittent doses of phenylephrine and ephedrine. The highest BIS index of 75.2 occurred near the start of surgery, about 15 min after induction. The patient was administered more fentanyl and propofol at that time, and the BIS index subsequently remained between 47 and 61 for the remainder of the two-hour case. Other than selection of the "Intraoperative Awareness" flag, there is no further documentation of awareness.

Case 7 occurred in an obese female patient in her 20's, with ASA-PS III, who presented for elective plastic surgery. The patient was premedicated with 2 mg of midazolam. General anesthesia was induced with 200 mg of propofol and 100 mg of lidocaine was given. Muscle paralysis was initiated with 10 mg of vecuronium and maintained with intermittent boluses. Maintenance of anesthesia was attempted with a TIVA approach utilizing infusions of propofol at 75 mcg/kg/min, dexmedetomidine at 0.6 mcg/kg/hr and intermittent boluses of midazolam (6 mg additional given). Vitals were notable for MAP ranges between 70 mmHg to 110 mmHg, sinus rhythm with heart rates 75 bpm to 100 bpm. Processed EEG monitoring was utilized during the case and notable BIS index ranging from 68 to 75 in the 25 min following incision. Despite additional intravenous (IV) medications including another 2 mg of midazolam, 150 mg of propofol bolus, and increased infusion dose of propofol to 125 mcg/kg/hr, the BIS index remained elevated above 70. An additional 10 mg dose of vecuronium was given and did not result in loss of TOF. It was then recognized that her IV access had been lost. The patient was started immediately on sevoflurane at 3.5%. A right internal jugular line was placed for definitive access. Additional midazolam was given and prior maintenance TIVA was continued. Notably, the BIS index ranged 30 to 40 for the remainder of the two-hour case. The awareness flag was selected by the anesthesiologist with concern for possible awareness. There is no further documentation of AWR.

Discussion

To our knowledge, this is the largest pool of cases systematically evaluated for adverse event data related to anesthetic AWR. Additionally, our use of electronic anesthesia records allowed for a more accurate assessment of important data including BIS index, end-tidal volatile concentration, and vitals, which would be inherently limited in any review of paper records, as demonstrated previously [20]. Even using conservative estimates for the incidences of AWR (0.01%), one might anticipate ~65 cases from a dataset of over 647,000 general anesthesia records. However, our actual results were an order of magnitude lower, consistent with lower estimates using some other non-prospective identification methodologies [9–11]. We strongly suspect that our health system's EAR adverse event data significantly underestimates the true incidence of AWR in our patient population. Thus, our case cohort is a potentially biased sample of early-presenting AWR cases, and we recognize that our identified cases have significant limitations in their predictive ability for AWR. Nonetheless, we are presenting the series of seven general anesthetic cases identified and have recognized some themes that are worthy of discussion.

Most well-known risk factors for AWR are based on descriptive data or case reports [21, 22]. The occurrence of AWR during cardiac, obstetric, and trauma surgical cases, seems intuitive, as these are situations in which it is likely to deliver lower anesthetic doses. Some patient-related risk factors are also not surprising, as they would predispose to anesthetic-resistance, including obesity and chronic alcohol or sedative use. Notably, most of these case- or patient- related risk factors did not emerge in our cohort, except that 4/7 were obese. In fact, all but one (case 3) were elective patients admitted from home.

Several risk factors for AWR related to medication choices have been variably reported in the literature. Relevant to our case series, the use of neuromuscular blocking drugs can mask patient movement that would likely provide an early clinical sign of light anesthesia. Correlation between pharmacologic paralysis and AWR has been suggested [23, 24], as well as increased distress of AWR patients who were unable to move during the awareness event [22]. It is notable that paralysis was used in all seven of our identified cases, substantiating this correlation. The pre-induction administration of benzodiazepines intuitively should be protective against AWR, by providing amnesia. In some studies, their administration has been anti-correlated to AWR risk [25, 26]. However, similar to larger studies [27], our series demonstrate that AWR can certainly still occur despite benzodiazepine premedication, as these were part of the anesthetic in all but case 4.

The use of TIVA has been correlated to AWR [27]. It makes intuitive sense that the use of TIVA may increase the risk, for two reasons related to specific favorable properties of volatile anesthetics. First, end-tidal gas monitoring allows breath to breath measurement of the dose of anesthetic delivered. If used in combination with processed EEG monitoring, expired anesthetic concentration provides potentially synergistic information that can be used to ensure an adequate dose and depth of anesthesia. Second, IV failure can cause an occult disruption of anesthetic delivery, and this is much more likely to go unrecognized than a breathing circuit disconnect. Only one case of IV infiltration was identified within the cohort of general anesthetics. However, it is worthy of note that one of the three sedation cases with AWR that were identified by our initial query also had IV infiltration noted as the suspected etiology. This highlights the importance of particular vigilance in assuring IV patency during TIVA cases to avoid AWR. Further, It has been previously demonstrated that lower-dose propofol TIVA with neuromuscular blockade and alfentanil, with or without midazolam premedication, resulted in a high incidence of AWR [28]. A TIVA technique with propofol ≤100 mcg/kg/min was used in cases 4, 5 and 7. Though cases 5 and 7 employed midazolam premedication, the lower propofol dosing strategy may have contributed to AWR in these three cases.

Improper or no use of depth of consciousness monitoring could play a role in AWR. The utility of processed EEG monitoring in preventing awareness has been shown not superior to end-tidal anesthetic gas concentration alarms, but is better than clinical signs alone [27]. It is also worthy of note that the previously-cited study on AWR with propofol TIVA [28] relied on clinical assessment to titrate anesthetic depth. This could seem to suggest that processed EEG monitoring should be applied in TIVA cases, whenever possible. However, notably the ASA's practice advisory only recommends that their use be considered on a case-by-case basis [21]. It does, however, stand to reason that, if a processed EEG monitor is employed, the anesthetic should be modified if index values are consistent with light anesthesia. In our series, cases 1 and 2 did not employ BIS monitoring, likely due to field avoidance concerns, but these cases did employ volatile anesthesia. Cases 4 and 6 (both TIVA) employed BIS monitoring, but index values were elevated ≥60 during most of the case. Though retrospective and anecdotal, this does raise the question as to whether additional or multimodal anesthetics would have both reduced the BIS index and/or prevented AWR. Case 3 illustrates the situation of reassuring BIS index, but a low anesthetic gas concentration. This suggests that clinicians should consider ensuring both adequate empiric anesthetic dose and reassuring depth of consciousness index values.

The timeline within the case in which AWR seemed to occur in our case series is also worthy of note. Cases 1, 4, and 5 document specific recall of events near the end of their surgical experiences. This serves as a reminder that AWR most often occurs with light anesthesia, and patients are most likely to experience light anesthesia during emergence. Providers must balance the desire for a timely wake-up against the risk of a patient becoming aware while still experiencing noxious stimulation. Though not suggested by events in our case series, this can also be an issue in cases with a prolonged time between IV induction and initiation of the maintenance anesthetic, as with difficult airway management. The administration of additional anesthetic should be considered during this initial period, as appropriate.

Finally, patients with a history of AWR are at 5-fold increased propensity for experiencing AWR again - even when they are enrolled in an AWR-prevention trial [29]. This seems to suggest that a subset of the population might show anesthetic resistance, even in the setting of reassuring depth of consciousness monitoring and clinical signs. This is illustrated by case 5, where the BIS index and vital signs were consistent with the appearance of adequate general anesthesia. An interesting population-based measure of this phenomenon is illustrated by the spread of data in the first figure of Aranake's previous study on AWR [29]. The top of the figure shows many data points with BIS indices above 60, despite being in a range of age-adjusted MAC that should be clinically adequate to ensure unconsciousness and amnesia. This unusual discordance in EEG response to anesthetics may be an area for future neuroscience investigation, to provide better, more personalized, anesthetic care for patients.

Limitations

This case series has several limitations. The retrospective nature of the study was not able to discern clinical decision-making details that may have been involved in each case, and this limits the ability to specifically determine causative factors for each AWR event. We also do not have long-term psychiatric follow-up documented for any of the patients. The design was also limited in ability to identify cases, relying on self-reporting by providers marking an event flag in the EAR. This inherently restricted the time window for identifying and reporting AWR to the immediate post-operative period. Previous studies have suggested that up to 2/3 of cases present only after PACU discharge [9]. These factors likely contributed to our lower incidence, compared to previous studies that employed longer follow-up periods in their methodology.

Future directions

We are implementing system-wide provider education surrounding anesthetic awareness prevention to reduce the occurrence of these potentially devastating events, including highlighting some of the important themes suggested by these cases. We are also reviewing our event reporting system, in general, with an aim to improve the capture rate of AWR and other rare, but important adverse events. Finally, the lack of specificity in documentation surrounding this series of AWR events suggests the need for a structured form to be used when both collecting data and offering follow-up to patients after an AWR event.

Conclusions

In a systematic, retrospective analysis of electronic anesthesia records, we have demonstrated that provider-reported adverse event data recorded in the immediate post-operative period is insensitive for detecting cases of intraoperative awareness. In the series of cases of awareness under general anesthesia that were identified, there are several important points for anesthesia providers to consider, including maintaining vigilance in monitoring both depth and dose of anesthesia, particularly with total intravenous anesthesia.

Abbreviations

ASA: American Society of Anesthesiologists; AWR: Awareness with recall; BMI: Body-mass index; bpm: beats per minute; EAR: Electronic anesthesia record; EEG: Electroencephalogram; IV: Intravenous; MAP: Mean arterial pressure; PACU: Post-anesthesia care unit; PS: Physical status; PTSD: Post-traumatic stress disorder; TIVA: Total intravenous anesthesia

Acknowledgments

The authors thank Dr. Steven L. Whitehurst for assistance in querying the electronic anesthetic record system to identify cases.

Author's contributions

ASD acquired, analyzed, and interpreted data and drafted the manuscript. MPS assisted with data acquisition, interpreted the data, and substantially revised the manuscript. JWI interpreted the data and substantially revised the manuscript. KMV conceived of the project, assisted with data acquisition, interpreted the data, and drafted and substantially revised the manuscript. All authors have read and approved the final manuscript.

Author details

[1]Department of Anesthesiology & Perioperative Medicine, University of Pittsburgh Medical Center, Pittsburgh, USA. [2]Department of Anesthesiology & Perioperative Medicine, University of Pittsburgh School of Medicine, 3459 Fifth Avenue, UPMC Montefiore, Suite 467, Pittsburgh, PA 15213, USA. [3]Clinical and Translational Science Institute, University of Pittsburgh, Pittsburgh, USA. [4]Department of Anesthesiology, Surgical Service Line, Veterans Affairs Pittsburgh Healthcare System, Pittsburgh, USA. [5]Department of Bioengineering, Swanson School of Engineering, University of Pittsburgh, Pittsburgh, USA. [6]Center for the Neural Basis of Cognition, Pittsburgh, USA.

References

1. Xu L, Wu AS, Yue Y. The incidence of intra-operative awareness during general anesthesia in China: a multi-center observational study. Acta Anaesthesiol Scand. 2009;53(7):873–82.
2. Avidan MS, Jacobsohn E, Glick D, Burnside BA, Zhang L, Villafranca A, Karl L, Kamal S, Torres B, O'Connor M, et al. Prevention of intraoperative awareness in a high-risk surgical population. N Engl J Med. 2011;365(7):591–600.
3. Avidan MS, Zhang L, Burnside BA, Finkel KJ, Searleman AC, Selvidge JA, Saager L, Turner MS, Rao S, Bottros M, et al. Anesthesia awareness and the bispectral index. N Engl J Med. 2008;358(11):1097–108.
4. Mashour GA, Shanks A, Tremper KK, Kheterpal S, Turner CR, Ramachandran SK, Picton P, Schueller C, Morris M, Vandervest JC, et al. Prevention of intraoperative awareness with explicit recall in an unselected surgical population: a randomized comparative effectiveness trial. Anesthesiology. 2012;117(4):717–25.
5. Zhang C, Xu L, Ma YQ, Sun YX, Li YH, Zhang L, Feng CS, Luo B, Zhao ZL, Guo JR, et al. Bispectral index monitoring prevent awareness during total intravenous anesthesia: a prospective, randomized, double-blinded, multi-center controlled trial. Chin Med J. 2011;124(22):3664–9.
6. Myles PS, Leslie K, McNeil J, Forbes A, Chan MT. Bispectral index monitoring to prevent awareness during anaesthesia: the B-aware randomised controlled trial. Lancet. 2004;363(9423):1757–63.

7. Messina AG, Wang M, Ward MJ, Wilker CC, Smith BB, Vezina DP, Pace NL. Anaesthetic interventions for prevention of awareness during surgery. Cochrane Database Syst Rev. 2016;10:CD007272.
8. Mashour GA, Wang LY, Turner CR, Vandervest JC, Shanks A, Tremper KK. A retrospective study of intraoperative awareness with methodological implications. Anesth Analg. 2009;108(2):521–6.
9. Pandit JJ, Andrade J, Bogod DG, Hitchman JM, Jonker WR, Lucas N, Mackay JH, Nimmo AF, O'Connor K, O'Sullivan EP, et al. 5th National Audit Project (NAP5) on accidental awareness during general anaesthesia: summary of main findings and risk factors. Br J Anaesth. 2014;113(4):549–59.
10. Jonker WR, Hanumanthiah D, O'Sullivan EP, Cook TM, Pandit JJ, th National Audit Project of the Royal College of A, Association of Anaesthetists of Great B, Ireland, College of Anaesthetists of I: A. national survey (NAP5-Ireland baseline) to estimate an annual incidence of accidental awareness during general anaesthesia in Ireland. Anaesthesia. 2014;69(9):969–76.
11. Pandit JJ, Cook TM, Jonker WR, O'Sullivan E, th National Audit Project of the Royal College of A, the Association of Anaesthetists of Great Britain I. A national survey of anaesthetists (NAP5 baseline) to estimate an annual incidence of accidental awareness during general anaesthesia in the UK. Br J Anaesth. 2013;110(4):501–9.
12. Whitlock EL, Rodebaugh TL, Hassett AL, Shanks AM, Kolarik E, Houghtby J, West HM, Burnside BA, Shumaker E, Villafranca A, et al. Psychological sequelae of surgery in a prospective cohort of patients from three intraoperative awareness prevention trials. Anesth Analg. 2015;120(1):87–95.
13. Leslie K, Chan MT, Myles PS, Forbes A, McCulloch TJ. Posttraumatic stress disorder in aware patients from the B-aware trial. Anesth Analg. 2010;110(3):823–8.
14. Osterman JE, Hopper J, Heran WJ, Keane TM, van der Kolk BA. Awareness under anesthesia and the development of posttraumatic stress disorder. Gen Hosp Psychiatry. 2001;23(4):198–204.
15. Schwender D, Kunze-Kronawitter H, Dietrich P, Klasing S, Forst H, Madler C. Conscious awareness during general anaesthesia: patients' perceptions, emotions, cognition and reactions. Br J Anaesth. 1998;80(2):133–9.
16. Samuelsson P, Brudin L, Sandin RH. Late psychological symptoms after awareness among consecutively included surgical patients. Anesthesiology. 2007;106(1):26–32.
17. Aceto P, Perilli V, Lai C, Sacco T, Ancona P, Gasperin E, Sollazzi L. Update on post-traumatic stress syndrome after anesthesia. Eur Rev Med Pharmacol Sci. 2013;17(13):1730–7.
18. Mashour GA, Esaki RK, Tremper KK, Glick DB, O'Connor M, Avidan MS. A novel classification instrument for intraoperative awareness events. Anesth Analg. 2010;110(3):813–5.
19. Nickalls RW, Mapleson WW. Age-related iso-MAC charts for isoflurane, sevoflurane and desflurane in man. Br J Anaesth. 2003;91(2):170–4.
20. Driscoll WD, Columbia MA, Peterfreund RA. Awareness during general anesthesia: analysis of contributing causes aided by automatic data capture. J Neurosurg Anesthesiol. 2007;19(4):268–72.
21. American Society of Anesthesiologists Task Force on Intraoperative A. Practice advisory for intraoperative awareness and brain function monitoring: a report by the american society of anesthesiologists task force on intraoperative awareness. Anesthesiology. 2006;104(4):847–64.
22. Ghoneim MM, Block RI, Haffarnan M, Mathews MJ. Awareness during anesthesia: risk factors, causes and sequelae: a review of reported cases in the literature. Anesth Analg. 2009;108(2):527–35.
23. Cook TM, Andrade J, Bogod DG, Hitchman JM, Jonker WR, Lucas N, Mackay JH, Nimmo AF, O'Connor K, O'Sullivan EP, et al. 5th National Audit Project (NAP5) on accidental awareness during general anaesthesia: patient experiences, human factors, sedation, consent, and medicolegal issues. Br J Anaesth. 2014;113(4):560–74.
24. Pollard RJ, Coyle JP, Gilbert RL, Beck JE. Intraoperative awareness in a regional medical system: a review of 3 years' data. Anesthesiology. 2007; 106(2):269–74.
25. Errando CL, Sigl JC, Robles M, Calabuig E, Garcia J, Arocas F, Higueras R, Del Rosario E, Lopez D, Peiro CM, et al. Awareness with recall during general anaesthesia: a prospective observational evaluation of 4001 patients. Br J Anaesth. 2008;101(2):178–85.
26. Wang Y, Yue Y, Sun YH, Wu AS, Wu QW, Zhang YQ, Feng CS. Investigation and analysis of incidence of awareness in patients undergoing cardiac surgery in Beijing, China. Chin Med J. 2005;118(14):1190–4.
27. Mashour GA, Avidan MS. Intraoperative awareness: controversies and non-controversies. Br J Anaesth. 2015;115(Suppl 1):i20–6.
28. Miller DR, Blew PG, Martineau RJ, Hull KA. Midazolam and awareness with recall during total intravenous anaesthesia. Can J Anaesthesia. 1996;43(9): 946–53.
29. Aranake A, Gradwohl S, Ben-Abdallah A, Lin N, Shanks A, Helsten DL, Glick DB, Jacobsohn E, Villafranca AJ, Evers AS, et al. Increased risk of intraoperative awareness in patients with a history of awareness. Anesthesiology. 2013;119(6):1275–83.

3

Effects of dexamethasone on post-operative cognitive dysfunction and delirium in adults following general anaesthesia

Li-Qin Li, Cong Wang, Mei-Dan Fang, Hong-Yu Xu, Hong-Liu Lu and Hou-Zhong Zhang*

Abstract

Background: Several studies have investigated the effects of dexamethasone on post-operative cognitive dysfunction (POCD) or post-operative delirium (POD); however, their conclusions have been inconsistent. Thus, we conducted a meta-analysis to determine the effects of dexamethasone on POCD and POD in adults following general anaesthesia.

Methods: The Cochrane Central Register of Controlled Trials (2018, Issue 11 of 12) in the Cochrane Library (searched 17 November 2018), MEDLINE OvidSP (1946 to 16 November 2018) and Embase OvidSP (1974 to 16 November 2018) were searched for randomised controlled trials that evaluated the incidence of POCD and POD following dexamethasone administration in adults (age ≥ 18 years) under general anaesthesia. We used the Grading of Recommendations, Assessment, Development and Evaluations framework to assess the quality of the evidence.

Results: Five studies were included (three studies with 855 participants in the dexamethasone group and 538 participants in the placebo group for the incidence of POCD, and two studies with 410 participants in the dexamethasone group and 420 participants in the placebo group for the incidence of POD). There was no significant difference between the dexamethasone group and the placebo group in terms of the incidence of POCD 30 days after surgery (RR [relative risk] 1.00; 95% CI [confidence interval: 0.51, 1.96], $P = 1.00$, $I^2 = 77\%$) or the incidence of POD (RR 0.96; 95% CI [0.68, 1.35], $P = 0.80$, $I^2 = 0\%$). However, both analyses had some limitations because of limited evidence and clinical heterogeneity, and we considered the quality of the evidence for the post-operative incidence of POCD and POD to be very low.

Conclusions: This meta-analysis revealed that prophylactic dexamethasone did not reduce the incidence of POCD and POD. Trials of alternative preventive strategies for POCD and POD, as well as a better understanding of the pathophysiology of those complex syndromes, are still needed to make progress in this field.

* Correspondence: 2994266687@qq.com
Department of Anesthesiology, Jilin University Second Hospital, No. 218 Ziqiang street, Changchun, Jilin 130021, People's Republic of China

Background

Post-operative cognitive dysfunction (POCD) and post-operative delirium (POD) are neuropsychological disorders that can occur following the administration of general anaesthesia. POCD is one of the most common complications in both young and elderly patients [1]. Evered et al. reported that the incidence rates of POCD at 7 days post-surgery were 17% for total hip joint replacement surgery and 43% for coronary artery bypass graft surgery. The incidence of POCD at 3 months post-surgery for both groups combined was 17% [2]. POCD is subtle and can only be detected by several neuropsychological tests, which are performed before and after surgery [3]. POD is a transient disturbance of a patient's consciousness, attention, cognition and perception, which can last from a few hours to a few days and can fluctuate in severity [4]. POCD and POD are serious complications that are associated with prolonged length of hospital stay, delayed recovery of function, decreased quality of life and increased risk of further complications and mortality [5–7].

Unfortunately, there are still many gaps in our knowledge regarding the pathophysiology of POCD and POD, which hinder our prevention and treatment attempts. At present, the prevention of POCD and POD is mainly based on non-pharmacological measures and comprehensive geriatric assessments focusing on risk factors [8, 9]. But the high prevalence of POCD and POD persists despite these attempts, and given the lack of human resources in hospitals, the idea that medication could prevent POCD and POD is interesting and potentially time-saving. There is growing evidence that the brain's reaction to a peripheral inflammatory process may play a role in the development of POD and POCD. Dillon et al. found that elevated preoperative and post-operative levels of C-reactive protein (CRP) are associated with POD [10]. A recent meta-analysis has suggested that high concentrations of inflammatory markers in the peripheral circulation and cerebrospinal fluid are associated with POCD and POD [11]. Dexamethasone is a long-acting glucocorticoid widely used in various inflammatory diseases [12, 13]. If the inflammatory response plays a role in the occurrence of POCD and POD, then inhibiting the inflammatory response through dexamethasone may prevent POCD and POD. In addition, several studies have investigated the effects of dexamethasone on POCD and POD; however, their conclusions have been inconsistent. Therefore, we have conducted a meta-analysis to evaluate the effects of prophylactic dexamethasone administration on the incidence of POCD and POD. Although the focus was on older adults after surgery, we were concerned that the existing study was too limited; hence, the search included all adults under general anaesthesia.

Methods

We adhered to the Preferred Reporting Items for Systematic Reviews and Meta-Analyses (PRISMA) statement [14], and we used the Grading of Recommendations, Assessment, Development and Evaluations (GRADE) framework to assess the quality of the evidence [15]. This study is registered with PROSPERO, 23 October 2018, number CRD42018114552.

Eligibility and exclusion criteria

We selected all of the studies that met the following eligibility criteria: (1) randomised controlled trials; (2) adults (≥18 years old) who underwent general anaesthesia; (3) perioperative administration of intravenous dexamethasone in order to prevent POCD and POD (including administration during the preoperative, intra-operative and post-operative periods) versus no interventions (no drug administered or placebo group), regardless of the dose administered; (4) the incidence of POCD and POD as a primary or secondary outcome and (5) availability of the full text in English. We excluded studies in which administration of another drug was used in the control group, dexamethasone was administered by another route, and no assessment tools were available to evaluate the incidence of POCD and POD.

Search strategy

We performed a systematic search of the Cochrane Central Register of Controlled Trials (2018, Issue 11 of 12) in the Cochrane Library (searched 17 November 2018), MEDLINE OvidSP (1946 to 16 November 2018) and Embase OvidSP (1974 to 16 November 2018). The search strategy is shown in Additional file 1: Appendix. We also manually searched the references of the included studies and reviews for additional studies. The following sources of ongoing and unpublished trials were screened: http://www.controlled-trials.com and http://www.clinicaltrials.gov.

Endpoints

The primary outcomes are the incidence of POCD or POD according to the author's own definition; however, there is a need for an objective assessment tool for POCD and POD.

The secondary outcomes are as follows: (1) all-cause mortality at 30 days, (2) any post-operative complications, (3) level of C-reactive protein (CRP) measured within the first 24 h post-operatively and (4) hospitalisation (measured in days) and intensive care unit (ICU; measured in hours) duration.

Study selection

After importing the search results into EndNote X9, two review authors (Li and Wang) independently screened the reports according to the predetermined inclusion criteria. Firstly, duplicate reports were removed, and the studies were selected on the basis of the title and abstract. Subsequently, the full text was screened for compliance with the inclusion criteria. A disagreement between Li and Wang was resolved through discussion and consensus with a third reviewer (Fang).

Extraction of data and assessment of risk of Bias in the included studies

Li and Wang extracted data independently from eligible studies using a predesigned form. A disagreement between the two review authors was resolved through discussion and consensus with a third reviewer (Fang). Two review authors (Li and Wang) independently assessed the risk of bias for each included study using the Cochrane Collaboration's tool [16]. We assessed each study according to the following seven domains: random sequence generation, allocation concealment, participant and personnel blinding, outcome assessment blinding, incomplete outcome data, selective reporting and other biases. We rated the overall risk of bias of a study as low if all of the domains were 'low risk', high if one or more of the domains were identified as 'high risk' and unclear if one or more of the domains were identified as 'unclear risk'.

Synthesis of results

We used the Cochrane Review Manager 5 for statistical analysis of the data. Only primary and secondary outcomes that we have defined in advance were used in our analysis. For those studies that did not report a mean and standard deviation (SD), we did not hand and transformate the date, because we did not know if it was normally distributed [17, 18]. Dichotomous variable data (e.g. POCD and POD incidence, all-cause mortality at 30 days and any post-operative complications) were expressed as relative risk (RR) with 95% confidence intervals (CIs), whereas continuous data (e.g. the level of CRP and length of hospital and ICU stay) were reported as weighted mean differences (WMD) with 95% CI.

Assessment of heterogeneity and data synthesis

We used the chi-square test and calculated the I2 statistic to assess the heterogeneity of the studies, and considered heterogeneity to be low (I2 < 50%), moderate (I2 = 50 to 75%) and high (I2 = 75 to 100%). We performed a subgroup analysis of cardiac surgery versus non-cardiac surgery and low-dose (≤0.2 mg/kg) versus high-dose (> 0.2 mg/kg) dexamethasone to explore clinical heterogeneity. We expected substantial clinical and methodological heterogeneity, so we used the randomised effect model [19]. A P-value < 0.05 was considered as statistically significant. If it was inappropriate to undertake the meta-analysis, we instead carried out a descriptive analysis of the study.

Assessment of publication Bias and sensitivity analysis

Where the number of included studies was more than 10, we assessed the risk of publication bias among the included studies based on a funnel plot. We performed the following sensitivity analysis to assess the stability of POCD and POD: (1) excluding reports with a high risk of bias and (2) using different models (the randomised effect model and the fixed effect model).

Results

Study selection

Details of the flow of retrieved results and study selection are shown in Fig. 1. According to the predefined search strategy, we retrieved 4850 studies. After removing the duplicate studies, we screened the remaining 3230 studies based on the title and abstract. We then read the full text of 23 studies for further assessment according to the inclusion criteria. No eligible studies were found by manual retrieval. Finally, five studies were included in our analysis. After searching the clinical trials registration platform, we identified two ongoing studies that will be assessed after they are completed [20, 21].

Study characteristics

Table 1 shows the characteristics of the included studies. Four of the included studies involved cardiac surgery [22–25], whereas the remaining one involved microvascular decompression surgery [26]. A larger, multicentre placebo-controlled randomised clinical trial was excluded because it did not report the occurrence of POCD, and not all patients had been assessed by the available delirium assessment tools [27]. The mean age of all the participants in the included studies was over 60 years, except for one study [26]. Four studies used a two-arm design in comparing dexamethasone with placebo except one, which used a three-arm design [26]. Three studies assessed the effects of dexamethasone on POCD [22, 24, 26], whereas two studies investigated the effects of dexamethasone on POD [23, 25]. Dexamethasone doses and administration time varied, as shown in Table 2. The definition and assessment tools for POCD and POD were also different (Table 2).

Risk of Bias in the included trials

The risk of bias in the included studies is summarised in Figs. 2 and 3. One study was identified as 'low risk' in all domains [22], three studies had an unclear risk of bias in one of the seven domains because of reporting bias [24–26] and one study had a high risk of bias in one of the seven domains [23].

Incidence of POCD

Three studies reported the incidence of POCD, in which data were reported as the number of participants

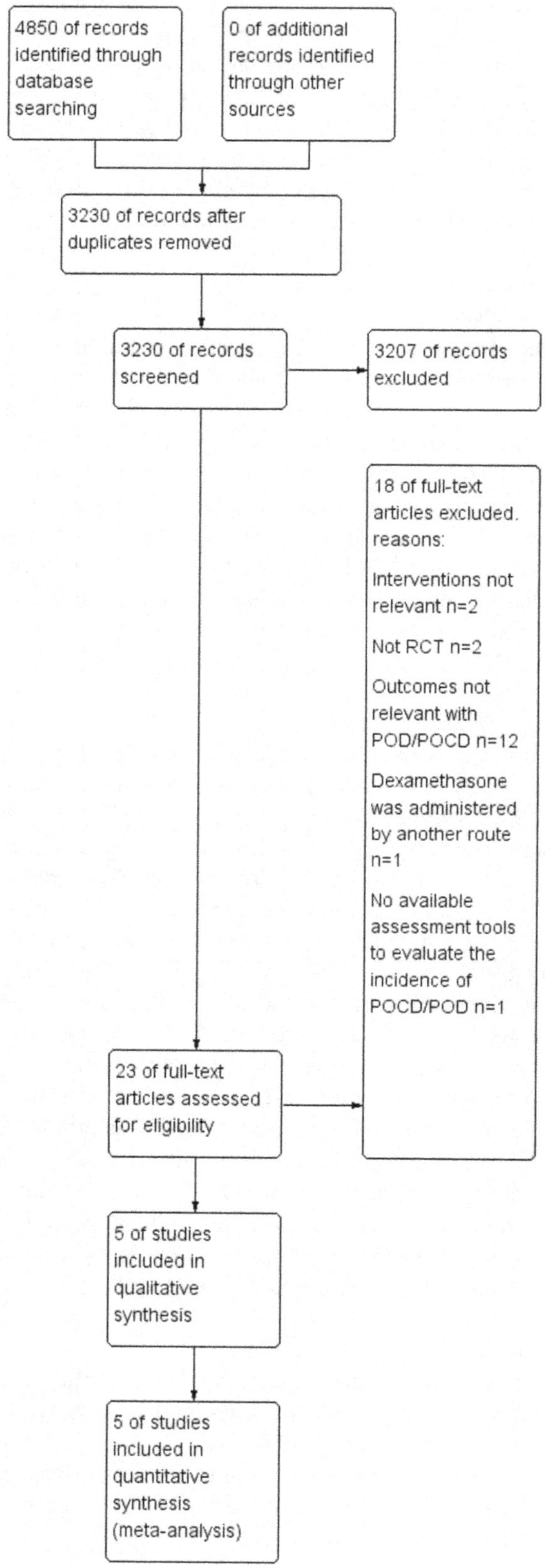

Fig. 1 Study flow diagram

[22, 24, 26]. Fang et al. reported the incidence of POCD at 5 days post-operatively [26], and Glumac et al. at 6 days post-operatively [22]. Ottens et al. assessed POCD at 1 and 12 months post-operatively [24], but we only selected the results reported 1 month after surgery in order to avoid double counting. Fang et al. used neurocognitive tests to assess the incidence of POCD, whereas Glumac et al. and Ottens et al. both used a battery of five neuropsychological tests, making their definitions of POCD different. This meta-analysis included 855 participants in the dexamethasone group and 538 participants in the placebo group, which accounted for 95% of the total 1460 enrolled participants. There was no significant difference in the incidence of POCD 30 days after surgery between the dexamethasone group and the control group (RR 1.00; 95% CI [0.51, 1.96], $P = 1.00$, $I^2 = 77\%$; Fig. 4). We judged, the quality of the evidence to be very low based on the GRADE framework: (1) two studies had a unclear risk of bias; (2) the definitions of the outcome and the assessment tools were different; (3) results were inconsistent and (4) the result was imprecise.

Incidence of POD

Two studies reported the incidence of POD, in which the data were reported as the number of participants [23, 25]. Mardani et al. reported the incidence of POD on the preoperative day, followed by the first, second and third post-operative days. In order to avoid double counting and given that POD typically occurs 2 to 3 days after surgery, we only selected the results reported on the third post-operative day [23]. Sauer et al. reported the incidence of the first four post-operative days [25]. Mardani et al. used the Mini-Mental State Examination (MMSE) to assess POD [23], whereas Sauer et al. used the Confusion Assessment Method (CAM) adapted for the ICU (CAM-ICU) [25]. The meta-analysis showed that there was no significant difference in the incidence of POD between the dexamethasone and placebo groups (RR 0.96; 95% CI [0.68, 1.35], $P = 0.80$, $I^2 = 0\%$; Fig. 5). We deemed the quality of the evidence to be very low because (1) the two studies had an 'unclear risk' of reporting bias and (2) the result was imprecise.

Secondary outcomes

No studies reported the all-cause mortality at 30 days post-surgery. One of the five included studies reported post-operative complications including deep sternal wound infection, leg infection, sepsis and pneumonia in addition to cardiac, cerebrovascular, respiratory and renal complications [23]. The study showed that there was no significant difference between the dexamethasone and control groups in post-operative complication

Table 1 The characteristics of the included studies

Studies ID	Design	Country	Age (min ± SD)		M/F		Type of surgery	Outcome
			Dex	Control	Dex	Control		
Fang 2014	3-arm RCT	China	48.9± 5.35[a]	48.0 ± 5.77	247/388	121/198	microvascular decompression	POCD
Glumac 2017	2-arm RCT	Croatia	63.7± 9.0	64.2± 9.4	63/22	64/20	Cardiac surgery	POCD
Mardani 2013	2-arm RCT	Iran	64.5± 11.10	60.04± 12.77	36/7	44/6	Cardiac surgery	POD
Ottens 2014[b]	2-arm RCT	The Netherla-nds	63.4± 12.3	65.4± 1.5	103/37	109/29	Cardiac surgery	POCD
Sauer 2014[b]	2-arm RCT	The Netherla-nds	67 ± 12	66 ± 12	255/112	225/145	Cardiac surgery	POD

SD = standard deviation, *POCD* = postoperative cognitive dysfunction, *POD* = postoperative delirium, *Dex* = dexamethasone. [a]This 3-arm RCT reported the age was 48.9 ± 5.35, 48.0 ± 5.60 in dexamethasone 0.1 mg/kg and dexamethasone 0.2 mg/kg respectively. [b]Ottens 2014 and Sauer 2014 were two substudies of a larger, multicenter placebo-controlled randomized clinical trial

rates [23]. We consider the quality of the evidence for this outcome to be very low because of the limited evidence available and the fact that the study was at high risk of bias.

Only one study reported the level of CRP [22], which was measured 12 h after surgery and on each of the first three post-operative days. The level of CRP in the dexamethasone group was lower compared with those in the placebo group at all-time points ($P < 0.001$). We deemed the evidence for this outcome to be of very low quality based on the limited evidence available.

Two studies reported the duration of hospitalisation (measured in days) [22, 23]. Our meta-analysis showed that the use of dexamethasone reduced the length of hospital stay (WMD − 0.57 days; 95% CI [− 1.08, − 0.07], $P = 0.03$, $I^2 = 0\%$; Fig. 6), but the difference was so small that it did not have a clinical significance. We considered the quality of the evidence for this outcome to be very low

Table 2 Characteristics of intervention and outcomes

Study ID	Dexamethas one doses	Control	Time of intervention or control	POCD/POD assessment method	POCD/POD definition	Assessment time
Fang 2014	D1:0.1 mg/kg D2:0.2 mg/kg	NS	before induction of anesthesia	Neuro-Psychologic-al test battery	An individual whose postoperative performance deteriorated by 1 or more SDs on 2 or more tests was classified as having experienced early POCD.	the day before and On the fifth postoperativ-e day
Glumac 2017	0.1 mg/kg	NS	10 h before the surgery	a battery of five neuropsychological tests	Authous calculated the Jacobson and Truax Reliable Change Index (RCI) for each patient in the dexamethasone and placebo groups. POCD in an individual is defined as an RCI equal to or less than S1.96 on at least one test	on the 6th day after the surgical procedure
Mardani 2013	8 mg DEX intravenous before induction of anesthesia followed by 8 mg every 8 h for 3 day.	NS	before induction of anesthesia followed every 8 h for 3 day	MMSE	delirium disorder was diagnosed if DSM-IV criteria were met in a patient	Preoperative day (PROD), first, second, andthird postoperativ-e day.
Ottens 2014	1 mg/kg (maximum 100 mg)	NS	shortly after induction of general anesthesia	a battery of five neuropsychological tests	Authous calculated the Jacobson and Truax Reliable Change Index (RCI), they defined POCD in an individual patient as an RCI equal to or less than −1.96, or Z-score equal to or less than − 1.96 in at least two different tests.	1 day before surgery and 1 month and 12 months after surgery
Sauer 2014	1 mg/kg (maximum 100 mg)	NS	at the time of induction of anesthesia	CAM-ICU	POD: diagnosed by the Confusion Assessment Method (CAM) adapted for the ICU (CAM-ICU) .	The primary study outcome was the presence of delirium on any of the first 4 postoperativ-e days. 7 days a week at a fixed time point

POCD = postoperative cognitive dysfunction, *POD* = postoperative delirium, *NS*: normal saline, *MSSE* = Mini-Mental State Examination, *SD* = standard deviation, *RCI* = Jacobson and Truax Reliable Change Index, *CAM* = Confusion Assessment Method, *CAM-ICU*=Confusion Assessment Method adapted for the ICU, *PROD* = Preoperative day

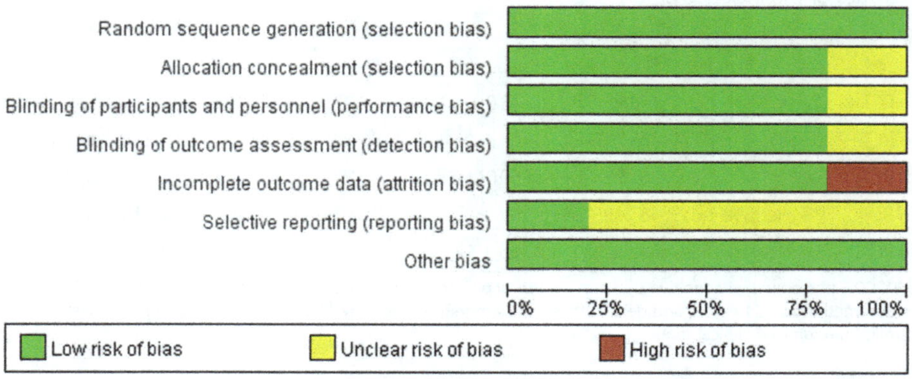

Fig. 2 Risk of bias graph. Review authors' judgements about each risk of bias item presented as percentages across all included studies

because of the limited availability of evidence and imprecision of the result.

Three studies reported the length of ICU stay [22, 23, 25]. Mardani et al. and Glumac et al. reported the duration as mean ± SD [22, 23]. Sauer et al. reported the duration as median (interquartile range); this was 23 (20–24) h in the dexamethasone group and 22 (20–24) h in the control group [25]. We excluded Sauer et al. and conducted a meta-analysis showing that the use of dexamethasone reduced the length of ICU stay (WMD − 13.75 h, 95% CI [− 23.82, − 3.68], $P = 0.007$, $I^2 = 34\%$; Fig. 7). We deemed the quality of the evidence for this outcome to be very low because of the limited availability of evidence and imprecision of the result.

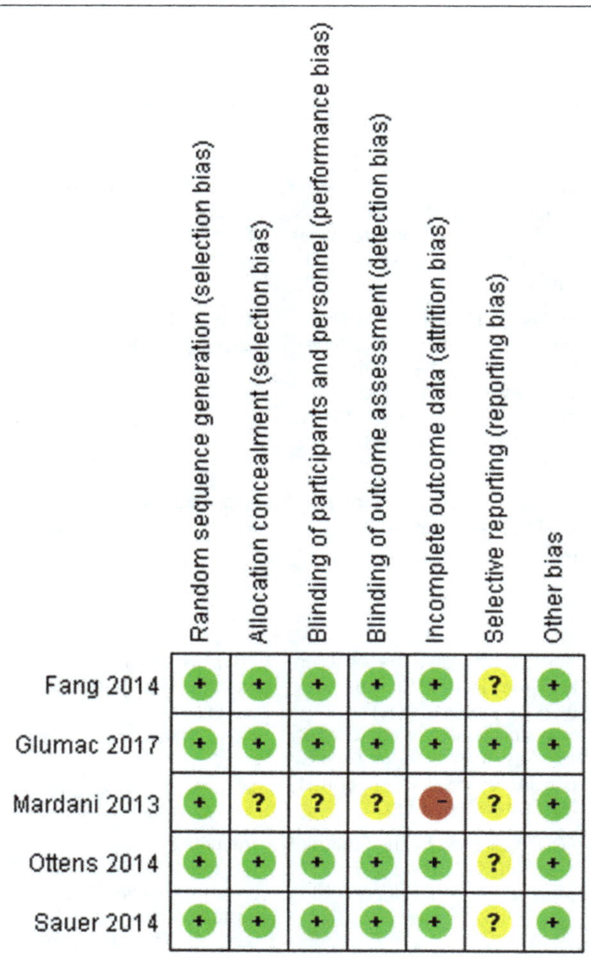

Fig. 3 Risk of bias summary: review authors' judgements about each risk of bias item for each included study

Subgroup analysis

For POCD, one study described non-cardiac surgery [26], whereas two studies described cardiac surgery [22, 24]. We performed a subgroup analysis of cardiac surgery versus non-cardiac surgery (as a subgroup of cardiac surgery only). We noted no difference in the incidence of POCD between the dexamethasone and control groups when non-cardiac surgery was excluded (RR 0.90, 95% CI [0.21, 3.77], $P = 0.89$, $I^2 = 87\%$; 439 participants, Fig. 8). We also found no significant difference between the subgroups ($P = 0.73$) as shown in Fig. 8. For POD, the participants of all the studies underwent cardiac surgery.

For POCD, two studies administered a low-dose of dexamethasone (≤0.2 mg/kg) [22, 26], and one study administered a dexamethasone dose of 1 mg/kg (maximum 100 mg) [24]. We also performed a subgroup analysis of low-dose (≤0.2 mg/kg) versus high-dose (> 0.2 mg/kg) dexamethasone (as a subgroup of low-dose ≤0.2 mg/kg only). This subgroup analysis showed no significant difference in the incidence of POCD between the low-dose dexamethasone (≤0.2 mg/kg) and control groups (RR 0.76, 95% CI [0.29, 1.98]; 1115 participants, Fig. 9). We noted no significant difference between the subgroups ($P = 0.14$) as shown in Fig. 9. For POD, one study administered 8 mg of dexamethasone before the induction of general anaesthesia and then followed by another 8 mg every 8 h [23]. In another study, dexamethasone was

Study or Subgroup	Favours dexamethasone Events	Favours dexamethasone Total	Favours control Events	Favours control Total	Weight	Risk Ratio M-H, Random, 95% CI
Fang 2014	165	635	71	319	41.7%	1.17 [0.92, 1.49]
Glumac 2017	9	80	21	81	29.3%	0.43 [0.21, 0.89]
Ottens 2014	19	140	10	138	29.0%	1.87 [0.90, 3.88]
Total (95% CI)		**855**		**538**	**100.0%**	**1.00 [0.51, 1.96]**
Total events	193		102			

Heterogeneity: Tau² = 0.27; Chi² = 8.74, df = 2 (P = 0.01); I² = 77%
Test for overall effect: Z = 0.00 (P = 1.00)

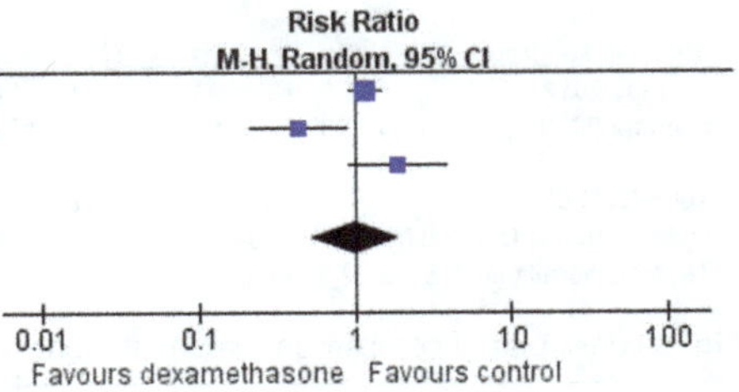

Fig. 4 Forest plot of comparison: Dexamethasone vs Control, Outcome: POCD in 30 days after surgery

administered at a dose of 1 mg/kg (maximum 100 mg) [25]; thus, we did not conduct a subgroup analysis.

Assessment of publication Bias and sensitivity analysis

Considering that the number of the included studies was small, we did not conduct an assessment of publication bias. Based on the prior definition, there was only one study with a low risk of bias, so we did not conduct the sensitivity analysis based on the risk of bias. Sensitivity analyses using the fixed effect model yielded stable overall results: (POCD: RR 1.10, 95% CI [0.89, 1.37]; POD: RR 0.96, 95% CI [0.68, 1.35]).

Discussion

This meta-analysis aimed to assess the effects of dexamethasone on POCD and POD in adults following general anaesthesia. We found that prophylactic intravenous administration of dexamethasone did not reduce the incidence of POCD 30 days following surgery or POD. Furthermore, our meta-analysis showed that the use of dexamethasone reduced the length of hospital stay, but the difference was so small that it did not have a clinical significance. Nevertheless, the results of our meta-analysis suggested that the length of ICU stay was shorter in the dexamethasone group than in the placebo group.

Although we included adults aged over 18 years, the mean age of all the participants in the included studies was over 60 years, except for one study [26]. It is likely that older patients are at higher risk of POCD and POD than younger patients; therefore, evidence related to the incidence of POCD and POD in younger patients (< 60 years old) is still lacking. All the studies recruited patients that were scheduled for cardiac surgery except for one [26], which included participants that underwent microvascular decompression; this may limit the applicability of the evidence. Consequently, we should be careful not to extrapolate its use to patients undergoing other types of surgery. However, when we excluded this study from the meta-analysis, we found that the direction of the evidence did not change. There are two ongoing studies that were found through the clinical trials registration platform that need to be followed-up once they are completed [20, 21]. They may change the conclusion of this meta-analysis.

Only one study was found to have a low risk of bias in all domains [22], whereas the other four studies had a high or unclear risk of bias in at least one of the seven domains [23–26]. Two studies did not register their clinical trials or have a published study protocol, so the risks of selective reporting bias were unclear [23, 26]. We used the GRADE framework to assess the quality of the evidence. We considered the quality of the evidence to be very low for the incidence of POCD because of inconsistencies in the results and imprecision of the result. The inconsistencies might be explained by the differences in the types of surgery performed, the dose of dexamethasone administered and the definitions and assessment tools used in the diagnosis of POCD. However, we found no reduction in heterogeneity when we conducted the subgroup analyses of cardiac surgery versus non-cardiac surgery and low-dose (≤0.2 mg/kg) versus high-dose (> 0.2 mg/kg) dexamethasone. We also deemed the quality of the evidence for the incidence of POD to be very low because (1) the two studies were at 'unclear risk' of reporting bias

Study or Subgroup	Favours dexamethasone Events	Favours dexamethasone Total	Favours control Events	Favours control Total	Weight	Risk Ratio M-H, Random, 95% CI
Mardani 2013	1	43	1	50	1.6%	1.16 [0.07, 18.04]
Sauer 2014	52	367	55	370	98.4%	0.95 [0.67, 1.35]
Total (95% CI)		**410**		**420**	**100.0%**	**0.96 [0.68, 1.35]**
Total events	53		56			

Heterogeneity: Tau² = 0.00; Chi² = 0.02, df = 1 (P = 0.89); I² = 0%
Test for overall effect: Z = 0.25 (P = 0.80)

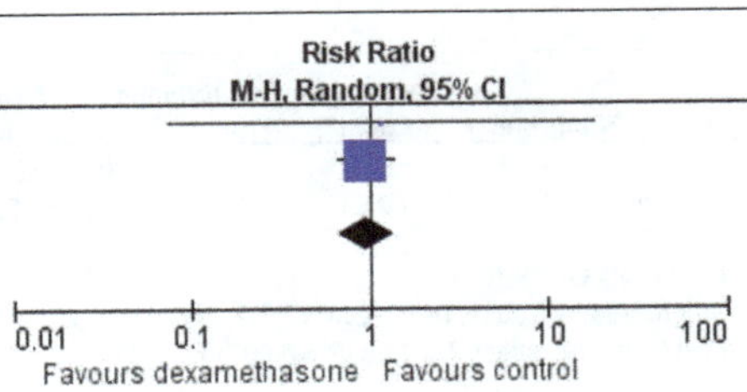

Fig. 5 Forest plot of comparison: Dexamethasone vs Control, Outcome: POD

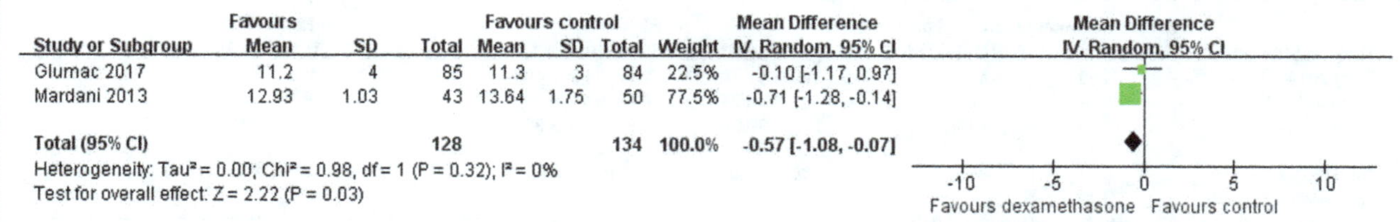

Fig. 6 Forest plot of comparison: Dexamethasone vs Control, Outcome: Duration of hospitalization (measured in days)

and (2) the result was imprecise. The result relating to the incidence of POD mainly came from one study (weight 98.4%) and has wide CI.

It is of note that three studies [22, 24, 26] used neuropsychological tests recommended in the Statement of Consensus on the Assessment of Neurobehavioral Outcomes after cardiac surgery to assess the incidence of POCD [28], which has proved to be of immense value in providing a sensitive means of assessing the change and in detecting beneficial results associated with specific interventions [29–31]. The incidence of POCD in the control group of our study is 19%. By using a battery of neuropsychological tests, Johnson [32] found that the incidence of POCD in those aged more than 60 years was 19.2%, which was comparable with our study. Mardani et al. used MMSE, and Sauer et al. utilised CAM-ICU to assess the occurrence of POD [23, 25]. Unfortunately, MMSE scores are not a very reliable diagnostic test of POD; the diagnostic sensitivity and specificity were 96 and 38%, respectively [33]. CAM-ICU had 93–100% sensitivities, 98–100% specificities and high interrater reliability in the detection of delirium [34]. The incidence of POD in the control group of our study was 13%. However, the reported incidence of POD varied widely depending on the clinical setting. A systematic review found that the incidence of POD was about 11–51%, and the incidence increased with age [35]; hence, it was difficult to compare the incidence of POD.

It was disappointing to find that dexamethasone could not reduce the occurrence of POCD and POD in our meta-analysis, particularly since increased studies have shown that inflammatory cytokines are associated with POCD and POD [10, 11, 36]. The reasons for this phenomenon may be as follows: (1) The occurrence of POCD and POD results from the interaction of many predisposing factors and susceptible factors [37], and a single intervention cannot fully influence the incidence of POCD and POD. (2) Although there is some evidence that inflammation is an important mechanism for POCD and POD, other factors that have not been identified might play a greater role in the development of POCD and POD.

Orena et al. performed a systematic review to explore the effect of anaesthesia on POD and found that dexamethasone may reduce the risk of POD [38]. However, dexamethasone did not reduce the incidence of POD in our meta-analysis. The reason for this difference was that Orena et al. only included one study [23], in which the results of the first post-operative day exhibited a significant reduction of delirium incidence in the dexamethasone group compared with the control group, but not in the second and third post-operative days. However, the number of patients included in this study was small (43 in the dexamethasone group and 50 in the control group), and the MMSE was used to evaluate the occurrence of POD, which is not a very reliable diagnostic test of POD, and the specificity was just 38%. Toner et al. assessed the safety of glucocorticoids in non-cardiac surgery patients and found no increase in the risk of infection, a clinically unimportant increase in the glucose value and a lower concentration of CRP, but there was no difference in the length of hospitalisation [39]. In our meta-analysis, only one study reported the level of CRP and found it to be lower in the dexamethasone group compared with the placebo group ($P < 0.001$). Two studies reported the length of hospitalisation (measured in days), which revealed that

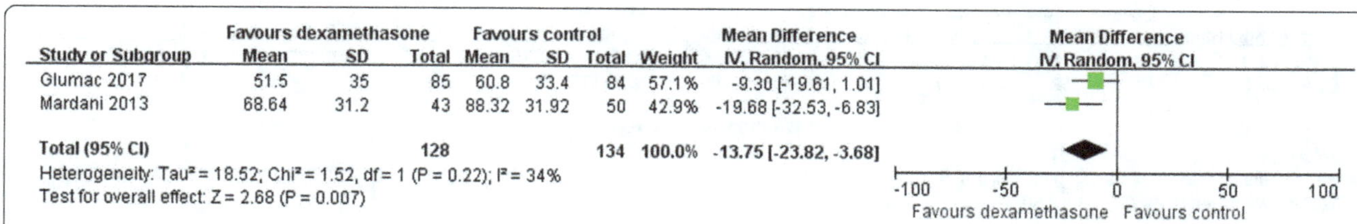

Fig. 7 Forest plot of comparison: Dexamethasone vs Control, Outcome: Length of ICU stay (measured in hours)

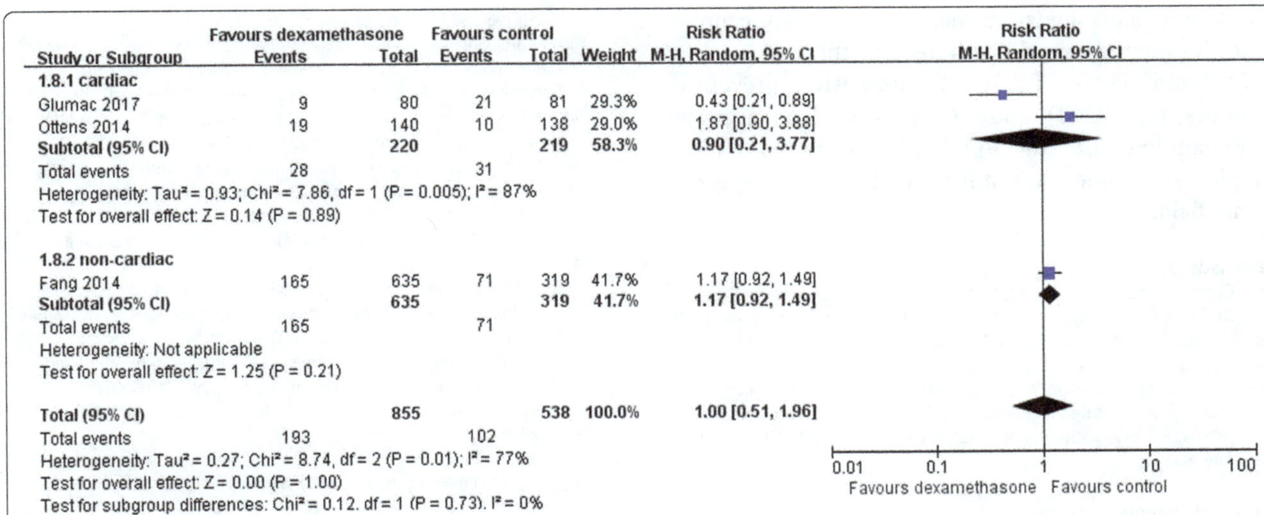

Fig. 8 Forest plot of comparison: Dexamethasone vs Control, Outcome: Subgroup analysis of cardiac surgery versus noncardiac surgery

the use of dexamethasone reduced the length of hospital stay (WMD − 0.57 days; 95% CI [− 1.08, − 0.07], $P = 0.03$, $I^2 = 0\%$), but the difference was so small that it did not have a clinical significance.

There are some limitations to this study. Firstly, we conducted a comprehensive search of the effect of dexamethasone on POCD and POD in several databases. However, these conclusions need to be interpreted with caution because of the limited number of evidence and the influence of the heterogeneity, especially the existing clinical heterogeneity, such as the type of surgery, the time and dose of dexamethasone administered and the different definition and evaluation tools of POCD and POD, which may limit the precision and reliability of the results. Secondly, since the incidence of POCD and POD was our primary outcome, randomised clinical trials that did not contain POCD and POD data were excluded. These studies may evaluate the secondary outcomes; thus, our meta-analysis of secondary outcomes raises no claim to completeness. Most studies excluded patients at high risk of POCD and POD; therefore, the application of conclusions may be limited.

Conclusion

Our meta-analysis is the first systematic review to confirm the effects of dexamethasone on the incidence of POCD and POD in adults following general

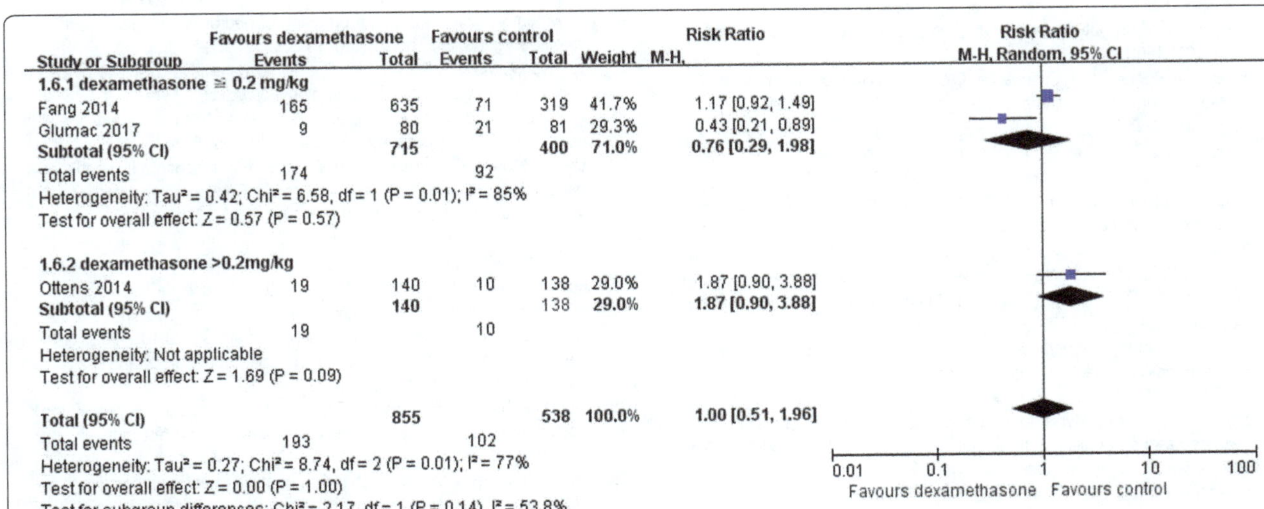

Fig. 9 Forest plot of comparison: Dexamethasone vs Control, Outcome: Subgroup analysis of low dose (≦ 0.2 mg/kg) versus high dose (> 0.2 mg/kg) dexamethasone

anaesthesia. This meta-analysis revealed that prophylactic dexamethasone did not reduce the incidence of POCD and POD. Trials of alternative preventive strategies for POCD and POD, as well as a better understanding of the pathophysiology of those complex syndromes, are still needed to make progress in this field.

Abbreviations

CABG: Coronary artery bypass graft; CAM: Confusion Assessment Method; CAM-ICU: Confusion Assessment Method adapted for the ICU; CI: Confidence intervals; CRP: C-reactive protein; GRADE: Grading of Recommendations, Assessment, Development and Evaluations; ICU: Intensive care unit; MMSE: Mini-Mental State Examination; POCD: Post-operative cognitive dysfunction; POD: Post-operative delirium; PRISMA: Preferred Reporting Items for Systematic Reviews and Meta-Analyses; RR: Relative risk; WMD: Weighted mean differences

Acknowledgements

Not applicable.

Authors' contributions

LLQ participated in the design, collected the data, performed the quality assessment and statistical analyses. ZHZ participated in the design and draft the manuscript. WC and FMD collected the data, performed the quality assessment, and helped to draft the manuscript. XHY, LHL helped to perform statistical analyses and search strategy. All authors read and approved the final manuscript.

References

1. Monk TG, Price CC. Postoperative cognitive disorders. Curr Opin Crit Care. 2011;17(4):376–81.
2. Evered L, Scott DA, Silbert B, et al. Postoperative cognitive dysfunction is independent of type of surgery and anesthetic. Anesth Analg. 2011;112(5):1179–85.
3. Steinmetz J, Rasmussen LS. Peri-operative cognitive dysfunction and protection. Anaesthesia. 2016;71(Suppl 1):58–63.
4. Robinson TN, Raeburn CD, Tran ZV, et al. Postoperative delirium in the elderly: risk factors and outcomes. Ann Surg. 2009;249(1):173–8.
5. Steinmetz J, Christensen KB, Lund T, et al. Long-term consequences of postoperative cognitive dysfunction. Anesthesiology. 2009;110(3):548–55.
6. Crocker E, Beggs T, Hassan A, et al. Long-term effects of postoperative Delirium in patients undergoing cardiac operation: a systematic review. Ann Thorac Surg. 2016;102(4):1391–9.
7. Gleason LJ, Schmitt EM, Kosar CM, et al. Effect of Delirium and other major complications on outcomes after elective surgery in older adults. JAMA Surg. 2015;150(12):1134–40.
8. Inouye SK, Bogardus ST, Charpentier PA. A multicomponent intervention to prevent delirium in hospitalized older patients [J]. N Engl J Med. 1999;340(9):669–76.
9. Marcantonio ER, Flacker JM, Wright RJ. Reducing delirium after hip fracture: a randomized trial [J]. J Am Geriatr Soc. 2001;49(5):516–22.
10. Dillon ST, Vasunilashorn SM, Ngo L, et al. Higher C-reactive protein levels predict postoperative Delirium in older patients undergoing major elective surgery: a longitudinal nested case-control study. Biol Psychiatry. 2017;81(2):145–53.
11. Liu X, Yu Y, Zhu S. Inflammatory markers in postoperative delirium (POD) and cognitive dysfunction (POCD): a meta-analysis of observational studies. PLoS One. 2018;13(4):e0195659.
12. Holte K, Kehlet H. Perioperative single-dose glucocorticoid administration: pathophysiologic effects and clinical implications. J Am Coll Surg. 2002;195(5):694–712.
13. Smith C, Erasmus PJ, Myburgh KH. Endocrine and immune effects of dexamethasone in unilateral total knee replacement. J Int Med Res. 2006; 34(6):603–11.
14. Liberati A, Altman DG, Tetzlaff J, et al. The PRISMA statement for reporting systematic reviews and meta-analyses of studies that evaluate healthcare interventions: explanation and elaboration. BMJ. 2009;339:b2700.
15. Guyatt GH, Oxman AD, Vist GE, et al. GRADE: an emerging consensus on rating quality of evidence and strength of recommendations. BMJ. 2008;336(7650):924–6.
16. Higgins JPT, Green S (editors). Cochrane Handbook for Systematic Reviews of Interventions Version 5.1.0 [updated March 2011]. The Cochrane Collaboration. 2011. Available from http://www.cochrane-handbook.org.
17. Hozo SP, Djulbegovic B, Hozo I. Estimating the mean and variance from the median, range, and the size of a sample. BMC Med Res Methodol. 2005;5:13.
18. Wan X, Wang W, Liu J, Tong T. Estimating the sample mean and standard deviation from the sample size, median, range and/or interquartile range. BMC Med Res Methodol. 2014;14:135.
19. Shuster JJ, Walker MA. Low-event-rate meta-analyses of clinical trials: implementing good practices. Stat Med. 2016;35(14):2467–78.
20. Glenn S. Dexamethasone and Postoperative Delirium. https://clinicaltrials.gov/ct2/show/NCT02109081?term=dexamethasone&cond=Delirium&rank=1 (first received 9 April , 2014). NCT02109081].
21. Wang DX. Dexamethasone, Flurbiprofen Axetil and Delirium After Lung Cancer Surgery. https://clinicaltrials.gov/ct2/show/NCT03200600?term=dexamethasone&cond=Delirium&rank=2 (first received 27 June , 2017). NCT03200600].
22. Glumac S, Kardum G, Sodic L, et al. Effects of dexamethasone on early cognitive decline after cardiac surgery: a randomised controlled trial. Eur J Anaesthesiol. 2017;34(11):776–84.
23. Mardani D, Bigdelian H. Prophylaxis of dexamethasone protects patients from further post-operative delirium after cardiac surgery: a randomized trial. J Res Med Sci. 2013;18(2):137–43.
24. Ottens TH, Dieleman JM, Sauer AM, et al. Effects of dexamethasone on cognitive decline after cardiac surgery: a randomized clinical trial. Anesthesiology. 2014;121(3):492–500.
25. Sauer AM, Slooter AJ, Veldhuijzen DS, et al. Intraoperative dexamethasone and delirium after cardiac surgery: a randomized clinical trial. Anesth Analg. 2014;119(5):1046–52.
26. Fang Q, Qian X, An J, et al. Higher dose dexamethasone increases early postoperative cognitive dysfunction. J Neurosurg Anesthesiol. 2014;26(3):220–5.
27. Dieleman JM, Nierich AP, Rosseel PM, et al. Intraoperative high-dose dexamethasone for cardiac surgery: a randomized controlled trial. JAMA. 2012;308(17):1761–7.
28. Murkin JM, Newman SP, Stump DA, et al. Statement of consensus on assessment of neurobehavioral outcomes after cardiac surgery. Ann Thorac Surg. 1995;59(5):1289–95.
29. Patel RL, Turtle MR, Chambers DJ, et al. Alpha-stat acid-base regulation during cardiopulmonary bypass improves neuropsychologic outcome in patients undergoing coronary artery bypass grafting. J Thorac Cardiovasc Surg. 1996;111(6):1267–79.
30. Murkin JM, Martzke JS, Buchan AM, et al. A randomized study of the influence of perfusion technique and pH management strategy in 316 patients undergoing coronary artery bypass surgery. II. Neurologic and cognitive outcomes. J Thorac Cardiovasc Surg. 1995;110(2):349–62.
31. Newman SP. Analysis and interpretation of neuropsychologic tests in cardiac surgery. Ann Thorac Surg. 1995;59(5):1351–5.
32. Johnson T, Monk T, Rasmussen LS, et al. Postoperative cognitive dysfunction in middle-aged patients. Anesthesiology. 2002;96(6):1351–7.
33. Wong CL, Holroyd-Leduc J, Simel DL, et al. Does this patient have delirium?: value of bedside instruments. Jama. 2010;304(7):779–86.
34. Ely EW, Inouye SK, Bernard GR, et al. Delirium in mechanically ventilated patients: validity and reliability of the confusion assessment method for the intensive care unit (CAM-ICU). JAMA. 2001;286(21):2703–10.
35. Inouye SK, Westendorp RG, Saczynski JS. Delirium in elderly people. Lancet. 2014;383(9920):911–22.
36. Burkhart CS, Dell-Kuster S, Gamberini M, et al. Modifiable and nonmodifiable risk factors for postoperative delirium after cardiac surgery with cardiopulmonary bypass. J Cardiothorac Vasc Anesth. 2010;24(4):555–9.
37. Steiner LA. Postoperative delirium. Part 1: pathophysiology and risk factors. Eur J Anaesthesiol. 2011;28(9):628–36.
38. Orena EF, King AB, Hughes CG. The role of anesthesia in the prevention of postoperative delirium: a systematic review. Minerva Anestesiol. 2016;82(6):669–83.
39. Toner AJ, Ganeshanathan V, Chan MT, et al. Safety of perioperative glucocorticoids in elective noncardiac surgery: a systematic review and meta-analysis. Anesthesiology. 2017;126(2):234–48.

4

Dezocine prevents sufentanil-induced cough during general anesthesia induction

Zhencheng Xiong[1,2†], Ping Yi[2†], Jipeng Song[1] and Mingsheng Tan[1,2*]

Abstract

Background: Sufentanil is one of the opioids currently used to induce general anesthesia, and cough is one of the most common complications. Many drugs have been used to prevent sufentanil-induced cough (SIC), and dezocine is one of them. Dezocine is an analgesic, acting as partial antagonist of κ-receptors and agonist of μ-receptors. The purpose of our meta-analysis is to evaluate the efficacy of dezocine on SIC.

Methods: We searched multiple databases including PubMed, Embase, ScienceDirect, the Cochrane Library, and China National Knowledge Infrastructure databases (CNKI) to identify studies that met the inclusion criteria. This meta-analysis focused on the incidence and severity of SIC after dezocine intervention, as well as adverse effects. This meta-analysis was registered on PROSPERO with reference number ID: CRD 42020144943.

Results: Five randomised controlled trials (RCTs) were identified, including 890 patients. Each study was a comparison of dezocine with an equal volume of 0.9% saline. When the injection dose of dezocine was 0.1 mg/kg, the incidence (pooled risk ratio (RR) = 0.03, [95% CI: 0.02 to 0.07], $P < 0.00001$, $I^2 = 0\%$) and severity (mild: RR = 0.07, [95% CI: 0.03 to 0.18], $P < 0.00001$, $I^2 = 0\%$; moderate: RR = 0.05, [95% CI: 0.02 to 0.16], $P < 0.00001$, $I^2 = 0\%$; severe: RR = 0.04, [95% CI: 0.01 to 0.16], $P < 0.00001$, $I^2 = 0\%$) of SIC were significantly decreased. There were no statistically significant differences in vital signs between the two groups based on the results of the pooled analysis.

Conclusion: This meta-analysis showed that dezocine significantly reduced the incidence and severity of SIC in the induction of general anesthesia, but had no significant effect on vital signs. More high-quality RCTs are needed to complement existing conclusions.

Keywords: Dezocine, Sufentanil, Cough, General anesthesia, Randomised controlled trials

* Correspondence: zrtanms@163.com
†Zhencheng Xiong and Ping Yi are equal contributors and co-first authors.
[1]Graduate School of Peking Union Medical College, Chinese Academy of Medical Sciences, Beijing 100730, People's Republic of China
[2]Department of Spine Surgery, China-Japan Friendship Hospital, No. 2 Yinghua Dongjie, Hepingli, Chaoyang District, Beijing 100029, People's Republic of China

Background

Opioids are widely used in the induction and maintenance of general anesthesia, mainly through the action of opioid receptors (μ, κ, δ), and opioids have a strong analgesic effect, fast onset, short duration, and reduction of cardiovascular response [1]. The most commonly used opioids in general anesthesia include fentanyl, sufentanil and remifentanil [2]. Due to different doses, routes of use, and population, opioids may have a series of adverse effects, such as nausea, vomiting, cough, addiction, urinary retention, and even respiratory depression [2]. Studies have shown that the incidence of cough caused by fentanyl, remifentanil, and sufentanil was 32% [3], 27.6% [4], and 28.5% [5], respectively. Coughing caused by the application of sufentanil is called sufentanil-induced cough (SIC) [6]. According to previous studies, independent risk factors for SIC include aging, body weight, smoking, injection time of opioid, and a priming dose of vecuronium, regardless of gender, the presence of either bronchial asthma or chronic obstructive pulmonary disease, or prior use of atropine [7].

SIC is generally transient, self-limiting, and benign in general anesthesia [8, 9]. According to the number of coughs recorded, the severity of cough was divided into mild (1–2), moderate (3–5) and severe (> 5) [6]. Studies have shown that SIC occurs mostly within 1 min of intravenous injection of opioids [6, 10, 11]. However, cough increases intracranial, intraocular and intra-abdominal pressures, which can cause a series of adverse effects [8]. SIC is more dangerous for patients with comorbidities such as increased intracranial pressure, brain hernia, brain trauma, cerebral aneurysm, increased ocular pressure, open eye injury, arterial aneurysm resection, a full stomach, pneumothorax, or hypersensitive airway disease [10]. It is necessary to take effective measures to suppress the occurrence of SIC in general anesthesia.

Many research teams had taken pharmacological or nonpharmacological measures to prevent SIC. Among them, nonpharmacological measures include slowing down the injection rate, diluting the drug concentration, reducing the drug dose, using the peripheral injection site, verifying the proper administration sequence of the drug, and instructing the patient to perform the huffing maneuver [12–15]. Pharmacological measures include ephedrine [16], dezocine [6, 10, 11, 17, 18], clonidine [19], ketamine [20], dexamethasone [20], and lidocaine [4, 9, 16].

Dezocine is a mixed agonist-antagonist opioid that is structurally similar to pentazocine [1]. Recent studies have shown that dezocine is an antagonist of κ-receptor and a partial agonist or antagonist of μ-receptor [1]. In recent years, several studies had shown that the administration of dezocine effectively prevented the occurrence and reflex degree of SIC in general anesthesia induction [6, 10, 11, 17, 18]. Moreover, the inhibitory effect of dezocine is related to the injected dose, and the effect is best when the dose is 0.1 mg/kg [21]. Dezocine, a member of opioids, also has similar side effects, such as postoperative nausea and vomiting (PONV), respiratory depression, and prolongation of anesthesia recovery time [10, 11]. Therefore, in clinical practice, we should also pay attention to the potential adverse effects of dezocine. We conducted a meta-analysis of randomised controlled trials (RCTs) to assess the efficacy of dezocine on SIC in order to provide a reference for clinical practice.

Methods

We carried out this meta-analysis according to the Preferred Reporting Items for Systematic Reviews and Meta-Analyses (PRISMA) statement [22].

Search strategy

In order to obtain all the literature related to our research, first of all, two researchers independently used the keywords combined with free words to search multiple databases according to Cochrane Collaboration guidelines, such as PubMed (1966 to May 1, 2020), Embase (1980 to May 1, 2020), ScienceDirect (1980 to May 1, 2020), Cochrane library (1966 to May 1, 2020), and CNKI (1980 to May 1, 2020). Next, potentially related literature was searched from a list of references in all included studies. We searched for the following terms "dezocine", "sufentanil-induced cough or SIC", "general anesthesia", "sufentanil", and "opioid" with the Boolean operators "AND or OR" by using Medical Subject Headings (MeSH) terms and corresponding keywords. Then, two researchers independently screened the above retrieved literature by reading the titles and abstracts. Finally, the selected literature was further filtered by reading the full text. After the discussion, all disagreeable literature was resolved.

Study selection

All trials included in our study meet the following criteria: (1) All patients included in these RCTs had an American Society of Anesthesiologists (ASA) physical status classification of I–II and scheduled for elective surgery under general anesthesia; (2) All included studies were original RCTs; (3) In all included studies, two groups were given either intravenous dezocine 0.1 mg/kg or a matching placebo (equal volume of 0.9% saline); (4) None of the patients received any premedication in all included studies; (5) The incidence and severity of cough for 2 min after opioids injection were recorded in all included studies; (6) The full text of the included literature can be obtained, and the measurement data of incidence and severity of SIC, systolic blood pressure (SBP), diastolic blood pressure (DBP), heart rate (HR), and pulse oximeter oxygen saturation (SpO_2) can be extracted.

Following studies were excluded from the meta-analysis: nonrandomized studies; the patients with a history of chronic cough, any sign of upper respiratory infection, asthma, smoking, clinical evidence of a difficult airway, bronchodilator or steroid therapy, use of pain medication (opioids or other drugs); studies not suitable with the inclusive criteria; and articles for which we were unable to obtain the full text and relevant data for pooled analysis.

Data extraction

Data were extracted independently by two researchers. After discussion, disagreements in the data extraction process were resolved, and then another researcher used the spreadsheet to collect the data. We extracted the following data: first author, publication year, country, study type, number of participants (dezocine: placebo), Weight (kg), age, gender, ASA physical status I/II, intervention (dezocine: placebo), application method, the time of intervention earlier than anesthesia induction, the time of coughing after opioid injection, and outcomes data.

Quality assessment

The risk of bias in each included RCT was assessed according to the Cochrane Handbook for Systematic Reviews [23]. The evaluation of bias can be divided into 7 sections: random sequence generation, allocation concealment, blinding of participant and personnel, blinding of outcome assessment, incomplete outcome data, selective reporting, and other bias. Each section can have a high risk of bias, low risk of bias and unclear risk of bias depending on the actual content of the included study [23].

Statistical analysis

Different studies compared dezocine and placebo groups according to the incidence and severity of SIC, as well as side effects. We pooled and calculated data for the same outcome measure in all studies and placed them on the same form. The severity was divided into subgroups according to the classification. We analyzed dichotomous data using risk ratio (RR) and their 95% confidence interval (CI), such as the incidence and severity of SIC [2]. And we analyzed continuous data using weighted mean differences (WMD) and their 95% CI, such as SBP, DBP, HR, and SpO_2. Statistical heterogeneity was calculated by using a chi-square test and I^2 test [24]. It is considered that the I^2 values of 25, 50, and 75% indicate low, moderate and high heterogeneity, respectively [25]. When $I^2 > 50\%$, $P < 0.1$, we performed a random-effect model; otherwise, a fixed-effect model was performed. If necessary, a sensitivity analysis was conducted to identify the origins of the significant heterogeneity. The funnel plot was often used to assess publication bias. In the current meta-analysis, publication bias and meta-regression were not assessable because they were usually only performed when at least 10 studies were included in the meta-analysis. The meta-analysis was performed using RevMan 5.3 for Windows (Cochrane Collaboration, Oxford, UK). If the result of the meta-analysis was a probability of $p < 0.05$, it was considered to be statistically significant.

Results

Study selection

Firstly, we searched in multiple databases by using keywords and free words, and finally confirmed 22 records. Then, a total of 9 records were screened out by reading titles and abstracts to remove duplicate records and irrelevant records. According to the inclusion criteria, records of non-RCT, letter or review, and records for which data could not be extracted were excluded. Finally, by reading the full text, a total of 5 RCTs were selected. Figure 1 showed the search strategy and the process of the study selection [6, 10, 11, 17, 18].

Study characteristics

This meta-analysis included a total of 5 RCTs published between 2014 and 2017. Characteristics of all the studies included in the meta-analysis are shown in Table 1. All studies compared the effect of dezocine on the incidence and severity of SIC compared with placebo. In these studies, the number of patients in the dezocine group was the same as that in the placebo group [6, 10, 11, 17, 18]. In four studies, the number of male patients (408 patients) was greater than the number of female patients (382 patients) [6, 10, 11, 18]. The dose and time of sufentanil injection in the five studies were different (0.3 μg /kg, 5 s; 0.5 μg/kg, 3 ~ 5 s; 0.3 μg /kg, 5 s; 0.5 μg/kg, 3 s; 0.5 μg/kg, 3 s) [6, 10, 11, 17, 18]. Table 1 shows that all patients included in 5 RCTs had an ASA physical status classification of I–II and scheduled for elective surgery under general anesthesia. All patients were randomly assigned to receive either dezocine 0.1 mg/kg or a matching placebo (equal volume of 0.9% saline) [6, 10, 11, 17, 18]. In all studies, the time interval between the intervention and the opioid injection was different. However, after the injection of opioids, the time to start recording cough was consistent, both at 2 min [6, 10, 11, 17, 18].

Risk of Bias

All five studies were considered to have a low risk of bias. Random sequence generation was found in 5 studies [6, 10, 11, 17, 18]. Allocation concealment and blinding of outcome assessment were found in one study [6]. Blinding of participants and personnel was found in 2 studies [6, 11]. As shown in Fig. 2, none of the five

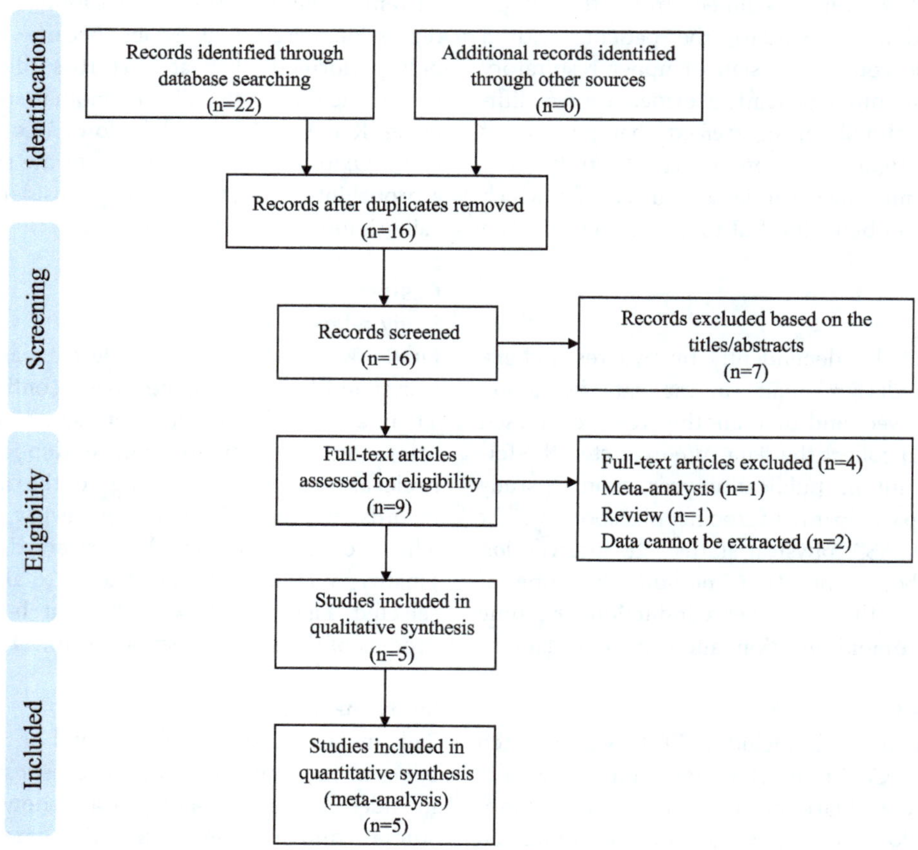

Fig. 1 Flow chart of the selection of studies

studies found incomplete results data, selective reports, and other bias [6, 10, 11, 17, 18].

Results of the meta-analysis

After carefully reading and analyzing the included articles, we summarized the evaluation tools used to measure the effect of patients after receiving dezocine or placebo treatment, including the incidence and severity of SIC, SBP, DBP, HR, and SpO_2. Among them, the incidence of SIC is the primary outcome measure.

The incidence of SIC

Five RCTs used the incidence of SIC as the primary outcome measurement [6, 10, 11, 17, 18]. As shown in Fig. 3, the forest plot shows the effect of dezocine on the incidence of SIC compared with placebo. A total of 5 studies (890 patients) provided data on the incidence of SIC for the dezocine and placebo groups [6, 10, 11, 17, 18]. In 2 studies, no cough occurred in the dezocine group 2 min after sufentanil injection [6, 11]. In all included studies, cough occurred 2 min after sufentanil injection in the placebo group [6, 10, 11, 17, 18]. Based on the results of the pooled analysis, there was a statistically significant difference between the two groups at the incidence of SIC (RR = 0.03, 95% CI: 0.02 to 0.07, $P <$ 0.00001, $I^2 = 0\%$) (Fig. 3). When $I^2 = 0\%$, it means that the three studies are highly homogenous, and the summary analysis results of the data are meaningful. The P value indicates that dezocine significantly inhibits the occurrence of SIC compared with an equal volume of 0.9% saline.

The severity of SIC

Five RCTs used the severity of SIC as the secondary outcome measurement [6, 10, 11, 17, 18]. As shown in Fig. 4, the forest plot shows the effect of dezocine on the severity of SIC compared with placebo. The severity of SIC was graded by cough frequency as mild (1–2) (Fig. 4a), moderate (3–4) (Fig. 4b), and severe (≥5) (Fig. 4c) [6]. A total of 5 studies (890 patients) provided data on the severity of SIC for dezocine and placebo groups [6, 10, 11, 17, 18]. In the dezocine group, there were 4 cases of mild SIC, 1 case of moderate SIC, and no coughing of severe SIC [6, 10, 11, 17, 18]. In the placebo group, 67 patients were in the mild SIC, 56 patients were in the moderate SIC, and 54 patients were in the severe SIC [6, 10, 11, 17, 18]. Based on the results of the pooled analysis, there was a statistically significant difference

Table 1 Characteristics of the studies included in the meta-analysis

Study	Country	Study type	Opioid	Opioid injection dose and time	Group	Weight (kg)	Age (years)	Gender M: F	ASA I/II	Intervention	Time 1	Time 2
Li et al., 2017 [10]	China	RCT	sufentanil	0.3 μg /kg, 5 s	Dezocine	62.2 ± 11.9	42.8 ± 11.5	80 (47/33)	55 /25	0.1 mg/kg, intravenous	10 min	2 min
					Placebo	64.1 ± 13.8	43.5 ± 10.4	80 (45/35)	56 /24	equal volume of 0.9% saline	10 min	2 min
Sun et al., 2015 [11]	China	RCT	sufentanil	0.5 μg/kg, 3 ~ 5 s	Dezocine	58 ± 9	51 ± 10	80 (36/44)	50 /30	0.1 mg/kg, 3 ~ 5 s, intravenous	3 min	2 min
					Placebo	59 ± 9	50 ± 9	80 (41/39)	55 /25	equal volume of 0.9% saline	3 min	2 min
Wang et al., 2015 [17]	China	RCT	sufentanil	0.3 μg /kg, 5 s	Dezocine	NP	NP	NP	NP	0.1 mg/kg, intravenous	10 min	2 min
					Placebo	NP	NP	NP	NP	equal volume of 0.9% saline	10 min	2 min
Liu et al., 2015 [6]	China	RCT	sufentanil	0.5 μg/kg, 3 s	Dezocine	62 ± 9	52 ± 13	185 (91/94)	125/60	0.1 mg/kg, 3 ~ 5 s, intravenous	2 min	2 min
					Placebo	60 ± 8	53 ± 11	185 (99/86)	117/68	equal volume of 0.9% saline	2 min	2 min
Xu et al., 2014 [18]	China	RCT	sufentanil	0.5 μg/kg, 3 s	Dezocine	61.2 ± 10.9	41.2 ± 14.3	50 (26/24)	NP	0.1 mg/kg, intravenous	5 min	2 min
					Placebo	62.1 ± 9.7	39.7 ± 16.1	50 (23/27)	NP	equal volume of 0.9% saline	5 min	2 min

RCT randomised controlled trial, *M* male, *F* female, *ASA* American Society of Anesthesiologists, *NP* not provided, *Time 1* record the time of intervention earlier than anesthesia induction, *Time 2* start recording the time of coughing after opioid injection

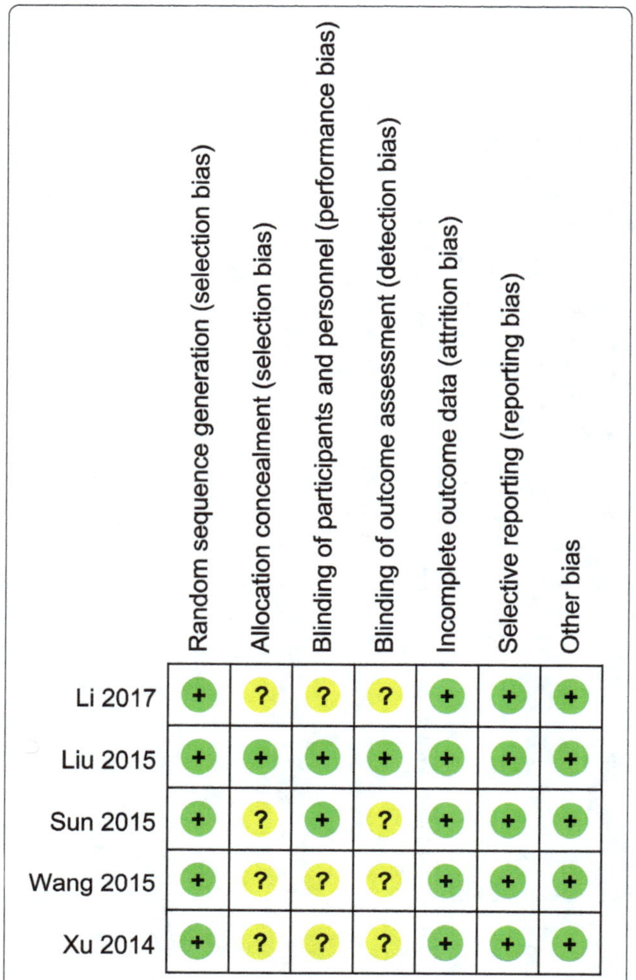

Fig. 2 Summary of Risk of Bias Assessment

between the two groups in the severity of SIC (mild: RR = 0.07, [95% CI: 0.03 to 0.18], $P < 0.00001$, $I^2 = 0\%$ (Fig. 4a); moderate: RR = 0.05, [95% CI: 0.02 to 0.16], $P < 0.00001$, $I^2 = 0\%$ (Fig. 4b); severe: RR = 0.04, [95% CI: 0.01 to 0.16], $P < 0.00001$, $I^2 = 0\%$ (Fig. 4c)). The above results indicated that dezocine not only significantly inhibited the occurrence of SIC, but also reduced the severity of SIC compared to an equal volume of 0.9% saline.

Adverse effects

As shown in Fig. 5, the forest plot shows the effect of dezocine on the vital signs compared with placebo. A total of 4 studies (730 patients) reported hemodynamic changes in SBP, DBP, and HR [6, 10, 17, 18]. However, only one study (160 patients) provided data on SpO_2 for dezocine and placebo groups [11]. We deleted one of the four studies because it provided the highest blood pressure and HR value 2 min after induction of anesthesia [6]. If the obvious changes in vital signs due to the application of dezocine or placebo affect the safety of anesthesia, it is called adverse effects [2]. We performed a pooled analysis of vital sign data after general anesthesia to compare the dezocine and placebo groups. After induction of anesthesia, there was no statistically significant difference in post-intervention vital signs between the two groups based on the results of the pooled analysis (SBP: MD = 0.06, [95% CI: − 3.22 to 3.35], $P = 0.97$, $I^2 = 58\%$ (Fig. 5a); DBP: MD = -0.54, [95% CI: − 2.55 to 1.46], $P = 0.60$, $I^2 = 0\%$ (Fig. 5b); HR: MD = 1.26, [95% CI: − 0.79 to 3.30], $P = 0.23$, $I^2 = 0\%$ (Fig. 5c)). The *P* value indicated that the vital signs are still at approximately the same level after the intervention in both groups. This result illustrates the effect of dezocine on vital signs, which is not significantly different from an equal volume of 0.9% saline. When $I^2 > 50\%$, this means that the included studies are highly heterogeneous. The heterogeneity of the above results is high and may be related to the inclusion of too few studies, requiring more high-quality RCTs.

Because only one study provided data on SpO_2 for dezocine and placebo groups, a pooled analysis could not be successfully performed. In one study, dizziness, lethargy, and respiratory depression were reported in the dezocine group [10]. In the future, more high-quality RCTs are needed to assess the adverse effects of dezocine.

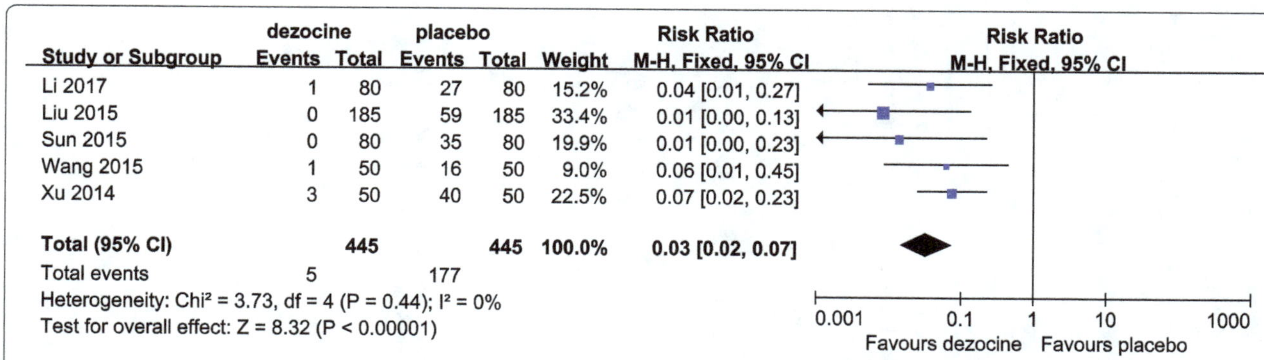

Fig. 3 Forest plot of the effect of dezocine compared with placebo on the incidence of SIC (SIC, sufentanil-induced cough)

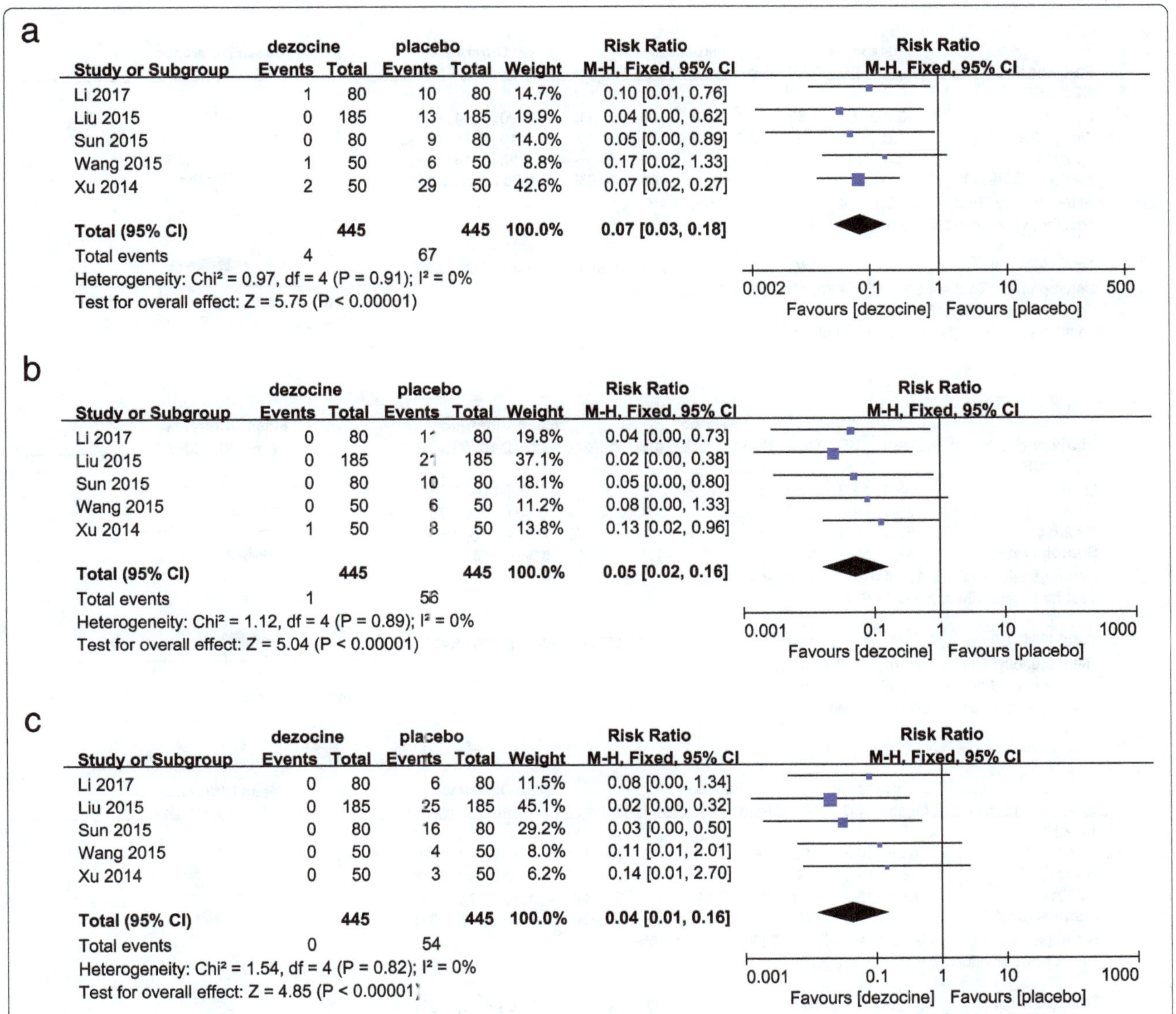

Fig. 4 Forest plot of the effect of dezocine compared with placebo on the severity of SIC. The severity of SIC was graded by cough frequency (**a**. mild (1–2), **b**. moderate (3–4), **c**. severe (≥5))

Publication bias

The funnel plot is often used to assess publication bias but is usually only performed when at least 10 studies are included. Five RCTs were included in this meta-analysis. Therefore, in the current meta-analysis, publication bias and meta-regression cannot be fully evaluated.

Sensitivity analysis

If necessary, a sensitivity analysis was conducted to identify the origins of the significant heterogeneity. Due to the high heterogeneity of SBP and HR before and after treatment, we performed a sensitivity analysis to assess the reliability of the results. However, there were only three studies that met the inclusion criteria, and the reliability of the results might be affected by the limited number of studies included.

Discussion

Opioids are primarily used in pain management due to morphine-like effects [1]. Opioids have good analgesic and sedative effects and are commonly used for the induction and maintenance of general anesthesia [6]. At the same time, opioids have many common side effects, including cough, in the induction of general anesthesia. The essence of cough is a defensive airway reflex [26]. Cough receptors are located in epithelial cells that are sensitive to both mechanical and chemical stimuli [26]. Among opioid-induced cough, SIC is not uncommon [6, 10]. The current mechanism for the occurrence of SIC is still controversial. Previous related studies have differed

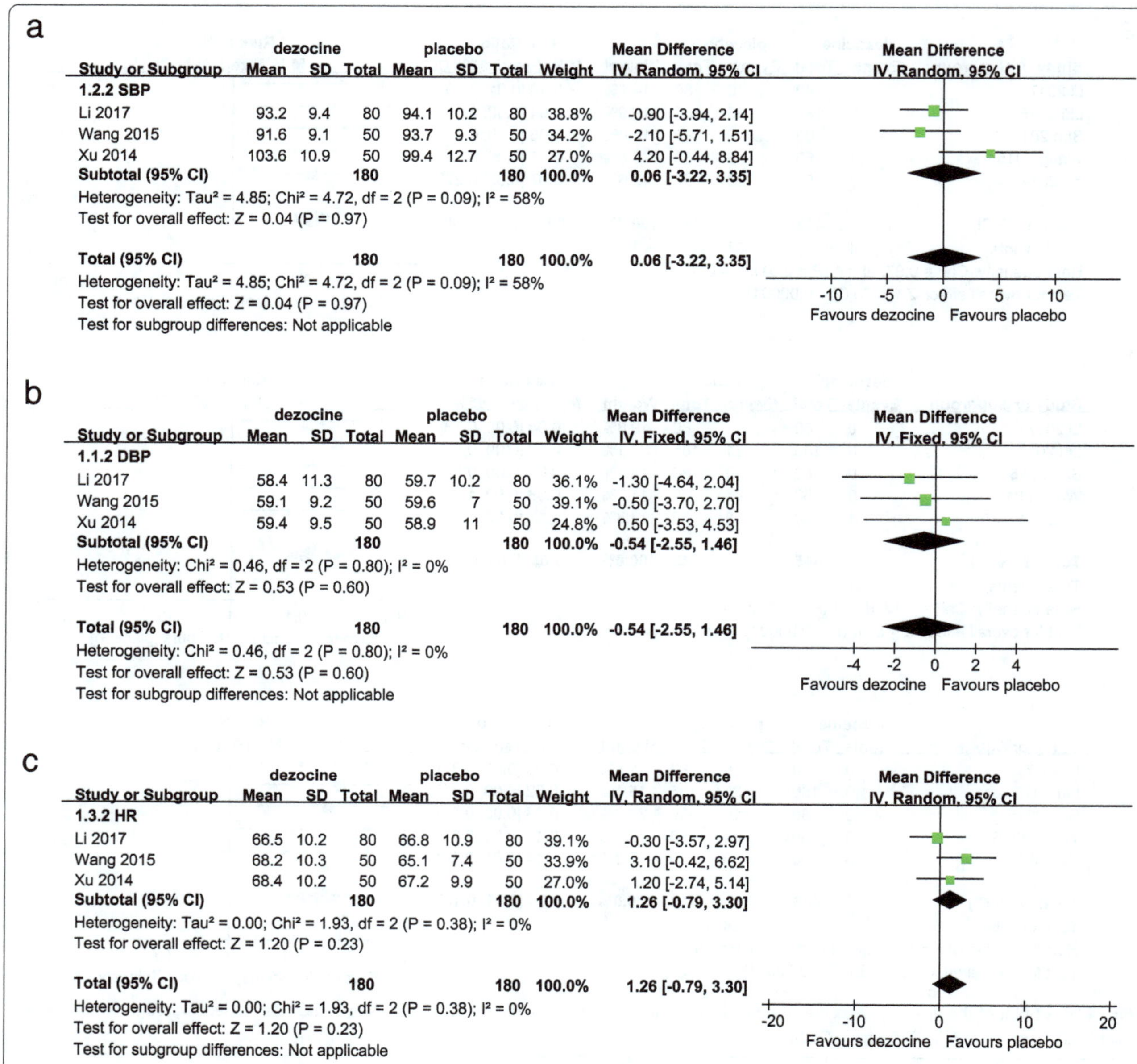

Fig. 5 Forest plot of the effect of dezocine compared with placebo on SBP (**a**), DBP (**b**), HR (**c**) after general anesthesia. (SBP, systolic blood pressure; DBP, diastolic blood pressure; HR, heart rate)

in the dose, injection rate or injection order of opioids, as well as pretreatment with different drugs during induction of general anesthesia, which can reduce SIC [2, 6]. Sufentanil, a thienyl analog of fentanyl, primarily activates μ-opioid receptors and also induces coughing during anesthesia induction like fentanyl [3, 27]. Studies have shown that fentanyl enhances the excitability of rapidly adapting receptors, and stimulates the release of histamine and neuropeptides in the airways to cause coughing [28]. Recent studies have shown that fentanyl-induced cough may contain a pulmonary chemoreflex mediated by rapidly adapting receptors (irritant receptors) or vagal C-fiber receptors (J-receptors) located in proximity to pulmonary vessels [29].

Studies have shown that SIC is generally transient, self-limiting, benign in general anesthesia, and more dangerous for patients with comorbidities such as increased intracranial pressure, arterial aneurysm resection, a full stomach, or hypersensitive airway disease [8–10]. The occurrence of SIC may bring challenges to the induction of general anesthesia, affecting the safety of patients. Therefore, there have been many studies in taking certain measures to prevent the occurrence of SIC [2]. The measures taken are generally divided into two types, pharmacological and nonpharmacological measures. Nonpharmacological measures are primarily achieved by modulating the dose and rate of opioid injection [21]. Pharmacological measures include a variety of drugs, including dexamethasone, lidocaine commonly used in local anesthesia, and even dezocine, which is also an opioid [2, 6]. Dezocine, a mixed opioid receptor partial agonist/antagonist, is an opioid that is structurally similar to pentazocine [1]. In previous studies, it was highly controversial whether dezocine was an agonist or antagonist of the kappa receptor. In the latest research, Liu et al. [1] found that dezocine is a partial mu receptor agonist, a kappa receptor antagonist, and has two new molecular targets (norepinephrine transporter, NET; and serotonin transporter, SERT). Studies have shown that dezocine effectively inhibits the incidence and severity of SIC [6, 10, 11, 17, 18].

Our meta-analysis summarizes the RCTs of dezocine in the prevention of SIC in general anesthesia induction. The indicators analyzed included the incidence and severity of SIC, as well as changes in vital signs. The pooled analysis showed that dezocine significantly inhibited the incidence and severity of SIC compared with an equal volume of 0.9% saline. All included studies recorded coughs occurring 2 min after opioid injection. We also compare changes in vital signs after the intervention. The pooled analysis also showed no difference in the changes in vital signs compared with an equal volume of 0.9% saline. However, the current specific mechanism for the prevention of SIC by dezocine is still unclear, and more relevant research is still needed.

Limitations

This meta-analysis still has some limitations. First, most studies lacked details of random sequence generation, allocation concealment, blinding of participant and personnel, and blinding of outcome assessment. Second, the injection dose and time of opioids were not exactly the same. Third, the time for starting the injection of dezocine is not uniform, the recording time of vital signs is not uniform, and the injection dose is single. Fourth, all trials were from the same country and might have an impact on the conclusions. Finally, the number of studies that met the inclusion criteria was very limited. Therefore, more high-quality RCTs need to be invested in the future.

Conclusions

The results of the above analysis indicated that the injection dose of 0.1 mg/kg of dezocine significantly inhibited the incidence and severity of SIC. There was no significant difference in the effects of dezocine on SBP, DBP, and HR compared with placebo. A number of publications have summarized the effects of dezocine on fentanyl-induced cough, but there are too few articles on SIC. This meta-analysis is the first to evaluate the efficacy of dezocine on SIC. However, more high-quality RCTs are needed to determine the optimal injection dose and time of dezocine in the future to supplement the existing conclusions.

Abbreviations

SIC: Sufentanil-induced cough; CNKI: China National Knowledge Infrastructure databases; RCTs: Randomised controlled trials; PONV: Postoperative nausea and vomiting; MeSH: Medical Subject Headings; PRISMA: Preferred Reporting Items for Systematic Reviews and Meta-Analysis; ASA: American Society of Anesthesiologists; SBP: Systolic blood pressure; DBP: Diastolic blood pressure; HR: Heart rate; SpO_2: Pulse oximeter oxygen saturation; RR: Risk ratio; CI: Confidence interval; WMD: Weighted mean differences; M-H: Mantel-haenszel; IV: Inverse variance

Acknowledgments

None.

Authors' contributions

ZCX, PY and MST conceived this review. ZCX, PY and JPS conducted the search, data screening and extraction. ZCX and JPS performed the data analysis. ZCX drafted the manuscript. ZCX, PY and MST revised the manuscript. All of the authors read and approved the final manuscript.

References

1. Liu R, Huang XP, Yeliseev A, Xi J, Roth BL. Novel molecular targets of dezocine and their clinical implications. Anesthesiology. 2014;120(3):714–23.
2. Li S, Li P, Ni J, Luo D. Different interventions in preventing opioid-induced cough: a meta-analysis. J Clin Anesth. 2016;34:440–7.
3. Agarwal A, Gautam S, Nath SS, Gupta D, Singh U. Comparison of the incidence and severity of cough induced by sufentanil and fentanyl: a prospective, randomised, double-blind study. Anaesthesia. 2007;62(12): 1230–2.
4. Kim JY, Park KS, Kim JS, Park SY, Kim JW. The effect of lidocaine on remifentanil-induced cough. Anaesthesia. 2008;63(5):495–8.
5. Wang J, Duan J, Wang QLY. Pretreatment with Nalbuphine prevents sufentanil-induced cough during the anesthesia induction: a randomized controlled trial. Ther Clin Risk Manag. 2020;16:281–6.
6. Liu X, Xu G, Shen Q, Zhao Q, Cheng XQ, Zhang J, Gu EW. Dezocine prevents sufentanil-induced cough during general anesthesia induction: a randomized controlled trial. Pharmacol Rep. 2015;67(1):52–5.
7. Oshima T, Kasuya Y, Okumura Y, Murakami T, Dohi S. Identification of independent risk factors for fentanyl-induced cough. Can J Anaesth. 2006; 53(8):753–8.
8. Lin JA, Yeh CC, Lee MS, Wu CT, Lin SL, Wong CS. Prolonged injection time and light smoking decrease the incidence of fentanyl-induced cough. Anesth Analg. 2005;101(3):670–4.
9. Sun L, Guo R, Sun L. The impact of prophylactic intravenous lidocaine on opioid-induced cough: a meta-analysis of randomized controlled trials. J Anesth. 2014;28(3):325–33.
10. Li Y, Li Y. Comparative study of intravenous different dose of dezocine premedication on sufentanil-induced cough. J Clin Pulmonary Med. 2017; 22(12):2219–22.
11. Sun J, Liu S, Lu H, Chen H, Yin M. The effects of different doses of dezocine on preventing sufentanil-induced cough. Int J Anesthesiol Resuscitation. 2015;36(7):602–4.
12. Yu H, Yang XY, Zhang X, Li Q, Zhu T, Wang Y, Liu B. The effect of dilution and prolonged injection time on fentanyl-induced coughing. Anaesthesia. 2007;62(9):919–22.
13. Min SK, Kim DH, Cho HB, Moon BK, Kim JY. Limited maximal flow rate of target-controlled remifentanil infusion and induced cough. Anaesthesia. 2012;67(2):145–8.
14. Shrestha SK, Bhattarai B, Shah RS. Preemptive use of small dose fentanyl suppresses fentanyl induced cough. Kathmandu Univ Med J (KUMJ). 2012; 10(40):16–9.

15. Ambesh SP, Singh N, Gupta D, Singh PK, Singh U. A huffing manoeuvre, immediately before induction of anaesthesia, prevents fentanyl-induced coughing: a prospective, randomized, and controlled study. Br J Anaesth. 2010;104(1):40–3.
16. Lin CS, Sun WZ, Chan WH, Lin CJ, Yeh HM, Mok MS. Intravenous lidocaine and ephedrine, but not propofol, suppress fentanyl-induced cough. Can J Anaesth. 2004;51(7):654–9.
17. Wang H, Qing E. Effect of intravenous dezocine premedication on sufentanil-induced cough. J Chin Pract Diagnosis Therapy. 2015;29(8):825–6.
18. Xu Q, Zhou D, Xiong S. The clinical observation of preinjection dezocine during induction of general anesthesia with sufentanil on different injection speed on induced cough reflex. J Clin Med Pract. 2014;16:137–9.
19. Horng HC, Wong CS, Hsiao KN, Huh BK, Kuo CP, Cherng CH, Wu CT. Pre-medication with intravenous clonidine suppresses fentanyl-induced cough. Acta Anaesthesiol Scand. 2007;51(7):862–5.
20. Saleh AJ, Zhang L, Hadi SM, Ouyang W. A priming dose of intravenous ketamine-dexmedetomidine suppresses fentanyl-induced coughing: a double-blind, randomized, controlled study. Ups J Med Sci. 2014;119(4): 333–7.
21. Xu Y, Zhu Y, Wang S, Ren Y, Miao C. Dezocine attenuates fentanyl-induced cough in a dose-dependent manner-a randomized controlled trial. Int J Clin Exp Med. 2015;8(4):6091–6.
22. Moher D, Liberati A, Tetzlaff J, Altman DG. Preferred reporting items for systematic reviews and meta-analyses: the PRISMA statement. BMJ. 2009; 339:b2535.
23. Higgins JP, Altman DG, Gotzsche PC, Juni P, Moher D, Oxman AD, Savovic J, Schulz KF, Weeks L, Sterne JA, et al. The Cochrane Collaboration's tool for assessing risk of bias in randomised trials. BMJ. 2011;343:d5928.
24. Higgins JP, Thompson SG. Quantifying heterogeneity in a meta-analysis. Stat Med. 2002;21(11):1539–58.
25. Higgins JP, Thompson SG, Deeks JJ, Altman DG. Measuring inconsistency in meta-analyses. BMJ. 2003;327(7414):557–60.
26. Yin N, Xia J, Cao Y, Lu X, Yuan J, Xie J. Effect of propofol combined with opioids on cough reflex suppression in gastroscopy: study protocol for a double-blind randomized controlled trial. BMJ Open. 2017;7(9):e014881.
27. Sun S, Huang SQ. Effects of pretreatment with a small dose of dexmedetomidine on sufentanil-induced cough during anesthetic induction. J Anesth. 2013;27(1):25–8.
28. Agarwal A, Azim A, Ambesh S, Bose N, Dhiraj S, Sahu D, Singh U. Salbutamol, beclomethasone or sodium chromoglycate suppress coughing induced by iv fentanyl. Can J Anaesth. 2003;50(3):297–300.
29. Kamei J, Nakanishi Y, Asato M, Ikeda H. Fentanyl enhances the excitability of rapidly adapting receptors to cause cough via the enhancement of histamine release in the airways. Cough (London, England). 2013;9(1):3.

5

Newborn infant parasympathetic evaluation (NIPE) as a predictor of hemodynamic response in children younger than 2 years under general anesthesia

Kan Zhang[1,2†], Siyuan Wang[3†], Lei Wu[1,2], Yun'an Song[1], Meihua Cai[1,2], Mazhong Zhang[1,2] and Jijian Zheng[1,2*]

Abstract

Background: It is still unknown whether newborn infant parasympathetic evaluation (NIPE), based on heart rate variability (HRV) as a reflection of parasympathetic nerve tone, can predict the hemodynamic response to a nociception stimulus in children less than 2 years old.

Methods: Fifty-five children undergoing elective surgery were analyzed in this prospective observational study. Noninvasive mean blood pressure (MBP), heart rate (HR) and NIPE values were recorded just before and 1 min after general anesthesia with endotracheal intubation as well as skin incision. The predictive performance of NIPE was evaluated by receiver-operating characteristic (ROC) curve analysis. A significant hemodynamic response was defined by a > 20% increase in HR and/or MBP.

Results: Endotracheal intubation and skin incision caused HR increases of 22.2% (95% confidence interval [CI] 17.5–26.9%) and 3.8% (2.1–5.5%), MBP increases of 18.2% (12.0–24.4%) and 10.6% (7.7–13.4%), and conversely, NIPE decreases of 9.9% (5.3–14.4%) and 5.6% (2.1–9.1%), respectively (all $P < 0.01$ vs. pre-event value). Positive hemodynamic responses were observed in 32 patients (62.7%) during tracheal intubation and 13 patients (23.6%) during skin incision. The area under the ROC curve values for the ability of NIPE to predict positive hemodynamic responses at endotracheal intubation and skin incision were 0.65 (0.50–0.78) and 0.58 (0.44–0.71), respectively.

Conclusions: NIPE reflected nociceptive events as well as anesthetic induction in children less than 2 years undergoing general anaesthetia. Nevertheless, NIPE may not serve as a sensitive and specific predictor to changes in hemodynamics.

Keywords: Newborn infant parasympathetic evaluation, Nociception, Analgesia, Pediatrics, Respiratory sinus arrythmia

* Correspondence: zhengjijian626@sina.com
†Kan Zhang and Siyuan Wang contributed equally to this work.
[1]Department of Anesthesiology, Shanghai Children's Medical Center, Shanghai Jiao Tong University School of Medicine & National Children's Medical Center (Shanghai), 1678 Dongfang Road, Shanghai 200127, China
[2]Pediatric Clinical Pharmacology Laboratory, Shanghai Children's Medical Center, Shanghai Jiao Tong University School of Medicine & National Children's Medical Center (Shanghai), Shanghai, China

Background

Endotracheal intubation and skin incision are two of the strongest noxious stimuli received by surgical patients under general anesthesia [1]. From one perspective, sufficient analgesic levels are critical to avoid unexpected movements, sympathetic reactions with consequent cardiovascular complications, and the development of pain memory. From another perspective, restriction to a minimum dosage of analgesic is desirable to avoid opioid-induced hyperalgesia, respiratory depression, and nausea as well as to achieve a shorter perioperative treatment period [2, 3]. Due to a lack of reliable tools for predicting and assessing the balance between analgesia and nociception during general anesthesia, clinicians mainly use classical symptoms of insufficient analgesia including increases in heart rate (HR), blood pressure, lacrimation, and sweating to tailor the administration of analgesic drugs, an approach that can reduce the side-effects of opioid overdosage but not underdosage [1, 4].

Subcortical-derived autonomic nervous system changes induced by nociceptive stimuli was shown to be reflective of the balance between nociception and analgesia [5–13]. Two parameters, the newborn infant parasympathetic evaluation (NIPE) and analgesia nociception index (ANI, MDoloris Medical Systems, Lille, France), were derived from a real-time reliable analysis of HR variability (HRV) in a time window of 64 s on a scale from 0 (maximum of nociception) to 100 (complete analgesia). NIPE is the neonatal version of the ANI used in adults [14, 15]. It has been shown that the autonomic nervous system responses to a noxious stimuli would change with the advancing age. As the nervous system matures, sympathetic HR modulation increases, while parasympathetic modulation decreases [16]. The ANI used in adult could not be adapted directly to children less than 2 years old due to the higher respiratory rate and heart rate in children [17]. The NIPE, on the other hand, reflects the parasympathetic tone. It was found that NIPE would decrease significantly in newborn infants after a painful surgical procedure [8]. The NIPE was also significantly reduced in babies borned by instrument-assisted delivery when compared to those delivered naturally [9].

In adult patients, the automomic index ANI had been used to predict hemodynamic changes associated with painful stimulation [10–13]. Study of the prediction ability of the NIPE in children has not yet been reported.

In this observational pilot study, two manuvors, namely endotracheal intubation and skin incision, were chosen as the noxious stimuli. As a primary endpoint, we evaluate whether the pre-event value of NIPE would be a good predictor of the hemodynamic responses of such stimulation.

Methods

Patients

This observational prospective study was approved by the ethics committee of Shanghai Children's Medical Center affiliated to Shanghai Jiao Tong University (SCMCIRB-K2018049) prior to its start and was registerated in the Chinese Clinical Trial website (http://www.chictr.org.cn/showproj.aspx?proj=27154, ChiCTR1800015973). Patients were enrolled over a 4-month period between June 2018 and September 2018. Full-term pediatric patients aged 1 month to 2 years with an American Society of Anesthesiologists physical status score I~II were included. Patients were scheduled for elective general or urinary surgery.

We excluded children who had a history of premature delivery or neurological, cardiac or respiratory conditions. Children who required prolonged resuscitation at birth, underwent general anaesthesia within the preceding week of study, experienced prolonged exposure to pain, and those who were currently receiving drugs with known effects on sympathetic and parasympathetic activity were also excluded. Written informed consents were obtained from the parents of study subjects.

Anesthetic technique and monitoring

All pediatric patients were fasted according to the relevant guidelines [18]. Crystalloid fluid (Ringer's acetate) containing 5% glucose was given in the ward by the attending surgeon or in the operating theater by the anesthesiologist in charge as appropriate. Oral midazolam 0.5 mg/kg as sedative premedication was administered to all children 30 min before patients were transferred to the operating room. All patients were accompanied by their parents or a senior nurse staff in our preparation room as they watched cartoon video or listened to stories for relaxation. Upon arrival in the operating theater, standard monitoring was applied using an anesthesia workstation (Datex-Ohmeda Aisys CS^2, GE Healthcare, USA) with a three-lead electrocardiogram (ECG), pulse oximetry and non-invasive blood pressure measured at the arm. After an intraveous line was secured, all patients received Ringer's acetate as maintenance fluid following the 4–2-1 rule.

Fentanyl 2–3 μg/kg was injected over a 15-s period. After 1 min, anesthesia was induced with propofol 2–3 mg/kg administered intravenously (i.v.) over 30 s. When the eyelash reflex was absent, the child was ventilated via a facemask with 100% oxygen. Rocuronium 0.6 mg/kg was administered i.v. for muscle relaxation, after adequate ventilation could be achieved via a facemask. A senior anesthesiologist (> 3 years experience) decided the timing of endotracheal intubation and performed intubation using video laryngoscope. The patients were then ventilated using pressure-controlled mode at a frequency of 20 breaths per minute (inhalation-to-exhalation ratio of 1:2). Peak inspiratory pressure would be adjusted to achieve tidal volume between 8 and 10 ml/kg and end-tidal carbon dioxide was maintained between 35 and 45 mmHg. Anesthesia was maintained with sevoflurane between 1.0–1.3 MAC according to the patient's age and the fentanyl boluse administered, as clinically required.

Study protocol

The MDoloris system (MDoloris Medical Systems, Loos, France) was integrated to the monitors of the anesthesia workstation for HRV analysis. After calibration, the instantaneous NIPE index was displayed on the monitor screen. The instantaneous NIPE was obtained based on four individual windows of 16 s. The R-R interval analysis for each 16-s block is based on a sliding window of 64 s. Continuous measurement of the indexes can be assumed by moving the 64-s window after each calculation. The sampling rate of the final parameters depends on the window moving period. In practice, a 1-s moving period is used [19].

The timing of endotracheal intubation was decided by the anesthesiologist who was blinded to the study protocol and the MDoloris monitoring system. The research team was responsible for recording the NIPE, HR and MBP measurements immediately before and 1 min after tracheal intubation and skin incision [20]. The changes in the MBP and HR during the observation were calculated by the following formula:

$$\text{change percent} = \frac{(\text{HR or MBP})_{\text{post-stimulus}} - (\text{HR or MBP})_{\text{pre-stimulus}}}{(\text{HR or MBP})_{\text{pre-stimulus}}} \times 100\%.$$

A hemodynamic response was considered significant and clinically relevant if an increase in either parameter (HR and/or MBP) of more than 20% was observed after the noxious event. We also calculated the dynamic NIPE to examine its ability to predict a hemodynamic response [21].

$$\text{NIPE}_{\text{dynamic}} = \frac{\text{NIPE}_{\text{post-stimulus}} - \text{NIPE}_{\text{pre-stimulus}}}{(\text{NIPE}_{\text{post-stimulus}} + \text{NIPE}_{\text{pre-stimulus}})/2} \times 100\%$$

Statistical analysis

Patient data was presented as the mean (95% confidence interval [CI]) or median (interquartile range [IQR]) as appropriate. All data were tested for normal distribution using the Kolmogorov-Smirnov test. Variables before and after stimulation were compared using paired t tests. Receiver operating characteristic (ROC) curves and the associated area under curve (AUC) values were computed to assess the ability of the NIPE (pre-stimulation values) to predict hemodynamic reactivity. GraphPad Prism 7 (GraphPad Software, Inc., San Diego, CA, USA) and MedCalc version 18.2 for Windows (MedCalc Software, Ostend, Belgium) were used for statistical analysis. P values < 0.05 were considered statistically significant.

Results

Seventy-one pediatric patients were initially recruited into this study. Of these, 16 patients were excluded due to a history of premature delivery, recent general anaesthesia, or arrythemia or a lack of parents' permission for participation. Finally, 55 patients met the inclusion criteria and parents or informed consents were obtained. The characteristics of these patients are presented in Table 1. Of these pediatric patients, 47 children were male, and 8 were female. Their mean age was 1.3 years (95% CI 1.1–1.5 years), and their mean weight was 10.6 kg (10.0–11.1 kg). During the period of tracheal intubation, the NIPE recordings for four patients were complicated by noise due to poor electrode–skin contact. Thus, the final analysis included NIPE data from 51 patients undergoing endoutracheal intubation and 55 patients undergoing skin incision (Fig. 1).

Induction of anaesthesia significantly changed the HR, MBP, and NIPE (all $P < 0.01$ vs. baseline). After induction of anaesthesia, in the absence of intubation, the HR and MBP decreased by 13% (95%CI 9–16%) and 15% (11–19%), respectively, while the NIPE increased by 19% (7–30%), as shown in Table 2.

A positive hemodynamic response was observed during tracheal intubation in 32 patients (62.7%) and during skin incision in 13 patients (23.6%). Endotracheal intubation resulted in significant changes in the patients' MBP, HR, and NIPE values (all $P < 0.01$ vs. before intubation). The average MBP and HR values increased by 18.2% (12.0–24.4%) and 22.2% (95%CI 17.5–26.9%), respectively, while the NIPE value decreased by 9.9% (5.3–14.4%). Skin incision also resulted in significant increases in the patients' MBP [by 3.8% (2.1–5.5%)] an HR [by

Table 1 Detailed characteristics of pediatric patients

	Patients (n = 55)
Gender (M/F)	47/8
Age (years)	1.3 (1.1–1.5)
Weight (kg)	10.6 (10.0–11.1)
Height (cm)	76.1 (72.7–79.5)
ASA (I/II)	50/5
Surgery (n)	
General surgery	20/55
Urinary surgery	20/55
Orthopedic surgery	15/55
Propofol dose (mg/kg)	3.1 (2.8–3.5)
Fentanyl dose (μg/kg)	2.3 (2.1–2.6)

ASA American Society of Anesthesiologists physical status. Data are mean (95% CI) or absolute numbers

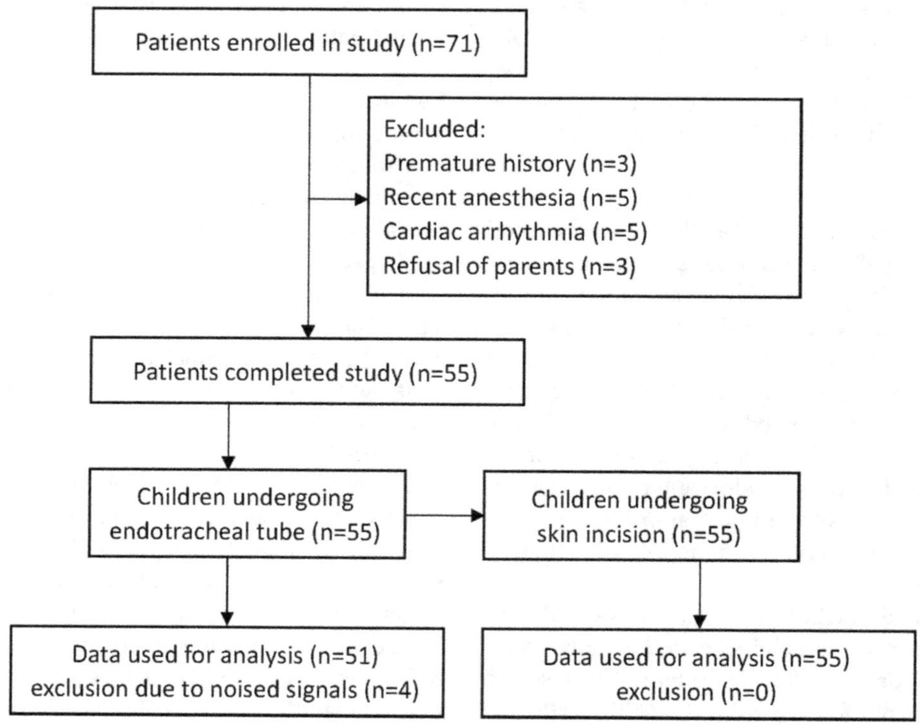

Fig. 1 Flow digram of patient/data inclusion in this observational study

10.6% (7.7–13.4%)] values and a decrease in the NIPE [by 5.6% (2.1–9.1%)] (all $P < 0.01$ vs. before incision). The MBP, HR, and NIPE values at each timepoint are presented in Table 2.

The AUC values for the ability of NIPE to predict a positive hemodynamic response at endotracheal intubation and at skin incision were 0.65 (95%CI 0.50–0.78) and 0.58 (0.44–0.71), respectively. The best cut-off values (the optimal threshold) for the NIPE index at the respective events were 42 (sensitivity 71.9% and specificity 52.6%) and 60 (sensitivity 69.2% and specificity 52.4%). These results indicate the probability of correctly predicting a positive hemodynamic response based on the NIPE was similar to that achieved with a random coin toss (Fig. 2).

The AUC values for the ability of $NIPE_{dynamic}$ to predict a positive hemodynamic response at endotracheal intubation and at skin incision were 0.68 (95%CI 0.53–0.80) and 0.54 (0.40–0.68), respectively. Thus, our results showed that the $NIPE_{dynamic}$ also was not sufficiently sensitive and specific to predict a hemodynamic response to these events.

Table 2 Change trends for mean blood pressure (MBP), heart rate (HR), and newborn infant parasympathetic evaluation (NIPE) at five time points

	T1	T2[#]	T3[*]	T4	T5[**]
MBP (mmHg)	73 ± 9	64 ± 11	75 ± 17	56 ± 9	62 ± 11
HR (bpm)	129 ± 23	111 ± 17	134 ± 17	111 ± 14	115 ± 15
NIPE	40 ± 12	45 ± 8	39 ± 7	60 ± 14	56 ± 13

#$P < 0.01$ T2 vs. T1; *$P < 0.01$ T3 vs. T2; **$P < 0.01$ T5 vs. T4. T1, before anesthesia induction; T2, immediately before intubation; T3, 1st min after intubation; T4, immediately before skin incision; T5, 1st min after skin incision

Data are shown as mean ± standard deviation

Discussion

In the present study, we observed (1) the NIPE as well as $NIPE_{dynamic}$ in children less than 2 years of age undergoing general anesthesia and found that these indexes failed to predict a hemodynamic response at tracheal intubation and skin incision. (2) The NIPE reflected nociceptive events as well as anesthetic induction in pediatric patients undergoing general anetshesia.

Several studies indicated ANI was able to predict movement and hemodynamic reactivity in adult patients [10–13]. Some studies observed hemodynamic response could not be anticipated based on the ANI [1, 21, 22]. Our study also did not find that the NIPE could predict a HR- or MBP-based response to nociceptive stimuli. The reason for this discrepancy of results are ultimately unclear. Patients in previous studies [10–13] did not receive neuromuscular blocking drugs before stimulation, whereas we used a regime with rocuronium. The previously described variation in autonomous stress response to tracheal intubation with and without neuromuscular blockade may partially explain the observed differences [23].

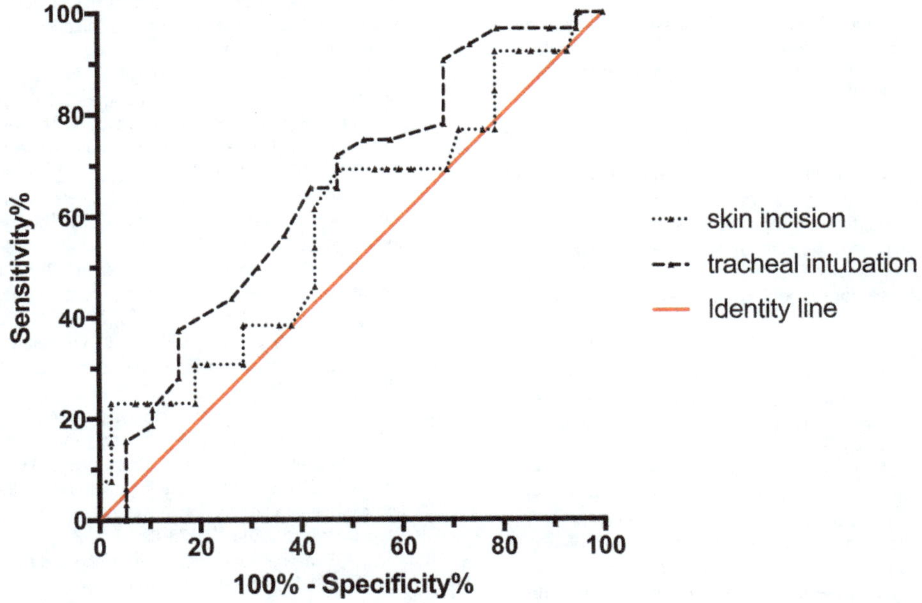

Fig. 2 Predictive ability of NIPE for a traditional hemodynamic change at tracheal intubation and skin incision. The area under receiver operating characteristic curve (AUC) values for this predictive ability of NIPE were 0.65 (95%CI 0.50–0.78) at endotracheal intubation and 0.58 (0.44–0.71) at skin incision

In consideration of perioperative safety, all children enrolled underwent ETT intubation after administration of a muscle relaxant. Children who were allowed to resume spontaneous breathing during surgery were not enrolled in order to avoid a statistical bias introduced by this anesthetic technique. The respiratory sinus arrythymia (RSA) was also affected by respiratory parameters (e.g., respiratory rate, tidal volume and inspiration-expiration ratio) [24, 25]. In the current study, the respiratory rate (RR) during mechanical ventilation was kept at a fixed number (20 breaths per minute), which was relatively lower than normal respiratory rate in awake children (~ 30 breaths per minute). Furthermore, in infants, the effects of different breathing rates with I:E ratios different from spontaneous breathing on HRV indices are unknown [26].

The pre-induction and pre-intubation NIPE values were low in our cohort (40 ± 12 and 45 ± 8, respectively). Absence of ventilation before intubation could explain the low NIPE values observed before intubation. NIPE is a measure for analyzing HRV that evaluates the parasympathetic activity by assessing RSA. Secondly, we speculate the a lower pre-intubation NIPE value may be associated with the injection pain and withdrawal response. Usually anesthesia for infants and children is induced with propofol and rocuronium. At last, HRV reflects the balance between parasympathetic and sympathetic nerve outflow from the central nervous system to the cardiac sinus node. Anxiety, which most likely plays a pathogenetic role, is associated with autonomic dysfunction [27]. Preoperative emotion (such as anxiety and fear) was shown to mediate RSA alteration in adults [28, 29]. Crying and struggling in older infants and toddlers may also lead to increased sympathetic nervous system activity. Acute stress, with subsequent release of catecholamines into the systemic circulation, causes abnormal HRV responses to acute pain [30]. In the pre-anesthesia period, although a series of strategies has been adopted, anxiety in children can be reduced but not eliminated, which also explains the low NIPE values that we observed prior to anesthesia induction.

Despite low pre-event values of NIPE in current study making a significant decline after noxious stimulus less likely, the NIPE showed a significanted change and reflected nociceptive events as well as anesthetic induction. Thus, NIPE may potentially aid the monitoring of nociception.

Finally, the present study has several limitations that should be noted. (1) NIPE evaluation requires ventilation, and NIPE analysis during apnea phases is questionable. (2) Under current sample size, weak response of hemodynamics to skin incision due to enough analgesia might have reduced the statistical power to detect prediction ability. A larger sample size is needed in further research.

Conclusion

In conclusion, the NIPE reflected nociceptive events as well as anesthetic induction in infants and young toddlers undergoing general anaesthetia. Nevertheless, NIPE may not serve as a sensitive and specific predictor to changes in hemodynamics.

Abbreviations

ANI: Analgesia nociception index; AUC: Area under curve; CI: Confidence interval; HR: Heart rate; MBP: Mean blood pressure; NIPE: Newborn infant parasympathetic evaluation; ROC: Receiver operating characteristic; RSA: Respiratory sinus arrythymia

Acknowledgements

We appreciate the efforts of all health-care providers and the patients and family for their participation in this study. We express special thanks to Dr. Chun yin WAT from the Department of Anesthesiology, the University of Hong Kong for professional language editing. We also acknowledge the Department of Anesthesiology team in Shanghai children's medical center of Shanghai Jiao Tong University for supporting the research.

Authors' contributions

This research was accomplished by seven co-authors; the contribution of each author are as follows: KZ was involved in designing the study, accomplishing the work of preoperative follow-up, collecting the most of the data, and drafting the manuscript; SYW was involved in designing the postoperative part of the research protocol and assisted KZ to finish postoperative follow-up; LW instructed the design of the research protocol; YAS performed the general anesthesia processes; MHC participated in designing the recruitment criteria and patient recruitment processes; MZZ gave some instructions in designing and writing the manuscript; JJZ gave some instructions in designing and writing the manuscript. All authors read and approved the final manuscript.

Author details

[1]Department of Anesthesiology, Shanghai Children's Medical Center, Shanghai Jiao Tong University School of Medicine & National Children's Medical Center (Shanghai), 1678 Dongfang Road, Shanghai 200127, China. [2]Pediatric Clinical Pharmacology Laboratory, Shanghai Children's Medical Center, Shanghai Jiao Tong University School of Medicine & National Children's Medical Center (Shanghai), Shanghai, China. [3]Department of Anesthesiology, 3201 Hospital, Xi'an Jiaotong University Health Science Center, Hanzhong, Shaanxi Province, China.

References

1. Defresne A, Barvais L, Clement F, Bonhomme V. Standardised noxious stimulation-guided individual adjustment of remifentanil target-controlled infusion to prevent haemodynamic responses to laryngoscopy and surgical incision: a randomised controlled trial. Eur J Anaesthesiol. 2018;35(3):173–83.
2. Fechner J, Ihmsen H, Schuttler J, Jeleazcov C. The impact of intra-operative sufentanil dosing on post-operative pain, hyperalgesia and morphine consumption after cardiac surgery. Eur J Pain. 2013;17(4):562–70.
3. Fletcher D, Martinez V. Opioid-induced hyperalgesia in patients after surgery: a systematic review and a meta-analysis. Br J Anaesth. 2014; 112(6):991–1004.
4. Daccache G, Jeanne M, Fletcher D. The analgesia nociception index: tailoring opioid administration. Anesth Analg. 2017;125(1):15–7.
5. Boselli E, Bouvet L, Begou G, Dabouz R, Davidson J, Deloste JY, Rahali N, Zadam A, Allaouchiche B. Prediction of immediate postoperative pain using the analgesia/nociception index: a prospective observational study. Br J Anaesth. 2014;112(4):715–21.
6. Logier R, Jeanne M, De Jonckheere J, Dassonneville A, Delecroix M, Tavernier B. PhysioDoloris: a monitoring device for analgesia / nociception balance evaluation using heart rate variability analysis. Conf Proc IEEE Eng Med Biol Soc. 2010;2010:1194–7.
7. Boselli E, Jeanne M. Analgesia/nociception index for the assessment of acute postoperative pain. Br J Anaesth. 2014;112(5):936–7.
8. Faye PM, De Jonckheere J, Logier R, Kuissi E, Jeanne M, Rakza T, Storme L. Newborn infant pain assessment using heart rate variability analysis. Clin J Pain. 2010;26(9):777–82.
9. Rakza T, Butruille L, Thirel L, Houfflin-Debarge V, Logier R, Storme L, De Jonckheere J. Short-term impact of assisted deliveries: evaluation based on behavioral pain scoring and heart rate variability. Clin J Pain. 2018; 34(5):445–9.
10. Boselli E, Bouvet L, Begou G, Torkmani S, Allaouchiche B. Prediction of hemodynamic reactivity during total intravenous anesthesia for suspension laryngoscopy using analgesia/nociception index (ANI): a prospective observational study. Minerva Anestesiol. 2015;81(3):288–97.
11. Funcke S, Sauerlaender S, Pinnschmidt HO, Saugel B, Bremer K, Reuter DA, Nitzschke R. Validation of innovative techniques for monitoring nociception during general anesthesia: a clinical study using tetanic and Intracutaneous electrical stimulation. Anesthesiology. 2017;127(2):272–83.
12. Gruenewald M, Herz J, Schoenherr T, Thee C, Steinfath M, Bein B. Measurement of the nociceptive balance by analgesia nociception index and surgical Pleth index during sevoflurane-remifentanil anesthesia. Minerva Anestesiol. 2015;81(5):480–9.
13. Jeanne M, Delecroix M, De Jonckheere J, Keribedj A, Logier R, Tavernier B. Variations of the analgesia nociception index during propofol anesthesia for total knee replacement. Clin J Pain. 2014;30(12):1084–8.
14. Cremillieux C, Makhlouf A, Pichot V, Trombert B, Patural H. Objective assessment of induced acute pain in neonatology with the newborn infant parasympathetic evaluation index. Eur J Pain. 2018;22(6):1071–9.
15. De Jonckheere J, Storme L. NIPE is related to parasympathetic activity. Is it also related to comfort? J Clin Monit Comput. 2019; https://doi.org/10.1007/s10877-019-00276-1.
16. Oberlander TF, Grunau RE, Pitfield S, Whitfield MF, Saul JP. The developmental character of cardiac autonomic responses to an acute noxious event in 4- and 8-month-old healthy infants. Pediatr Res. 1999;45(4 Pt 1):519–25.
17. Constant I, Sabourdin N. Monitoring depth of anesthesia: from consciousness to nociception. A window on subcortical brain activity. Paediatr Anaesth. 2015;25(1):73–82.
18. Practice Guidelines for Preoperative Fasting and the Use of Pharmacologic Agents to Reduce the Risk of Pulmonary Aspiration. Application to healthy patients undergoing elective procedures: an updated report by the American Society of Anesthesiologists Task Force on preoperative fasting and the use of pharmacologic agents to reduce the risk of pulmonary aspiration. Anesthesiology. 2017;126(3):376–93.
19. De Jonckheere J, Rakza T, Logier R, Jeanne M, Jounwaz R, Storme L. Heart rate variability analysis for newborn infants prolonged pain assessment. Conf Proc IEEE Eng Med Biol Soc. 2011;2011:7747–50.
20. Xue FS, Liu KP, Liu Y, Xu YC, Liao X, Zhang GH, Li CW, Yang QY, Sun HT. Assessment of small-dose fentanyl and sufentanil blunting the cardiovascular responses to laryngoscopy and intubation in children. Paediatr Anaesth. 2007;17(6):568–74.
21. Boselli E, Logier R, Bouvet L, Allaouchiche B. Prediction of hemodynamic reactivity using dynamic variations of analgesia/nociception index (ANI). J Clin Monit Comput. 2016;30(6):977–84.
22. Ledowski T, Averhoff L, Tiong WS, Lee C. Analgesia nociception index (ANI) to predict intraoperative haemodynamic changes: results of a pilot investigation. Acta Anaesthesiol Scand. 2014;58(1):74–9.
23. Janda M, Bajorat J, Kudlik C, Pohl B, Schubert A, Noldge-Schomburg G, Hofmockel R. Comparison of heart rate variability response in children undergoing elective endotracheal intubation with and without neuromuscular blockade: a randomized controlled trial. Paediatr Anaesth. 2013;23(12):1153–9.
24. Billman GE. The effect of heart rate on the heart rate variability response to autonomic interventions. Front Physiol. 2013;4:222.
25. Reyes del Paso GA, Langewitz W, Mulder LJ, van Roon A, Duschek S. The utility of low frequency heart rate variability as an index of sympathetic cardiac tone: a review with emphasis on a reanalysis of previous studies. Psychophysiology. 2013;50(5):477–87.
26. Lin IM, Tai LY, Fan SY. Breathing at a rate of 5.5 breaths per minute with equal inhalation-to-exhalation ratio increases heart rate variability. Int J Psychophysiol. 2014;91(3):206–11.
27. Miu AC, Heilman RM, Miclea M. Reduced heart rate variability and vagal tone in anxiety: trait versus state, and the effects of autogenic training. Auton Neurosci. 2009;145(1–2):99–103.
28. Sleigh JW, Henderson JD. Heart rate variability and preoperative anxiety. Acta Anaesthesiol Scand. 1995;39(8):1059–61.
29. Ledowski T, Bein B, Hanss R, Tonner PH, Roller N, Scholz J. Pseudocholinesterase activity increases and heart rate variability decreases with preoperative anxiety. Eur J Anaesthesiol. 2005;22(4):289–92.
30. Terkelsen AJ, Molgaard H, Hansen J, Andersen OK, Jensen TS. Acute pain increases heart rate: differential mechanisms during rest and mental stress. Auton Neurosci. 2005;121(1–2):101–9.

6

Evaluation of alveolar recruitment maneuver on respiratory resistance during general anesthesia

Junko Nakahira*, Shoko Nakano and Toshiaki Minami

Abstract

Background: Alveolar recruitment maneuvers enable easily reopening nonaerated lung regions via a transient elevation in transpulmonary pressure. To evaluate the effect of these maneuvers on respiratory resistance, we used an oscillatory technique during mechanical ventilation. This study was conducted to assess the effect of the alveolar recruitment maneuvers on respiratory resistance under routine anesthesia. We hypothesized that respiratory resistance at 5 Hz (R5) after the maneuver would be decreased after the lung aeration.

Methods: After receiving the ethics committee's approval, we enrolled 33 patients who were classified with an American Society of Anesthesiologists physical status of 1, 2 or 3 and were undergoing general anesthesia for transurethral resection of a bladder tumor within a 12-month period from 2017 to 2018. The recruitment maneuver was performed 30 min after endotracheal intubation. The maneuver consisted of sustained manual inflation of the anesthesia reservoir bag to a peak inspiratory pressure of 40 cmH_2O for 15 s, including 5 s of gradually increasing the peak inspiratory pressure. Respiratory resistance was measured using the forced oscillation technique before and after the maneuver, and the mean R5 was calculated during the expiratory phase. The respiratory resistance and ventilator parameter results were analyzed using paired Student's t-tests, and $p < 0.05$ was considered statistically significant.

Results: We analyzed 31 patients (25 men and 6 women). R5 was 7.3 ± 1.6 cmH_2O/L/sec before the recruitment maneuver during mechanical ventilation and was significantly decreased to 6.4 ± 1.7 cmH_2O/L/sec after the maneuver. Peak inspiratory pressure and plateau pressure were significantly decreased, and pulmonary compliance was increased, although the values were not clinically relevant.

Conclusion: The recruitment maneuver decreased respiratory resistance and increased lung compliance during mechanical ventilation.

(Continued on next page)

* Correspondence: ane052@osaka-med.ac.jp
Department of Anesthesiology, Osaka Medical College 2-7 Daigaku-machi, Takatsuki, Osaka 569-8686, Japan

(Continued from previous page)
Keywords: Respiratory resistance, Alveolar recruitment maneuver, Forced oscillation technique

Background

Lung-protective ventilation using a low tidal volume is the standard of care for mechanically ventilated patients with acute respiratory distress syndrome [1] and was recently demonstrated to significantly improve postoperative outcomes in patients undergoing surgery [2–5]. Alveolar recruitment maneuvers (ARMs), which are used to reopen collapsed lungs, and positive end-expiratory pressure (PEEP) are lung-protective ventilation strategies [6–8]. Using recruitment maneuvers to open the lungs improves the effectiveness of PEEP for gas exchange during mechanical ventilation [9–11]. Although many studies have reported the effectiveness of low tidal volume ventilation and ARMs [2–4, 12–15], no studies have evaluated ARMs independently of the PEEP level [16]. The definition of ARMs varies among studies. An automatic ARM is an automated stepwise recruitment maneuver with PEEP-titration [17]. Although automatic ARMs are widely used, most hospitals use ventilators without an automatic ARM mode. We routinely use a sustained inflation ARM, which transiently applies a high-pressure static increase in airway pressure for 10–15 s.

The forced oscillation technique (FOT) is used to measure respiratory impedance by measuring the relationship between pressure waves applied externally to the respiratory system and the resulting respiratory airflow. The FOT device measures respiratory resistance at 5 Hz (R5), which includes the resistance in the oropharynx, larynx, trachea, bronchi, pulmonary alveolus, and chest wall tissue. Exertional breathing maneuvers are not required during FOT measurement. MostGraph-01® (Chest MI, Tokyo, Japan) is a noninvasive device that measures respiratory resistance using broadband frequency FOT. We previously reported using this device to measure increased respiratory resistance after general anesthesia [18–21].

Because few studies have evaluated ARMs independently of the PEEP level, we investigated the effect of ARMs on respiratory status during surgery. We hypothesized that compared with respiratory compliance, tidal volume and partial pressure of oxygen in the arterial blood (PaO_2), respiratory resistance would be a better parameter for detecting the effects of ARMs in patients with mostly intact respiratory systems. This study was conducted to assess the effect of ARMs on respiratory resistance during routine anesthesia. We hypothesized that the R5 would be decreased after the ARM because of the lung aeration and that the tidal volume would be increased, even under volume-controlled ventilation.

Methods

The ethics committee of Osaka Medical College, Japan (approval reference number 1252) approved the study, which was conducted in accordance with the declaration of Helsinki (1964). All participants provided written informed consent. The study was registered at the Japan Medical Association Center for Clinical Trials (reference JMA-IIA00136). We enrolled 33 patients who were classified as American Society of Anesthesiologists physical status 1, 2 or 3 and undergoing general anesthesia for transurethral resection of a bladder tumor within a 12-month period from 2017 to 2018. Exclusion criteria included substantive abnormalities in spirometry (forced expiratory volume in 1 s < 50% of predicted volume; forced vital capacity < 50% of predicted volume), active asthma (requiring bronchodilator therapy or coughing or wheezing at rest), preoperative fractional nitric oxide concentration in exhaled breath (FeNO) > 50 ppb [22], previous lung surgery, history of chronic obstructive pulmonary disease requiring bronchodilator therapy, home oxygen therapy or having had a respiratory tract infection within the previous 3 months. The primary outcome was the difference between the pre-ARM R5 and post-ARM R5 during ventilation. The secondary outcome was the difference in tidal volume and lung compliance.

Preoperative measurements

Respiratory examinations were performed, including spirometry without bronchodilation and FeNO measurement. Spirometry was performed within a month before surgery using a spirometer (System 21 device®, Minato Igkagaku, Osaka, Japan) and FeNO was measured using NIOX VERO® (Aerocrine, Aolna, Sweden) the day before surgery. Respiratory resistance was measured using the MostGraph-01® the day before and the day after surgery. Patients sat with a nose clip and their cheeks supported firmly during the respiratory resistance measurements.

Anesthetic management

A standardized anesthetic technique was used. Anesthesia was induced with 1.0–1.5 mg/kg intravenous propofol, 0.7–0.9 mg/kg rocuronium, a continuous infusion of 0.4 μg/kg/min remifentanil and 2.0–3.0% inhaled sevoflurane. The trachea was intubated with a tube that had an internal diameter of 7.0 mm for women and 8.0 mm for men (Portex Soft Seal®, Smiths Medical, Kent, UK). Anesthesia was maintained with inhaled sevoflurane, intravenous remifentanil and intravenous rocuronium at 4–6 µg/kg/min. The sevoflurane concentration was titrated over 1.5% at the discretion of the attending anesthetist according to a bispectral index monitor that was controlled between 40 and 60. At the end of the surgery, patients were administered 1000 mg intravenous acetaminophen for pain relief, followed by 1.5–2.0 mg/kg (maximum 200 mg) intravenous sugammadex. Tracheal suctioning was performed once or twice before patients were extubated. The endotracheal tube was removed when patients could communicate and breathe spontaneously with sufficient tidal volume. Supplementary oxygen at 6 L/min was administered via facemask immediately after extubation.

Devices and measurement procedures during anesthesia

After inducing anesthesia, all patients were mechanically ventilated using the volume-controlled mode with an inspiratory/expiratory ratio of 1:2, an inspiratory pause time/total inspiratory time ratio of 0.1, tidal volume of 8 mL/kg ideal body weight with a PEEP of 5 cmH_2O, a respiratory frequency of 10–12 breaths/min to maintain the end-tidal carbon dioxide from 35 to 45 mmHg, and an oxygen inspiratory fraction of 0.4 (Drägel Fabius®, Dragel Medical, Lubeck, Germany). The ARM was performed 30 min after tracheal intubation and consisted of sustained manual inflation of the anesthesia reservoir bag to a peak inspiratory pressure of 40 cmH_2O for 15 s, including gradually increasing the peak inspiratory pressure for 5 s. Before the ARM, the peak airway pressure, plateau pressure, PEEP, and tidal volume were obtained from the ventilation monitor. Dynamic respiratory compliance (Cdyn) and static pulmonary compliance (Cst) were calculated as Cdyn = tidal volume/(peak pressure – PEEP) and Cst = tidal volume/(plateau – PEEP).

We modified this device to measure the R5 during ventilation using an endotracheal tube under general anesthesia. We used the MostGraph-01®, which was modified to measure respiratory resistance during mechanical ventilation (Figs. 1, 2) as previously described [23]. We put a connection on the vent to connect a loud speaker to the ventilator and endotracheal tube. The company that made and sold this device (Chest MI) made this modification after giving us their permission. Thirty minutes after inducing anesthesia, we measured the respiratory resistance using the modified device. During this measurement, the ventilator setting was changed to a tidal volume of 16 mL/kg ideal body weight with zero PEEP and an oxygen inspiratory fraction of 0.6. We measured the respiratory resistance again using the MostGraph-01® immediately after the ARM, changed the ventilator setting back to the previous setting and measured the peak airway pressure, plateau pressure, PEEP, and tidal volume again. Offline data from the MostGraph-01® were analyzed after each operation (Fig. 3). The mean respiratory resistance at 5 Hz was calculated after baseline adjustment using the mean value of the latter half of the inspiratory phase.

Statistical analysis

Our preliminary measurements for the pre-ARM R5 and post-ARM R5 were 5.49 ± 1.25 cm H_2O/L/s (mean ± SD) and 4.88 ± 1.35 cm H_2O/L/s, respectively; therefore, the standard deviation was considered to be 1.25, and the expected difference in R5 was considered to be 1.25 cm

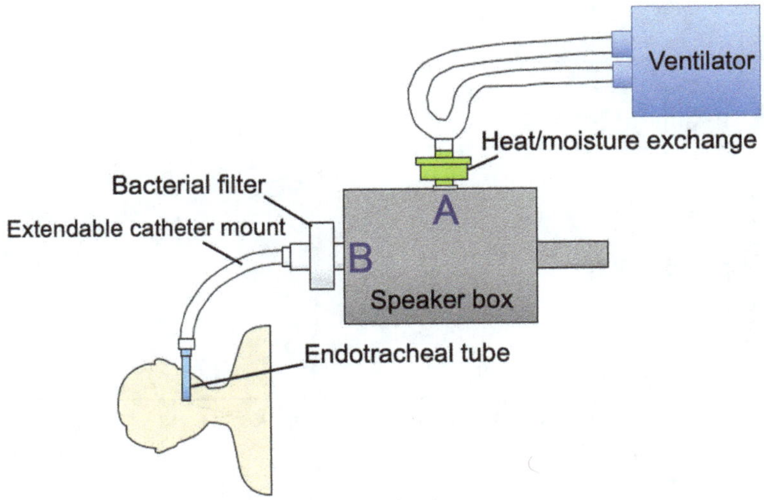

Fig. 1 Schema of respiratory resistance measurements using the MostGraph-01® during mechanical ventilation. A is the connection between the speaker box and ventilator circuit. B is the connection between the speaker box and examinee. The speaker box is composed of a loud speaker and a pressure and flow sensor

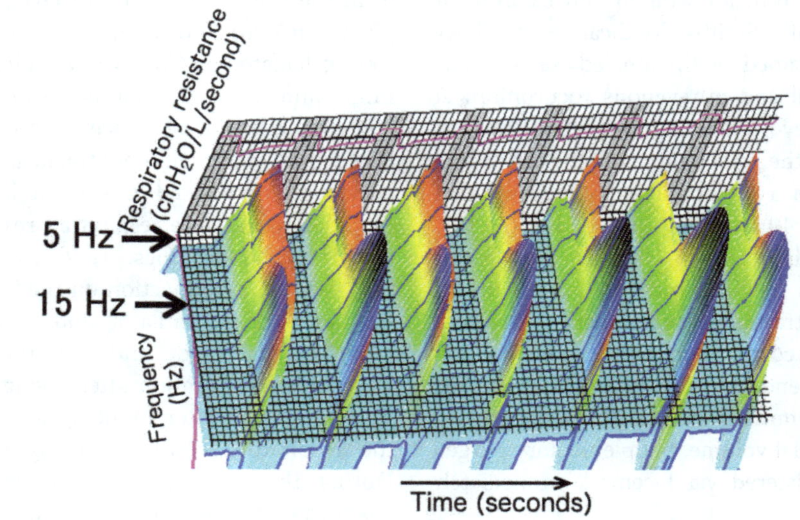

Fig. 2 Example of respiratory resistance during mechanical ventilation. Three-dimensional graph of respiratory resistance with a frequency range from 4 to 35 Hz is shown. High respiratory resistance over 15 Hz indicates fluttering of a check valve in the ventilator

H_2O/L/sec. The sample size was determined from our preliminary R5 study of 8 patients using a subglottic airway device. A sample size of 33 patients was required to obtain 80% power between the pre-ARM and post-ARM at an α error level of 5% and an intragroup difference of 1.25 cm H_2O/L/s in R5. Data are expressed as the mean ± SD or median (interquartile range, 25–75%) according to the variable distribution. Normality was analyzed using the Shapiro-Wilk test. The MostGraph-01® and ventilator parameter results were analyzed using paired Student's *t*-tests; $p < 0.05$ was considered statistically significant. All statistical analyses were performed using GraphPad Prism 6 software (GraphPad Software, La Jolla, CA, USA).

Results

For two of the 33 patients, the respiratory resistance measurement during mechanical ventilation was saved incorrectly; therefore, 31 patients (25 men and 6 women) were included in the final analysis. No patients experienced any serious perioperative events. No patient showed a preoperative FeNO > 50 ppb. No patient had < 96% oxygen saturation as measured by pulse oximetry. Table 1 shows the patients' characteristics. The preoperative R5 was 2.6 ± 0.9 cmH_2O/L/sec; the postoperative R5 was 2.8 ± 0.9 cmH_2O/L/sec.

R5 was significantly decreased after the post-ARM during mechanical ventilation (Table 2). The R5 was 7.3 ± 1.6 cmH2O/L/sec during mechanical ventilation before the

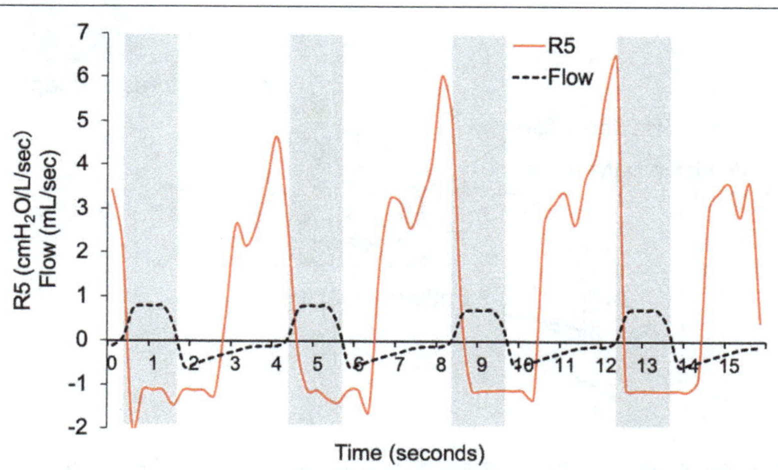

Fig. 3 Example of respiratory resistance at 5 Hz during mechanical ventilation. Gray zones represent the inspiratory phase. The mean respiratory resistance at 5 Hz was calculated after baseline adjustment using the mean value of the latter half of the inspiratory phase

Table 1 Patient characteristics and operative results (n=31)

Characteristics	
Male/female (n)	25/6
Age (years)	69 (63-78)
Height (cm)	164.7±7.7
Body weight (kg)	65.8±10.9
Ideal body weight (kg)	59.8±5.5
Body mass index	24.2±3.0
Body surface area (m^2)	1.72±0.17
ASA physical status I/II/III (n)	1/23/7
Comorbidities (n)	
Hypertension	10
Diabetes	6
Dyslipidemia	3
Atrial fibrillation	2
Dialysis	1
Coronary artery disease	1
Ex-/current smoker (n)	15
Brinkman index	300 (0-700)
VC (L)	3.4±0.8
%VC (% predicted)	97.5±11.6
FVC (L)	3.3±0.8
%FVC (% predicted)	98.4±12.1
FEV1.0 (L)	2.5±0.6
%FEV1.0 (% predicted)	76.2 (71.6-79.8)
FEV1.0/FVC (%)	73.0±11.0
FeNO (ppb)[a]	17 (15-21)
Preoperative R5 (cmH_2O/L/second)	2.6±0.9
Postoperative R5 (cmH_2O/L/second)	2.8±0.9
Operation time (minutes)	31 (21-55)
Anesthesia time (minutes)	79 (65-93)
Fluid infusion (mL)	400 (250-550)
Internal diameter of tracheal tube 7/7.5/8 mm (n)	6/1/24

Values are the mean±SD or median (percentile, 25%–75%) or number (n). Brinkman index, defined as the number of cigarettes smoked per day multiplied by smoking years, was calculated only for smokers and ex-smokers. *ASA* American Society of Anesthesiologists, *VC* Vital capacity, *FVC* Forced vital capacity, *FEV1.0* Forced expiratory volume in the first second.
[a]Data were detected in 17 cases.

recruitment maneuver; the R5 was significantly decreased to 6.4 ± 1.7 cmH_2O/L/sec after the maneuver. Peak inspiratory airway pressure and plateau pressure were significantly decreased. Pre- and post-ARM lung compliance (Cdyn) were 47.0 ± 8.8 mL/cmH_2O and 50.0 ± 8.9 mL/cmH_2O, respectively. Pre- and post-ARM Cst were 58.3 ± 13.9 mL/cmH_2O and 63.1 ± 13.3 mL/cmH_2O, respectively. Lung compliance significantly increased after the ARM. Post-ARM tidal volume on the ventilator measurement

Table 2 Respiratory effects of the alveolar recruitment maneuver (n=31)

	Pre-ARM	Post-ARM	*P* value
MostGraph® measurement			
Tidal volume (mL)	447±55	458±53	0.077
R5 (cmH_2O/L/second)	7.3±1.6	6.4±1.7	0.001
Ventilator measurement			
Tidal volume setting (mL)	497±53	497±53	NA
Actual tidal volume (mL)	480±56	488±56	0.026
Peak inspiratory pressure (cmH_2O)	15.5±1.7	15.0±1.5	<0.001
Plateau pressure (cmH_2O)	13.6±1.6	13.0±1.4	<0.001
PEEP (cmH_2O)	5±0	5±0	NA
Cdyn (mL/cmH_2O)	47.0±8.8	50.0±8.9	<0.001
Cst (mL/cmH_2O)	58.3±13.9	63.1±13.3	<0.001

ARM Alveolar recruitment maneuver, *Cdyn* Dynamic respiratory compliance, *Cst* Static pulmonary compliance, *NA* Not applicable, *PEEP* Positive end-expiratory pressure.

was significantly increased compared with the pre-ARM tidal volume but not on the MostGraph measurement.

Discussion

This was the first study to evaluate the effect of ARMs on respiratory resistance. R5 represents respiratory resistance, including resistance in the oropharynx, larynx, trachea, bronchi, lungs, and chest wall tissue. This study showed that ARMS improved the R5 under general anesthesia, increased the lung compliance, and reduced the peak and plateau pressures. An increase in lung compliance immediately after applying the ARM might reflect a reduced atelectasis. A decrease in R5 suggests an improved Cdyn. Although the effect of ARMs on lung compliance is controversial [13], many studies have reported a statistically significant increase in lung compliance after ARMs in patients undergoing surgery [2, 12–15]. We hypothesized that respiratory resistance would be a better parameter for measuring the effects of ARMs in patients with intact respiratory systems; however, this hypothesis was incorrect.

A 2006 multicenter observational study in France reported that ARMs were only used in 7% of patients [24]; however, ARMs are widely used to improve arterial oxygenation [6]. Various ARMs have been proposed, including 1) sustained high-pressure inflation, 2) high tidal volumes and inspiratory pressures delivered intermittently, and 3) stepwise increases in PEEP and/or airway plateau inspiratory pressure [25]. However, the optimal method for ARMs remains uncertain. ARM use is not standardized and is left to the individual physician based on their experience. In this study, no automatic ARM was available for our ventilation machine; therefore, we performed sustained inflation as the ARM. Briefly, the manual ARM consisted of applying a continuous positive

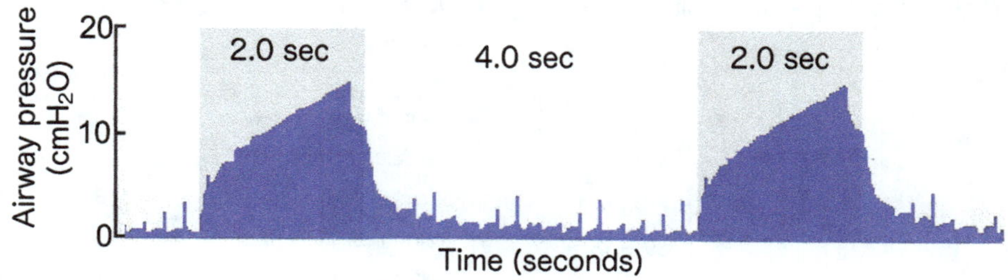

Fig. 4 Airway pressure wave detected using a ventilator sensor during the respiratory resistance measurement. Airway pressure including oscillation pressure is shown. The ventilator settings were as follows: respiratory rate: 10/min, inspiratory/expiratory ratio: 0.5, and inspiratory pause time/total inspiratory time ratio: 10%. Gray zones represent the inspiratory phase. Respiratory resistance could not be detected in the first 0.4 s of the expiratory phase because high airway pressure (> 4 cmH_2O) prevents detecting respiratory resistance

airway pressure of 30 cmH_2O for 30 s [26]. A study reported that a plateau "opening pressure" of 40 cmH_2O for 7–8 s effectively opened all alveoli in a nonobese patient with healthy lungs [27]. We used a continuous positive airway pressure of 40 cmH_2O for 10 s in this study, primarily to prevent significant hemodynamic changes. ARM refers to a transient increase in transpulmonary pressure induced by increased intrathoracic pressure and decreased venous return, leading to a decrease in left ventricular end-diastolic areas and stroke volume [26, 28]. Importantly, automatic ARMs can cause hypotension [2, 13].

Contemporary anesthetic ventilators often include options to display the pressure-volume loop and calculated dynamic compliance values. Comparing the pre- and post-ARM lung compliance enables easier detection of the ARM's effectiveness [26]. Automatic ARMs can be scheduled using the latest ventilation machine models. Previous studies performed the ARM as soon as mechanical ventilation was initiated, which was repeated after any discontinuation from the ventilator [13, 29]. Measuring respiratory resistance enables determining the best ARM for specific situations when patients are undergoing surgery.

Some studies have reported beneficial effects from ARMs. A randomized controlled trial revealed fewer incidences of postoperative nausea and vomiting after gynecological laparoscopic surgery [30]. Additionally, ARMs may reduce the incidence of shoulder pain following laparoscopic surgery [31, 32]. Our results showed no clinical significance regarding postoperative complications.

This study had some limitations. This was the first study to detect respiratory resistance during mechanical ventilation using the MostGraph-01®. We followed previously described methods to measure the respiratory resistance through an endotracheal tube [23]. There were limitations in evaluating respiratory resistance during mechanical ventilation. Respiratory resistance cannot be detected during the initial 0.4 s of the expiratory phase because the high airway pressure (> 4 cmH_2O) prevents it (Fig. 4). This delays the increased respiratory resistance. Establishing the respiratory resistance measurement under high airway pressure requires increasing the size of the oscillation speaker.

Another limitation was that PEEP was not applied when measuring respiratory resistance using the MostGraph-01® because adding a positive expiratory pressure made it difficult to detect respiratory resistance. In normal clinical situations, PEEP is needed directly after ARMs to prevent lung collapse; therefore, a better technique is required.

We did not measure PaO_2 to evaluate the effect of the ARMs. We could not perform blood gas analyses during the transurethral resection surgeries performed during this study. This surgery was chosen to prevent the influence of respiratory status under well-controlled anesthesia. We showed that respiratory resistance was statistically significant but could not show its clinical relevance. A new study, including clinical parameters, is needed.

Conclusions

The ARM decreased respiratory resistance and increased lung compliance during mechanical ventilation. The ARM caused the airways to reopen. Although some difficulties were noted, measuring the FOT using the MostGraph-01® is a straightforward method to evaluate changes in respiratory resistance. We showed that respiratory resistance was statistically significant but could not show its clinical relevance. This measurement may help determine the best ARM type for patients under general anesthesia.

Abbreviations

ARMs: Alveolar recruitment maneuvers; Cdyn: Dynamic respiratory compliance; Cst: Static pulmonary compliance; FeNO: Fractional nitric oxide concentration in exhaled breath; FOT: Forced oscillation technique; PEEP: Positive end-expiratory pressure; R5: Respiratory resistance at 5 Hz

Acknowledgments

We thank Traci Raley, MS, ELS, from Edanz Group (https://en-author-services.edanzgroup.com/ac) for editing a draft of this manuscript.

Authors' contributions

JN participated in designing and coordinating the study and drafted the manuscript. SN made substantial contributions by performing statistical analyses and helping to draft the manuscript. TM made substantial contributions to the study conception and helped draft the manuscript. All authors have read and approved the final manuscript.

References

1. Acute Respiratory Distress Syndrome Network, Brower RG, Matthay MA, Morris A, Schoenfeld D, Thompson BT, et al. Ventilation with lower tidal volumes as compared with traditional tidal volumes for acute lung injury and the acute respiratory distress syndrome. N Engl J Med. 2000;342:1301–8.
2. PROVE Network Investigators for the Clinical Trial Network of the European Society of Anaesthesiology, Hemmes SN, Gama de Abreu M, Pelosi P, Schultz MJ. High versus low positive end-expiratory pressure during general anaesthesia for open abdominal surgery (PROVHILO trial): A multicentre randomised controlled trial. Lancet. 2014;384:495–503.
3. Serpa Neto A, Hemmes SN, Barbas CS, Beiderlinden M, Biehl M, Binnekade JM, et al. Protective versus conventional ventilation for surgery: a systematic review and individual patient data meta-analysis. Anesthesiology. 2015;123: 66–78.
4. Neto AS, Hemmes SN, Barbas CS, Beiderlinden M, Fernandez-Bustamante A, Futier E, et al. Association between driving pressure and development of postoperative pulmonary complications in patients undergoing mechanical ventilation for general anaesthesia: a meta-analysis of individual patient data. Lancet Respir Med. 2016;4:272–80.
5. Writing Committee for the PROBESE Collaborative Group of the PROtective VEntilation Network (PROVEnet) for the Clinical Trial Network of the European Society of Anaesthesiology, Bluth T, Serpa Neto A, Schultz MJ, Pelosi P, Gama de Abreu M, et al. Effect of intraoperative high positive end-expiratory pressure (PEEP) with recruitment maneuvers vs low PEEP on postoperative pulmonary complications in obese patients: A randomized clinical trial. JAMA. 2019;321:2292–305.
6. Futier E, Constantin JM, Paugam-Burtz C, Pascal J, Eurin M, Neuschwander A, et al. A trial of intraoperative low-tidal-volume ventilation in abdominal surgery. N Engl J Med. 2013;369:428–37.
7. Futier E, Marret E, Jaber S. Perioperative positive pressure ventilation: an integrated approach to improve pulmonary care. Anesthesiology. 2014;121: 400–8.
8. Hedenstierna G. Small tidal volumes, positive end-expiratory pressure, and lung recruitment maneuvers during anesthesia: good or bad? Anesthesiology. 2015;123:501–3.
9. Rothen HU, Sporre B, Engberg G, Wegenius G, Reber A, Hedenstierna G. Prevention of atelectasis during general anaesthesia. Lancet. 1995;345:1387–91.
10. Girgis K, Hamed H, Khater Y, Kacmarek RM. A decremental PEEP trial identifies the PEEP level that maintains oxygenation after lung recruitment. Respir Care. 2006;51:1132–9.
11. Maisch S, Reissmann H, Fuellekrug B, Weismann D, Rutkowski T, Tusman G, et al. Compliance and dead space fraction indicate an optimal level of positive end-expiratory pressure after recruitment in anesthetized patients. Anesth Analg. 2008;106:175–81.
12. Weingarten TN, Whalen FX, Warner DO, Gajic O, Schears GJ, Snyder MR, et al. Comparison of two ventilatory strategies in elderly patients undergoing major abdominal surgery. Br J Anaesth. 2010;104:16–22.
13. Severgnini P, Selmo G, Lanza C, Chiesa A, Frigerio A, Bacuzzi A, et al. Protective mechanical ventilation during general anesthesia for open abdominal surgery improves postoperative pulmonary function. Anesthesiology. 2013;118:1307–21.
14. Acosta CM, Sara T, Carpinella M, Volpicelli G, Ricci L, Poliotto S, et al. Lung recruitment prevents collapse during laparoscopy in children: a randomised controlled trial. Eur J Anaesthesiol. 2018;35:573–80.
15. Lovas A, Németh MF, Trásy D, Molnár Z. Lung recruitment can improve oxygenation in patients ventilated in continuous positive airway pressure/ pressure support mode. Front Med (Lausanne). 2015;2:25.
16. Miskovic A, Lumb AB. Postoperative pulmonary complications. Br J Anaesth. 2017;118:317–34.
17. Tusman G, Böhm SH, Melkun F, Staltari D, Quinzio C, Nador C, et al. Alveolar recruitment strategy increases arterial oxygenation during one-lung ventilation. Ann Thorac Surg. 2002;73:1204–9.
18. Nakahira J, Nakano S, Sawai T, Ishio J, Ono N, Minami T. Factors causing post-anesthetic high respiratory resistance in patients undergoing transurethral resection of bladder tumors. Anesth Pain Med. 2017;7:e44553.
19. Nakano S, Nakahira J, Kuzukawa Y, Sawai T, Minami T. The effects of endotracheal tube and i-gel® supraglottic airway device on respiratory impedance: a prospective observational study. Anesth Pain Med. 2016;7:e42964.
20. Nakano S, Nakahira J, Sawai T, Kuzukawa Y, Ishio J, Minami T. Perioperative evaluation of respiratory impedance using the forced oscillation technique: a prospective observational study. BMC Anesthesiol. 2016;16:32.
21. Kuzukawa Y, Nakahira J, Sawai T, Minami T. A perioperative evaluation of respiratory mechanics using the forced oscillation technique. Anesth Analg. 2015;121:1202–6.
22. Dweik RA, Boggs PB, Erzurum SC, Irvin CG, Leigh MW, Lundberg JO, et al. An official ATS clinical practice guideline: interpretation of exhaled nitric oxide levels (FENO) for clinical applications. Am J Respir Crit Care Med. 2011;184:602–15.
23. Peslin R, Felicio da Silva J, Duvivier C, Chabot F. Respiratory mechanics studied by forced oscillations during artificial ventilation. Eur Respir J. 1993;6:772–84.
24. Jaber S, Coisel Y, Chanques G, Futier E, Constantin JM, Michelet P, et al. A multicentre observational study of intra-operative ventilatory management during general anaesthesia: tidal volumes and relation to body weight. Anaesthesia. 2012;67:999–1008.
25. Chiumello D, Algieri I, Grasso S, Terragni P, Pelosi P. Recruitment maneuvers in acute respiratory distress syndrome and during general anesthesia. Minerva Anestesiol. 2016;82:210–20.
26. Biais M, Lanchon R, Sesay M, Le Gall L, Pereira B, Futier E, et al. Changes in stroke volume induced by lung recruitment maneuver predict fluid responsiveness in mechanically ventilated patients in the operating room. Anesthesiology. 2017;126:260–7.
27. Rothen HU, Neumann P, Berglund JE, Valtysson J, Magnusson A, Hedenstierna G. Dynamics of re-expansion of atelectasis during general anaesthesia. Br J Anaesth. 1999;82:551–6.
28. Thonnerieux M, Alexander B, Binet C, Obadia JF, Bastien O, Desebbe O. The ability of esCCO and ECOM monitors to measure trends in cardiac output during alveolar recruitment maneuver after cardiac surgery: a comparison with the pulmonary thermodilution method. Anesth Analg. 2015;121:383–91.
29. Futier E, Constantin JM, Jaber S. Protective lung ventilation in operating room: a systematic review. Minerva Anestesiol. 2014;80:726–35.
30. Phelps P, Cakmakkaya OS, Apfel CC, Radke OC. A simple clinical maneuver to reduce laparoscopy-induced shoulder pain: a randomized controlled trial. Obstet Gynecol. 2008;111:1155–60.
31. Tsai HW, Wang PH, Yen MS, Chao KC, Hsu TF, Chen YJ. Prevention of postlaparoscopic shoulder and upper abdominal pain: a randomized controlled trial. Obstet Gynecol. 2013;121:526–31.
32. Sharami SH, Sharami MB, Abdollahzadeh M, Keyvan A. Randomised clinical trial of the influence of pulmonary recruitment manoeuvre on reducing shoulder pain after laparoscopy. J Obstet Gynaecol. 2010;30:505–10.

7

Effect of sevoflurane on systemic and cerebral circulation, cerebral autoregulation and CO_2 reactivity

Marianna Juhász[1], Levente Molnár[1], Béla Fülesdi[1,3*], Tamás Végh[1,3], Dénes Páll[2] and Csilla Molnár[1]

Abstract

Background: Sevoflurane is one of the most frequently used inhaled anesthetics for general anesthesia. Previously it has been reported that at clinically used doses of sevoflurane, cerebral vasoreactivity is maintained. However, there are no data how sevoflurane influences systemic and cerebral circulation in parallel. The aim of our study was to assess systemic and cerebral hemodynamic changes as well as cerebral CO_2-reactivity during sevoflurane anesthesia.

Methods: Twenty nine patients undergoing general anesthesia were enrolled. Anesthesia was maintained with 1 MAC sevoflurane in 40% oxygen. Ventilatory settings (respiratory rate and tidal volume) were adjusted to reach and maintain 40, 35 and 30 mmHg $EtCO_2$ for 5 min respectively. At the end of each period, transcranial Doppler and hemodynamic parameters using applanation tonometry were recorded.

Results: Systemic mean arterial pressure significantly decreased during anesthetic induction and remained unchanged during the entire study period. Central aortic and peripherial pulse pressure and augmentation index as markers of arterial stiffness significantly increased during the anesthetic induction and remained stable at the time points when target CO_2 levels were reached. Both cerebral autoregulation and cerebral CO_2-reactivity was maintained at 1 MAC sevoflurane.

Discussion: Cerebral autoregulation and CO_2-reactivity is preserved at 1 MAC sevoflurane. Cerebrovascular effects of anesthetic compounds have to be assessed together with systemic circulatory effects.

Keywords: Sevoflurane, Cerebral blood flow, cerebral autoregulation, CO_2-reactivity, applanation tonometry, Transcranial Doppler

Background

The most important vasoregulatory mechanisms determining brain circulation are cerebral autoregulation and cerebral vasoreactivity. Cerebral autoregulation is the inherent ability of the brain circulation to maintain constant cerebral blood flow during alterations of systemic blood pressure and cerebral perfusion pressure. Cerebral vasoreactivity is responsible for enabling to change the blood flow (either globally or locally) according to the metabolic needs of the brain tissue [1]. Ideally, anesthetic agents should not have any significant impact on cerebral autoregulation and cerebral vasoreactivity during general anesthesia, which is especially important in the neurosurgical practice. There are data indicating that volatile anesthetics may alter both autoregulation and cerebral vasoreactivity to carbon-dioxide [2–4] under general anesthesia. Inhalational agents are usually characterized by dose-dependent depressive effect on cerebral autoregulation, with the exception of sevoflurane [3]. Sevoflurane, the most widely used inhalational agent does not influence cerebral vasoreactivity at MAC levels

* Correspondence: fulesdi@med.unideb.hu
[1]Faculty of Medicine, Department of Anesthesiology and Intensive Care, University of Debrecen, Nagyerdei krt. 98, Debrecen, Hungary
[3]Hungarian Center, Outcomes Research Consortium, Cleveland, USA

between 0.3 and 1.5 in healthy individuals [5]. There are reports suggesting that the autoregulatory plateau is shortened under sevoflurane anesthesia with MAC 1, and the upper and lower limits of autoregulation were independent of the age of the patients [5].

During induction and maintenance of general anesthesia different systemic and cerebral effects of the anesthetic agents have to be taken into account to have a global view on the anesthetic's effect and for the interpretation of the results. Thus, in the present study we aimed to assess changes in cerebral circulation and peripheral systemic hemodynamic changes in parallel during induction and maintenance of anesthesia with sevoflurane and the effect of different hypocapnic levels.

Applanation tonometry, a new, non-invasive method has been recently reported to be accurate for non-invasive intraoperative assessment of systemic hemodynamic changes during general anesthesia [6]. In line with this, for our measurements we used parallel assessment of systemic and cerebral circulation with the combination of applanation tonometry and transcranial Doppler.

We aimed to answer the following study questions:

- What is the effect of anesthetic induction and reaching the steady state sevoflurane anesthesia on systemic hemodynamics and cerebral blood flow measurements?
- Is cerebral autoregulation maintained at normocapnic steady state 1 MAC sevoflurane anesthesia?
- What are the cerebral and systemic hemodynamic effects of induced hypocapnia at 1 MAC sevoflurane?

Methods

Study population

After approval from the local Ethics Committee (DEOEC RKEB/IKEB 3584–2012;), written informed consent was obtained from 35 ASA I-II patients scheduled for varicectomy and inguinal hernial repair surgery. The study was registered at http://www.clinicaltrials.gov, identifier: NCT02054143, retrospectively registered. Exclusion criteria were age < 18 years or > 60 years, severe cardiovascular disease, severe carotid artery stenosis, cerebrovascular disease, smoking, diabetes mellitus, renal disease, hyperlipidemia, left ventricular hypertrophy and severe alteration of the preoperative pulmonary function, characterized as FEV1 < 70% and FEV1/FVC ≤70% of the predicted value.

Devices and measurements

For applanation tonometry SphygmoCor (AtCor Medical, Sydney, Australia) device was used. During applanation tonometry the sensor was placed on the patient's skin over the radial artery. This placement applies pressure on the radial artery and the pressure of the sensor flattens (i.e., 'applanates') the radial artery. Under optimal 'applanation conditions', the transmural pressure of the radial artery wall is zero and the intraluminal applanation tonometry can be recorded by the sensor. In the present study applanation tonometry parameters were recorded at the left radial artery. Using applanation tonometry we registered systolic and diastolic aortic pressure, aortic pulse pressure, peripherial pulse pressure, augmentation pressure, augmentation index normalized on actual heart rate (Alx@HR) and ejection duration. All measurements were performed by the same experienced operator (DP).

Transcranial Doppler (TCD) measurements were performed using Rimed Digilite transcranial Doppler sonography (Rimed Ltd., Israel). The temporal window was used for insonation of the middle cerebral artery at 45–55 mm depth, depending on the best signal. A fixed probe was used to register systolic, diastolic and mean blood flow velocities; pulsatility indices were calculated by the device.

Study protocol

Preoperative measurements were recorded one hour before anesthetic induction in supine position in quiet environment. Patients were then premedicated with 7.5 mg midazolam orally 60 min before entering the operating room. Anaesthesia was induced with a combination of 2 $mg.kg^{-1}$ propofol and 2 $\mu g.kg^{-1}$ fentanyl. Intubation was facilitated by administration of 0.6 $mg.kg^{-1}$ rocuronium. Fentanyl and rocuronium were repeated as needed. Anesthesia was maintained with sevoflurane in 40% oxygen. The concentration of sevoflurane was titrated to a target Bispectral Index (BIS) between 40 and 60 (Covidien, Dublin, Ireland) and it was targeted at 1 MAC. Neuromuscular block was monitored with acceleromyography (TOF Watch SX, NV Organon, Oss, the Netherlands). Standard monitoring included five-leads ECG, NIBP, core temperature at the tympanic membrane, and pulse oximetry. Normothermia was maintained with forced-air system (Bair Hugger 750, 3 M, Eden Prairie, MN, USA).

Patients were ventilated using volume-controlled square-wave flow pattern ventilation with 6–8 $mL.kg^{-1}$ TV, 5 cmH_2O PEEP, 2 $L.min^{-1}$ fresh gas flow and with a respiratory rate adjusted to reach and maintain 40 mmHg $EtCO_2$ (Draeger Primus anesthesia workstation, Draeger Lübeck, Germany).

After induction of general anaesthesia and intubation, lungs were ventilated in supine position for 20 min as described above. At this stage, hemodynamic, transcranial Doppler, applanation tonometry and ventilatory parameters were simultaneously recorded.

In the second phase of the study minute ventilation (respiratory rate and tidal volume) was changed to reach and maintain 35 mmHg $EtCO_2$. After 5 min stabilisation period all measurements were repeated.

At the next stage of measurement series ventilatory settings were again changed to reach and maintain 30 mmHg $EtCO_2$ After a 5 min stabilisation period, applanation tonometry and transcranial Doppler measurements were repeated. The flow chart of the study is summarized in Fig.1.

During each measurement pulse oxygen saturation (SpO_2), heart rate, systolic and diastolic blood pressure, bispectral index values, systolic, diastolic and mean blood flow velocities and pulsatility indices in the middle cerebral artery, systolic and diastolic aortic pressure, aortic pulse pressure, peripherial pulse pressure, augmentation pressure, Alx@HR, ejection duration and operation index were registered.

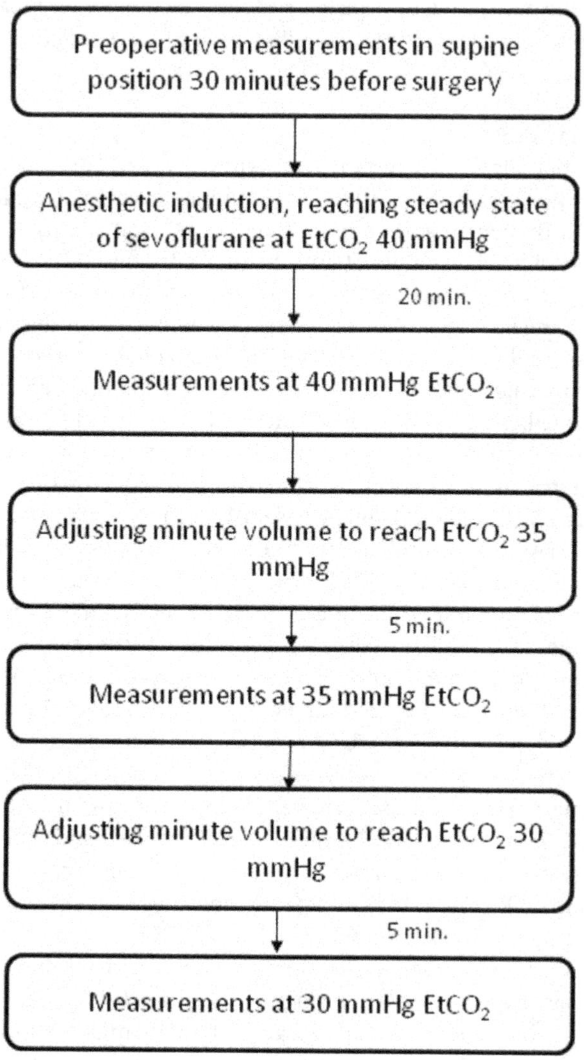

Fig. 1 Flow chart of the study

The entire study and its interpretation follows the CONSORT guidelines.

Statistical methods

Before starting the study, a power analysis was performed to calculate the necessary number of patients to be included. We hypothesized that sevoflurane will not affect cerebral CO_2-reactivity at 1 MAC (primary end point). Based on our previous study performed among non-anesthetized individuals, we found that hyperventilation lasting for 1 min results in a decrease of PCO_2 by 7 mmhHg, accompanied by a 26.7 cm/s decrease of the middle cerebral artery mean blood flow velocity [7]. Accordingly, we calculated that 1 mmHg decrease of PCO_2 results in a 3.84 cm/s change in blood flow velocity. As per protocol we intended to decrease CO_2 by 10 mmHg in 2 steps, we calculated with a 38.4 cm/s (30 cm/s standard deviation) change, with a power of 0.9 and with an alpha of 0.01. Our power calculation indicated that 12 patients need to be included to test our hypothesis. As both registration methods may be operator-dependent, for sake of clarity we decided to include 30 patients. The normality of distribution of data was tested by Shapiro–Wilks test. Thereafter, differences were analyzed with the Repeated Measures Analysis of Variance (ANOVA) with Bonferroni post hoc correction. Values of $p < 0.05$ were accepted as statistically significant. Data are presented as mean (SD). MedCalc Statistical Software version 18.2.1. (MedCalc Software bvba, Ostend, Belgium) was used for statistical analy.

Results

Demographic data

Twenty-nine patients were enrolled aged 19–58 (mean 37), 17 female, 12 male. 7 patients underwent inguinal hiatal repair surgery, while 22 varicetomy. 1 patient was excluded due to inapproriate temporal window for TCD.

Respiratory parameters and anesthetic depth during the procedure

During the course of the study ventilatory settings were changed at different stages of the study to reach and maintain different levels of $EtCO_2$ (40, 35 and 30 mmHg respectively). Accordingly, there were significant differences in values of tidal volumes, respiratory rates. BIS values were stable during the entire procedure indicating adaequate depth of anesthesia (Table 1).

Hemodynamic parameters

There were no significant differences neither in systolic blood pressure values, nor in heart rate during the course of the study. In contrast, there were significant differences in diastolic blood pressure: preoperative

Table 1 Hemodynamic parameters during the course of the study

	$ETCO_2$ 40	$ETCO_2$ 35	$ETCO_2$ 30	p
Tidal volume	516 (64)	550 (63)‡‡‡	570 (88)‡‡‡	$p < 0.001$
Respiratory rate	9 (2)†††	12 (13) ‡‡‡	15 (3)$^{‡‡‡, -††}$	$p < 0.001$
BIS	42 (2)	42 (1)	42 (2)	$p = 0.75$

Data are presented as mean (SD) *: Significant difference compared to preoperative values ‡: Significant difference compared to $EtCO_2$ 40 values †: Significant difference compared to $EtCO_2$ 35 values, $^{\#}$: Significant difference compared to $EtCO_2$ 30 values, $^{*, †, \#, ‡}$ indicates $p < 0.05$; $^{**, ††, \#\#, ‡‡}$ indicates $p < 0.01$; $^{***, †††, \#\#\#, ‡‡‡}$ indicates $p < 0.001$

values were significantly higher than values measured in any other timepoints (Table 2).

Applanation tonometry parameters

Mean arterial pressure significantly decreased during induction of anesthesia, reaching a steady state and remained stable during the entire course of the study. In parallel, aortic and peripheral pulse pressures both increased during the induction phase as did the augmentation index. All parameters remained unchanged during the next phases of the study (Fig. 2).

Transcranial Doppler sonography parameters

Preoperative middle cerebral artery mean blood flow velocity values were not significantly different from values measured at steady state sevoflurane stage under normocapnic conditions ($EtCO_2$ 40 mmHg). However, mean blood flow velocity values measured during $EtCO_2$ 35 and 30 mmHg were significantly different form each other as well as from preoperative and values measured at $EtCO_2$40 (Fig. 3). Pulsatility index values did not change during induction phase and reaching the steady state, however they significantly increased along with the decreased $EtCO_2$ values (Fig. 4.). There was a strong significant correlation between Vmean and $EtCO_2$ values ($p < 0.001$, Pearson's $r = 0.79$).

Relationship between mean arterial pressure and cerebral blood flow velocity changes after induction and stabilisation of anesthesia

We assessed the percent change between mean arterial pressure and middle cerebral artery mean blood flow velocity before anesthetic induction and 20 min after anesthesia was induced and a steady state of sevoflurane anesthesia was reached at normocapnic PCO_2 (40 mmHg). As shown in Fig. 5, there was a significant linear relationship between the two parameters, indicating preserved static autoregulation of the cerebral circulation at normocapnic steady state of sevoflurane anesthesia.

Discussion

Anesthetic agents may have various effects on systemic circulation determining the cerebral perfusion pressure. Additionally, whyle using some agents, direct cerebral effect has also to be taken into account. Both effects are dose-dependent and are exerted through vasodilation or vasoconstriction of the cerebral vessels (medium-size vessels and arterioles), as well as through decreasing $CMRO_2$ - thus influencing flow-metabolism coupling of the brain tissue. The main actors of this systemic and cerebral effects are cerebral arterioles, that are responsible for autoregulatory reactions during changes of cerebral blood flow and vasoreactivity related to metabolic changes [1]. Consequently, for sake of clarity, all the possible influencing factors (systemic and metabolic factors) have to be assessed in parallel while it is intended to test the effect of an anesthetic agent on cerebral blood flow, cerebral autoregulation and cerebral vasoreactivity. The proposed mechanisms of action of general anesthetics on cerebral circulation are summarized at Fig. 6.

Previous reports indicated that sevoflurane between 0.5–1.0 MAC has minimal direct vasodilatory effect on the brain arteries [8, 9] and has no systemic hemodynamic effects (cardiac contractility and/or peripheral vascular resistance) at the most frequently used 1 MAC sevoflurane [10]. In the present study, during the induction phase, the combination of propofol-fentanyl-rocuronium and adding sevoflurane resulted in a decreased mean arterial pressure (mainly due to the decrease of the diastolic pressure) and an increase in aortic and pulse pressure. During the later phases of anesthesia, however no significant changes occurred in any of the hemodynamic parameters (mean arterial pressure, aortic pressure, pulse pressure and augmentation index), indicating no systemic effects of sevoflurane. It is conceivable that the peripheral vasodilation oserved during the induction phase can be mainly ascribed to the use of propofol.

We found that reaching the stady state under sevoflurane anesthesia resulted in a decrease of the mean arterial pressure leading to non significant change in the

Table 2 Hemodynamic parameters during the course of the study

	Preop	$ETCO_2$ 40	$ETCO_2$ 35	$ETCO_2$ 30	p
Systolic blood pressure	109 (29)	106 (8)	108 (9)	108 (9)	$p = 0.46$
Diastolic blood pressure	81 (9)	65 (10)***	67 (10)***	66 (11)***	$p < 0.001$
Heart rate	67 (10)	70 (12)	67 (11)	69 (12)	$p = 0.38$

Data are presented as mean (SD), *: Significant difference compared to preoperative measured values, *** indicates $p < 0.001$

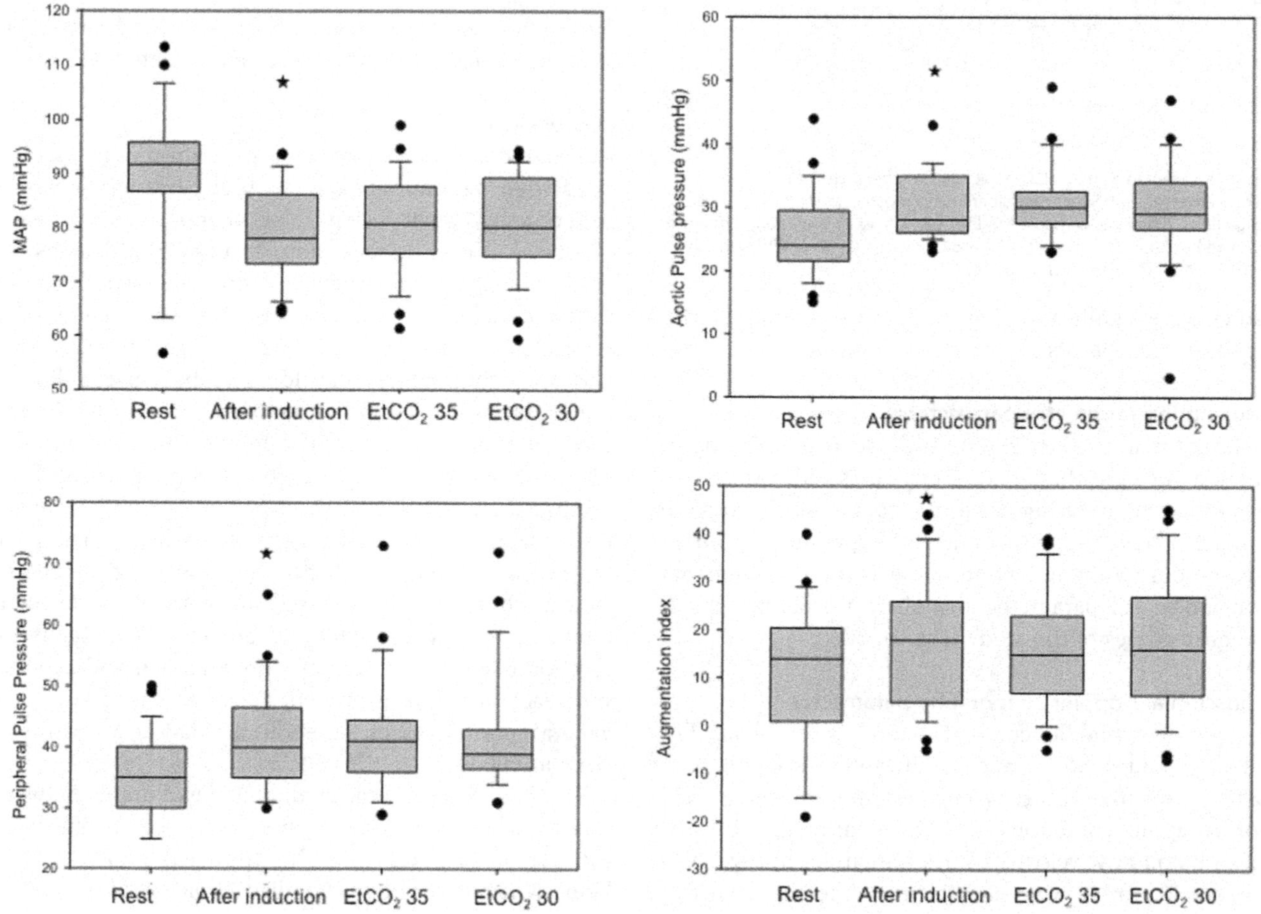

Fig. 2 Applanation tonometry parameters at rest and during the course of the study. Medians and CI values are shown. * indicates $p < 0.05$ difference as compared to steady state values

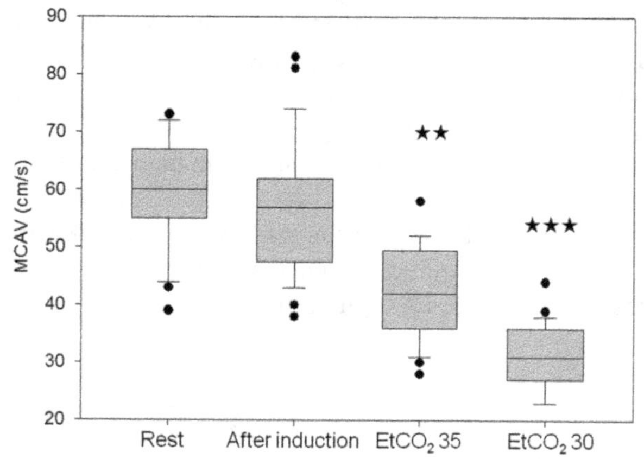

Fig. 3 Changes of middle cerebral artery mean blood flow velocity (MCAV) during the course of the study. Medians and CI values are shown. ** indicates $p < 0.01$, *** indicates $p < 0.001$ differences as compared to steady state values

cerebral blood flow velocity. Cerebral autoregulation is defined as the inherent ability of the brain circulation to maintain a constant cerebral blood flow during changes of cerebral perfusion pressure [1]. In line with this, we checked the relationship between %-changes of MAP and cerebral blood flow velocity values and found a linear relationship between the two factors, indicating preserved autoregulation. While mean arterial pressure decreased, cerebral blood flow velocity remained unchanged during the induction phase and reaching the steady state. As demonstrated in Fig. 5., pulsatility index (representing the vascular resistance of the cerebral arterioles) significantly decreased during this period enabling unchanged cerebral blood flow during the decrease of MAP.

Carbon-dioxide reactivity of the cerebral circulation is defined as the change in cerebral blood flow velocity per mmHg change in PCO_2. In previous volunteer studies it has been demonstrated that forced hyperventilation lasting for 60 s results in a 38% percent decrease of the middle cerebral artery mean flood flow velocity

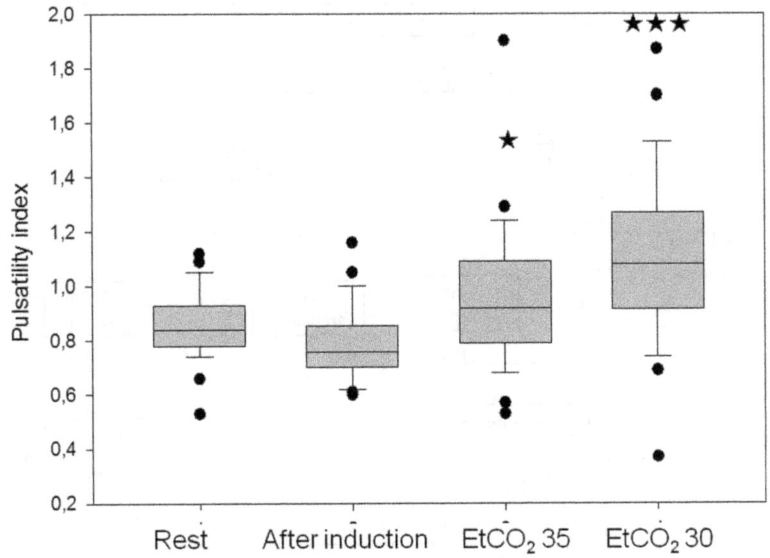

Fig. 4 Changes of pulsatility index during the course of the study. Medians and CI values are shown. * indicates $p < 0.05$, *** indicates $p < 0.001$ differences as compared to steady state values

compared to the resting BFV [7]. The accepted normal values for CO_2-reactivity is 2–5 cm/s/mmHg [4]. In the present study a decrease of PCO_2 from 40 mmHg to 35 mmHg resulted in an average decrease of mean blood flow velocity of 4 cm/s/mmHg, whereas to 30 mmgHg PCO_2 resulted in a decrease of 8 cm/s/mmHg. These values correspond to the previous observations and indicate preserved CO_2-reactivity during sevoflurane anesthesia at MAC 1 concentrations.

Both cerebral autoregulation and cerebral vasoreactivity are multifactorially determined defending mechanisms of the brain that aim to optimize global and cerebral circulation according to the actual metabolic needs. The main actors of these two mechanisms are cerebral arterioles, roughly 200 μm in diameter [1]. The patency of autoregulatory and vasoreactivity reactions depends on systemic factors (such as cerebral perfusion pressure), local metabolic demands as well

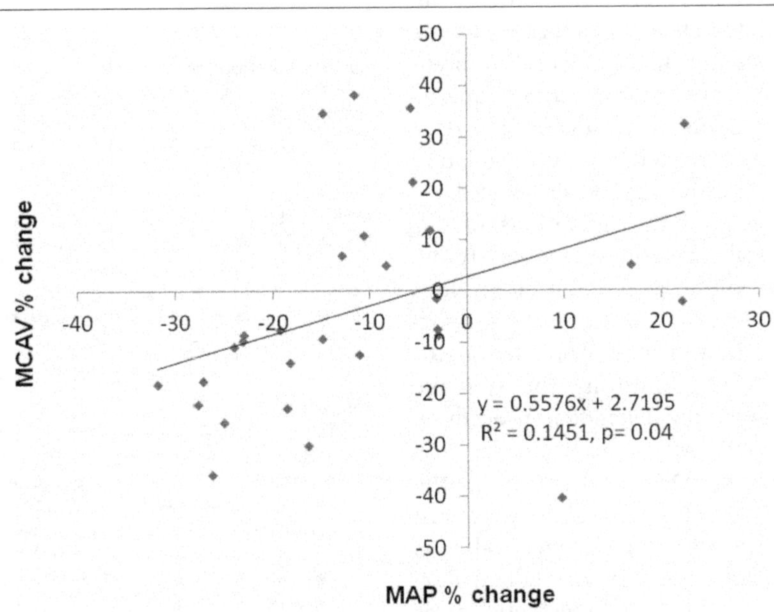

Fig. 5 Relationship between the %change of mean arterial pressure (MAP) and middle cerebral artery mean blood flow velocity (MCAV) after anesthetic induction and reaching the steady state

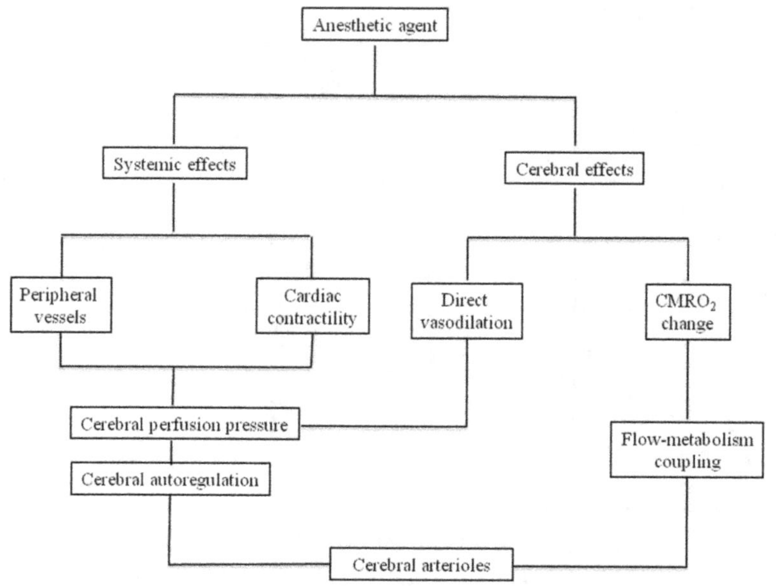

Fig. 6 The proposed mechanism of action of anesthetics on cerebral blood flow regulation

as underlying diseases of the patients. Previously it has been demonstrated that cerebral autoregulation and reactivity of the cerebral vessels to induced hypocapnia may be impaired in patients with certain underlying diseases, such as hypertension and diabetes mellitus [11–14]. As a consequence, sudden intraoperative changes of cerebral perfusion pressure and/or carbon-dioxide concentration may challenge the autoregulatory and metabolic regulatory responses and thus may result in critical brain tissue oxygenation. In line with our observations, previous studies in humans also demonstrated that sevoflurane at ≤1 MAC concentrations does not affect cerebral autoregulation [15–17]. In a very recent study Sperna Weiland and co-workers found that sevoflurane does not affect the already impaired cerebral autoregulation in diabetic patients at clinicially applied doses [18].

Finally, we have to mention the limitations of our study. The methodological limitations are that transcranial Doppler does not measure cerebral blood flow, only changes of the blood flow velocities are proportional to cerebral blood flow values. Applanation tonometry that was used for monitoring the systemic hemodynamic effect is operator-dependent procedure. Therefore all measurements were performed by the same, experienced physician (DP). And finally, in the present study we only tested CO_2-reactivity toward hypocapnic direction. This was done intentionally, as in the usual practice normocapnia is maintained during anesthesia and in specific neuroanesthetic cases only induced hypocapnia is used as the part of the intracranial pressure decreasing strategy.

Conclusion

Sevoflurane at clinically administered doses does not have any significant systemic hemodynamic effects and does not influence static cerebral autoregulation and cerebrovascular reactivity.

Abbreviations

CMRO2: Cerebral metabolic rate of oxygen; CO2: Carbon dioxide; EtCO2: End-tidal CO2; MAC: Minimum alveolar concentration; MAP: Mean arterial pressure

Acknowledgements

None.

Authors' contributions

MJ, LM, BF, DP, TV: performing intraoperative measurements, statistical analysis, drafting the manuscript, BF, CM: concept of the study, drafting the manuscript. All authors read and approved the final version of the manuscript.

Author details

[1]Faculty of Medicine, Department of Anesthesiology and Intensive Care, University of Debrecen, Nagyerdei krt. 98, Debrecen, Hungary. [2]Faculty of Medicine, Department of Medicine, University of Debrecen, Debrecen, Hungary. [3]Hungarian Center, Outcomes Research Consortium, Cleveland, USA.

References

1. Settakis G, Molnár C, Kerényi L, Kollár J, Legemate D, Csiba L, Fülesdi B. Acetazolamide as a vasodilatory stimulus in cerebrovascular diseases and in conditions affecting the cerebral vasculature. Eur J Neurol. 2003;10(6):609–20.
2. Nishiyama T, Matsukawa T, Yokoyama T, Hanaoka K. Cerebrovascular carbon dioxide reactivity during general anesthesia: a comparison between sevoflurane and isoflurane. Anesth Analg. 1999;89:1437–41.
3. Dagal A, Lam AM. Cerebral autoregulation and anesthesia. Curr Opin Anaesthesiol. 2009;22:547–52.
4. Mariappan R, Mehta J, Chui J, Manninen P, Venkatraghavan L. Cerebrovascular reactivity to carbon dioxide under anesthesia: a qualitative systematic review. J Neurosurg Anesthesiol. 2015;27(2):123–35.

5. Goettel N, Patet C, Rossi A, Burkhart CS, Czosnyka M, Strebel SP, Steiner LA. Monitoring of cerebral blood flow autoregulation in adults undergoing sevoflurane anesthesia: a prospective cohort study of two age groups. J Clin Monit Comput. 2016;30:255–64.
6. Sárkány P, Lengyel S, Nemes R, Orosz L, Páll D, Molnár C, Fülesdi B. Non-invasive pulse wave analysis for monitoring the cardiovascular effects of CO2 pneumoperitoneum during laparoscopic cholecystectomy--a prospective case-series study. BMC Anesthesiol. 2014;14:98.
7. Settakis G, Lengyel A, Molnár C, Bereczki D, Csiba L, Fülesdi B. Transcranial Doppler study of the cerebral hemodynamic changes during breath-holding and hyperventilation tests. J Neuroimaging. 2002;12:252–8.
8. Kadoi Y, Takahashi K, Saito S, Goto F. The comparative effects of sevoflurane versus isoflurane on cerebrovascular carbon dioxide reactivity in patients with diabetes mellitus. Anesth Analg. 2006;103:168–72.
9. Matta BF, Heath KJ, Tipping K, Summors AC. Direct cerebral vasodilatory effects of sevoflurane and isoflurane. Anesthesiology. 1999;91:677–80.
10. Ebert TJ, Harkin CP, Muzi M. Cardiovascular responses to sevoflurane: a review. Anesth Analg. 1995;81(6 Suppl):S11–22.
11. Fülesdi B, Limburg M, Bereczki D, Michels RP, Neuwirth G, Legemate D, Valikovics A, Csiba L. Impairment of cerebrovascular reactivity in long-term type 1 diabetes. Diabetes. 1997;46:1840–5.
12. Páll D, Lengyel S, Komonyi E, Molnár C, Paragh G, Fülesdi B, Katona E. Impaired cerebral vasoreactivity in white coat hypertensive adolescents. Eur J Neurol. 2011;18:584–9.
13. Settakis G, Páll D, Molnár C, Bereczki D, Csiba L, Fülesdi B. Cerebrovascular reactivity in hypertensive and healthy adolescents: TCD with vasodilatory challenge. J Neuroimaging. 2003;13:106–12.
14. Siró P, Molnár C, Katona É, Antek C, Kollár J, Settakis G, Fülesdi B. Carotid intima-media thickness and cerebrovascular reactivity in long-term type 1 diabetes mellitus. J Clin Ultrasound. 2009;37:451–6.
15. Molnár C, Settakis G, Sárkány P, Kálmán S, Szabó S, Fülesdi B. Effect of sevoflurane on cerebral blood flow and cerebrovascular resistance at surgical level of anaesthesia: a transcranial Doppler study. Eur J Anaesthesiol. 2007;24:179–84.
16. Gupta S, Heath K, Matta BF. Effect of incremental doses of sevoflurane on cerebral pressure autoregulation in humans. Br J Anaesth. 1997;79:469–72.
17. Summors AC, Gupta AK, Matta BF. Dynamic cerebral autoregulation during sevoflurane anesthesia: a comparison with isoflurane. Anesth Analg. 1999;88:341–5.
18. Sperna Weiland NH, Hermanides J, van der Ster BJP, Hollmann MW, Preckel B, Stok WJ, van Lieshout JJ, Immink RV. Sevoflurane based anaesthesia does not affect already impaired cerebral autoregulation in patients with type 2 diabetes mellitus. Br J Anaesth. 2018;121:1298–307.

8

Lung injury induced by short-term mechanical ventilation with hyperoxia and its mitigation by deferoxamine in rats

Xiao-Xia Wang[1†], Xiao-Lan Sha[1†], Yu-Lan Li[1*], Chun-Lan Li[1], Su-Heng Chen[1], Jing-Jing Wang[1] and Zhengyuan Xia[2,3]

Abstract

Background: Long-term mechanical ventilation with hyperoxia can induce lung injury. General anesthesia is associated with a very high incidence of hyperoxaemia, despite it usually lasts for a relatively short period of time. It remains unclear whether short-term mechanical ventilation with hyperoxia has an adverse impact on or cause injury to the lungs. The present study aimed to assess whether short-term mechanical ventilation with hyperoxia may cause lung injury in rats and whether deferoxamine (DFO), a ferrous ion chelator, could mitigate such injury to the lungs and explore the possible mechanism.

Methods: Twenty-four SD rats were randomly divided into 3 groups ($n = 8$/group): mechanical ventilated with normoxia group (MV group, $FiO_2 = 21\%$), with hyperoxia group (HMV group, $FiO_2 = 90\%$), or with hyperoxia + DFO group (HMV + DFO group, $FiO_2 = 90\%$). Mechanical ventilation under different oxygen concentrations was given for 4 h, and ECG was monitored. The HMV + DFO group received continuous intravenous infusion of DFO at 50 $mg{\bullet}kg^{-1}{\bullet}h^{-1}$, while the MV and HMV groups received an equal volume of normal saline. Carotid artery cannulation was carried out to monitor the blood gas parameters under mechanical ventilation for 2 and 4 h, respectively, and the PaO_2/FiO_2 ratio was calculated. After 4 h ventilation, the right anterior lobe of the lung and bronchoalveolar lavage fluid from the right lung was sampled for pathological and biochemical assays.

Results: PaO_2 in the HMV and HMV + DFO groups were significantly higher, but the PaO_2/FiO_2 ratio were significantly lower than those of the MV group (all $p < 0.01$), while PaO_2 and PaO_2/FiO_2 ratio between HMV + DFO and HMV groups did not differ significantly. The lung pathological scores and the wet-to-dry weight ratio (W/D) in the HMV and HMV + DFO groups were significantly higher than those of the MV group, but the lung pathological score and the W/D ratio were reduced by DFO ($p < 0.05$, HMV + DFO vs. HMV). Biochemically, HMV resulted in significant reductions in Surfactant protein C (SP-C), Surfactant protein D (SP-D), and Glutathion reductase (GR) levels and elevation of xanthine oxidase (XOD) in both the Bronchoalveolar lavage fluid and the lung tissue homogenate, and all these changes were prevented or significantly reverted by DFO.

(Continued on next page)

* Correspondence: east_tale@aliyun.com; 1203401211@qq.com
†Xiao-Xia Wang and Xiao-Lan Sha contributed equally to this work.
[1]Department of Anesthesiology, First Hospital of Lanzhou University, Lanzhou 730000, People's Republic of China

(Continued from previous page)

Conclusions: Mechanical ventilation with hyperoxia for 4 h induced oxidative injury of the lungs, accompanied by a dramatic reduction in the concentrations of SP-C and SP-D. DFO could mitigate such injury by lowering XOD activity and elevating GR activity.

Keywords: Hyperoxia acute lung injury, Mechanical ventilation, Deferoxamine, Lung surfactant protein, Xanthine oxidase, Glutathion reductase

Background

During the course of general anesthesia, inhalation of high fraction of inspired oxygen (FiO_2) is usually used to prevent hypoxaemia in emergencies and to enhance patients' tolerance to apnea and hypopnea [1]. However, excessively high concentration of oxygen supplied during the surgery may sometimes lead to hyperoxaemia [2, 3]. A multi-center clinical study showed that the incidence of hyperoxaemia during general anesthesia reaches up to 83% [4]. Although the effect of hyperoxia in critical illness is still inconclusive [5], and the risk of hyperoxaemia in craniocerebral trauma or stroke was also ambiguous,observational studies showed a close relationship between hyperoxaemia and increased mortality in critically ill patients [6, 7], and it can also lead to poor prognosis in patients with hypoxic-ischemic encephalopathy [8]. Besides, as shown in the animal experiments, long-term exposure to the hyperoxic environment caused oxidative injury of the lungs [9], and another clinical study indicated that long-term hyperoxia increased the risks of lung complications in humans, including pneumonia, atelectasis and pulmonary edema [10]. However, it remains unclear whether or not short-term hyperoxia also exerts an adverse impact on the lung tissues. Since most of the surgeries under general anesthesia are accomplished over relatively a short time, this study was concerned whether mechanical ventilation with hyperoxia for 4 h would cause oxidative injury of the lungs.

Pulmonary surfactant (PS) is a lipoprotein secreted by alveolar epithelial type II cells (AECII), and its main bioactive components are surfactant proteins (SPs), including SP-A, SP-B, SP-C and SP-D. Among them, SP-C is a hydrophobic polypeptide derived from AECII and involved in the adjustment of alveolar surface tension. SP-C-deficient mice are found to be susceptible to bacterial and viral infections [11, 12]. SP-D regulates the immune and inflammatory responses and serves as a marker for alveolar integrity. Changes in SP-D content are positively correlated to the severity of lung injury [13, 14]. Experiments have shown [15] that long-term exposure ($t > 24$ h) to atmospheric oxygen concentration above 90% will lead to dynamic changes of SP. At present, there have been no relevant reports as to the potential influence of short-term mechanical ventilation with hyperoxia on SP.

Deferoxamine (DFO) is a ferrous ion chelator, which is currently used to treat the diseases caused by iron overload, for example, acute iron poisoning and chronic iron allergy. Animal studies have shown that [16, 17] DFO can alleviate the oxidative stress induced by reactive oxygen species (ROS) in rat pulmonary contusion, which is further related to an increase in the activity of xanthine oxidase (XOD). In addition, DFO can also increase the content of glutathione (GSH), clearing excessive ROS and reducing the injury done by ROS to the cells [18]. Britt et al. reported [19, 20] that the regulation of GSH level had a protective effect against the hyperoxia-induced lung injury. Glutathion reductase (GR) is a key enzyme regulating the GSH level and helping protect the cells from the oxidative stress injury. In the present, we aimed to clarify whether DFO had a protective effect against the lung injury caused by mechanical ventilation with hyperoxia and whether DFO worked by influencing the activities of XOD and GR.

Mechanical ventilation with hyperoxia was implemented to the rats for 4 h. Then we discussed whether short-term hyperoxia could induce the oxidative stress injury of the lungs or the associated changes in SP. Furthermore, continuous infusion of DFO was performed during mechanical ventilation so as to verify whether DFO had a protective effect against the lung injury induced by mechanical ventilation with hyperoxia.

Methods

Section of animals

Twenty-four healthy adult male SD rats, each weighing 200 ± 10 g on average, were provided by the Laboratory Animal Center of Lanzhou University School of Medicine. Before the formal experiment began, the rats were acclimatized for 1 week in a quiet environment, with natural illumination, temperature 20–26 °C, diurnal range of temperature ≤ 4 °C, and humidity 40–60%. The experimental design conformed to the ethical standards for animal experiments at the First Hospital of Lanzhou University.

Animal model and treatment

Using a random number table, the rats were divided into 3 groups, with 8 rats in each group, namely, mechanical ventilation with normoxia group (MV group), mechanical ventilation with hyperoxia group (HMV group) and mechanical ventilation with hyperoxia+DFO group (HMV + DFO group). Anesthesia was induced by intraperitoneal injection of 2% Phenobarbital sodium (0.2 ml/100 g). The rats were immobilized to the operating table in a supine position. Heart rate (HR) was monitored. Tail vein puncture and cannulation were performed to prepare for the transfusion. The neck was fully exposed. The left carotid artery was punctured and cannulated under a sterile condition. Posterior to the exposed trachea a T-shaped incision about 2–3 mm long was made and the endotracheal tube was inserted and connected to the ventilator for small animals (HX-100E, Chengdu, China) for mechanical ventilation. The respiratory parameters were configured [21]: tidal volume 10 ml/kg, frequency 40–60 times/min, and inspiration-to-expiration ratio 1:1. The MV group received mechanical ventilation with 21% oxygen in air. The HMV and HMV + DFO groups received mechanical ventilation with 90% oxygen concentration, for 4 h continuously.

During mechanical ventilation, rats in the HMV + DFO group received continuous infusion of DFO via the tail vein ($50\,mg{\cdot}kg^{-1}{\cdot}h^{-1}$, Novartis, Shanghai, China) for 4 h. The MV and HMV groups were given an equal volume of normal saline (1 ml/h). At 2 and 4 h, 0.2 ml of blood was drawn from the carotid artery for blood gas analysis. The respiratory rate was adjusted based on the results of blood gas analysis to maintain $PaCO_2$ at 35–45 mmHg. Anesthetic maintenance was achieved by intermittent intraperitoneal injection of 2% phenobarbital sodium and using fentanyl (12 μg/kg) according to the changes in HR during the ventilation. At the completion of the experiments, the rats were euthanized with over dose of phenobarbital sodium injection.

Blood gas analysis

At 2 and 4 h of mechanical ventilation, blood samples were collected from the carotid artery for blood gas analysis. PH, $PaCO_2$ and PaO_2 were recorded, and PaO_2/FiO_2 ratio was calculated.

Lung wet/dry ratio (W/D)

After mechanical ventilation for 4 h, the rats were euthanized. The chest was opened, and the right posterior lobe of the lung was harvested. The dry weight (W) of the lung tissue was determined using a precision electronic balance. Then the lung tissues were immediately placed into a drying oven for constant temperature drying at 80 °C for 72 h. After that, the lung tissues were weighed again until constant weight, which was the dry weight (D). The wet/dry weight ratio was calculated by (W/D) = W (g)/D (g) × 100%, and its changes were monitored.

Histological evaluation

The right anterior lobe of the lung was harvested and fixed inflated, and prepared into slices 4 μm thick. HE staining was performed, and histological changes were observed under the optical microscope. Pathological scoring was performed by a pathologist who was blinded with the group assignment or experiment design. The scoring criteria [22] was as follows: 0 point, normal alveolar structure, mesenchyme and pulmonary vessels; 1 point, mild damage of the alveolar structure, small amount of inflammatory cells in the mesenchyme, and the scope of bleeding and edema in the mesenchyme and alveolar spaces less than 25%; 2 points: moderate damage of the alveolar structure, a large amount of inflammatory cells in the mesenchyme and some alveolar spaces, widened mesenchyme, congestion in the capillaries, and scope of bleeding and edema in the alveolar spaces 25–50%; 3 points: severe damage of the alveolar structure, agglomeration of inflammatory cells in most alveoli and mesenchyme, apparently widened mesenchyme, and the scope of bleeding and edema in the alveolar spaces 50–75%.

Assessment of SP-C, SP-D, XOD and GR

Tissue preparation

The upper end of the trachea and right hilum were ligated. The sterile endotracheal tube was replaced and connected to a 5 ml needle. Next, 2.5 ml of pre-cooled phosphate-buffered saline (PBS) was injected into the needle for left alveolar lavage. After two aspirations, the lavage fluid was drawn into a centrifuge tube. The lavage was repeated for 3 times, and it was considered successful if the recovery rate was above 80% [23]. The collected bronchoalveolar lavage fluid (BALF) was centrifuged at 3000 r/min at 4 °C for 10 min, and the supernatant was collected. Meanwhile, 110 mg of right middle lobe of the lung was harvested and washed with PBS previously preserved at 4 °C. Impurities were removed from the lung tissues. The lung tissues were weighed and added with PBS 9 times the mass of the lung tissues. Lung tissue homogenate was prepared in an ice-water bath using a homogenizer and centrifuged at 3000 r/min at 4 °C for 15 min. The supernatant was collected.

Detection of SP-C, SP-D, XOD and GR in BALF and lung tissue homogenate

Enzyme Linked ImmunoSorbent Assay (ELISA) was performed to detect the concentrations of SP-C, SP-D, XOD and GR in BALF and lung tissue homogenate. All detection procedures were undertaken according to the instruction manual of the ELISA kits (Mlbio, Shanghai, China) for SP-C (sensitivity, <0.1 pg/ml), SP-D (sensitivity, < 0.1 pg/ml), XOD (sensitivity, < 0.1 U/L) and GR (sensitivity, < 1.0 mIU/ml) in rats.

Statistical analysis

All statistical analyses were performed using SPSS 22.0 software. It was verified by the Shapiro-Wilks normality test that all original data obeyed a normal distribution. Next, Bartlett's test was used to determine whether the independent samples satisfied homogeneity of variances. The pathological scores of lung tissues and the data on W/D ratio and concentrations of SP-C, SP-D and GR satisfied homogeneity of variances. One-way ANOVA was performed to compare three groups of data. SNK test was performed for multiple comparisons. Data on XOD concentration did not satisfy homogeneity of variances, and so Tamhane's T2 was performed. The results of arterial blood gas analysis were compared by the repeated measures ANOVA. Data were expressed as mean ± standard deviation ($\bar{x} \pm s$). $P < 0.05$ was taken to indicate significant difference.

Results

Data of blood gases

At 2 and 4 h of mechanical ventilation, blood gas analysis showed that as compared with the MV group, PaO_2 increased in the HMV and HMV + DFO groups ($P<$ 0.001), while PaO_2/FiO_2 ratio decreased ($P<0.001$). There were no significant differences in PaO_2 and PaO_2/FiO_2 ratio between the HMV and HMV + DFO groups ($P>0.05$). At 2 and 4 h, there were no significant differences in PH and $PaCO_2$ between the three groups ($P > 0.05$) (Table 1).

Lung tissue observation results and pathology score

As to the pathological changes of the lung tissues, the alveolar structure was distinctively visualized and was basically intact in the MV group. There were few inflammatory cells in the pulmonary mesenchyme and alveolar spaces; the alveolar septum was not widened, and neither was there apparent dilation of the pulmonary vessels. In the HMV group, some of the alveolar walls fractured, with mild alveolar fusion. This mainly presented with widening of alveolar septa and congestion and dilation of the pulmonary vessels. There was exudation of inflammatory cells and fluid from the pulmonary mesenchyme and alveolar spaces. Abnormalities in the alveolar structure, morphology and size and the degree of exudation of inflammatory cells in the HMV + DFO group were significantly alleviated as compared with HMV group (Fig. 1). As compared with the MV group, the pathological scores of the lung tissues in the HMV and HMV + DFO groups increased significantly ($P<0.001$, $P<0.05$). As compared with the HMV group, the pathological scores of the lung tissues in the HMV + DFO group decreased significantly ($P<0.005$) (Fig. 2).

Lung W/D ratio

As compared with the MV group, the W/D ratio of the lung tissues in the HMV and HMV + DFO groups increased significantly ($P<0.001$), while the W/D ratio of the lung tissues in the HMV + DFO group decreased significantly ($P<0.001$) (Fig. 3).

Changes of SP-C, SP-D, XOD and GR levels in BALF

As compared with the MV group, the concentrations of SP-C, SP-D and GR in the BALF of the HMV and HMV + DFO group decreased significantly ($P<0.001$), while the XOD concentration increased significantly ($P<$ 0.001). As compared with the HMV group, the concentrations of SP-C, SP-D and GR in the BALF increased significantly in the HMV + DFO group ($P<$ 0.001), while the XOD concentration decreased significantly ($P<0.001$) (Fig. 4).

Changes of SP-C, SP-D, XOD and GR levels in lung tissue homogenate

As compared with the MV group, the concentrations of SP-C, SP-D and GR in the lung tissue homogenate of the HMV and HMV + DFO group decreased significantly ($P<0.001$), while the XOD concentration increased significantly ($P<0.001$). As compared with the HMV group, the concentrations of SP-C, SP-D and GR in the lung tissue homogenate increased significantly in the HMV + DFO group ($P<0.001$), while the XOD concentration decreased significantly ($P<0.001$). (Fig. 5).

Table 1 Arterial blood gas analysis results at 2 and 4 h (mean ± SD)

Groups	Time (h)	PaO_2 (mmHg)	$PaCO_2$ (mmHg)	PH	PaO_2/FiO_2 (mmHg)
MV	2	89.25 ± 3.85	34.13 ± 3.76	7.35 ± 0.05	425.00 ± 18.31
	4	90.25 ± 4.53	37.13 ± 3.18	7.38 ± 0.04	429.76 ± 21.56
HMV	2	204.88 ± 7.57*	33.38 ± 5.01	7.33 ± 0.05	227.64 ± 8.41*
	4	208.75 ± 7.44*	36.63 ± 3.38	7.35 ± 0.03	231.94 ± 8.26*
HMV + DFO	2	205.50 ± 9.64*	36.50 ± 4.07	7.34 ± 0.04	228.33 ± 10.70*
	4	208.00 ± 6.95*	37.88 ± 4.88	7.36 ± 0.04	231.11 ± 7.72*

Table 1 Data of blood gases. Values are displayed as means ± SD
Group MV Mechanical ventilation with normoxia group, *Group HMV* Mechanical ventilation with hyperoxia group, *Group HMV + DFO* Mechanical ventilation with hyperoxia+DFO group
*$P = 0.000$ as compared with the MV group

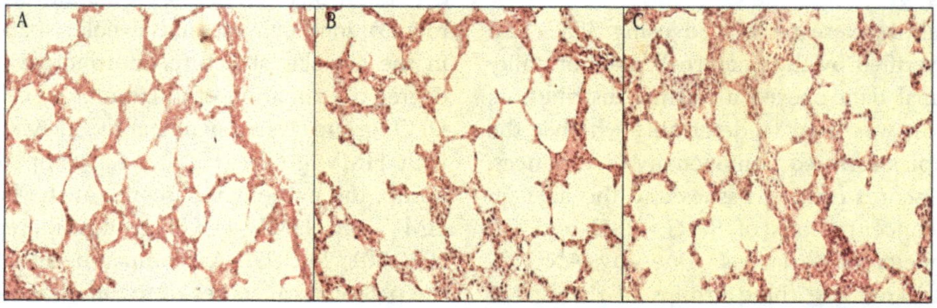

Fig. 1 Lung tissue observation results. **a** shows the pathological changes of lung tissues in the MV group (mechanical ventilation with normoxia group); **b** shows the pathological changes of lung tissues in the HMV group (mechanical ventilation with hyperoxia group); **c** shows the pathological changes of lung tissues in the HMV + DFO group (mechanical ventilation with hyperoxia group+DFO). As compared with the HMV group, the lung injury was greatly alleviated

Discussion

In the present study, lung tissue pathology and the increase of lung tissue W/D ratio suggested that mechanical ventilation with hyperoxia for 4 h caused lung injury. The arterial blood gas analysis results obtained at 2 and 4 h of ventilation showed that the rats were in a state of hyperoxemia evidenced as elevated PaO_2.The decreases in the concentrations of SP-C, SP-D and GR in the BALF and lung tissue homogenate along with a considerable increase in the XOD concentration were evidences that hyperoxia affected the secretions of SP-C, SP-D, GR and XOD. After DFO treatment, the lung injury of rats was alleviated, while concentrations of SP-C, SP-D and GR increased as compared to those under hyperoxia without DFO treatment, accompanied with a reduction of the increased XOD. This indicated that DFO had a protective effect against the lung injury caused by short-term hyperoxia, and its working mechanism might be related to an increase in the activity of GR and a decrease in the activity of XOD.

Long-term exposure to a hyperoxic environment may lead to lung injury [9, 24]. Kawamura showed that continuous exposure of rats to 98% atmospheric oxygen for 60 h would cause oxidative injury of the lungs. Another meta-analysis pointed out that critically ill patients after mechanical ventilation with hyperoxia usually had poor outcome associated with the lungs [25, 26]. However, whether short-term mechanical ventilation with hyperoxia will cause lung injury remains a topic not getting enough attention. Here, PaO_2/FiO_2 ratio, W/D ratio and

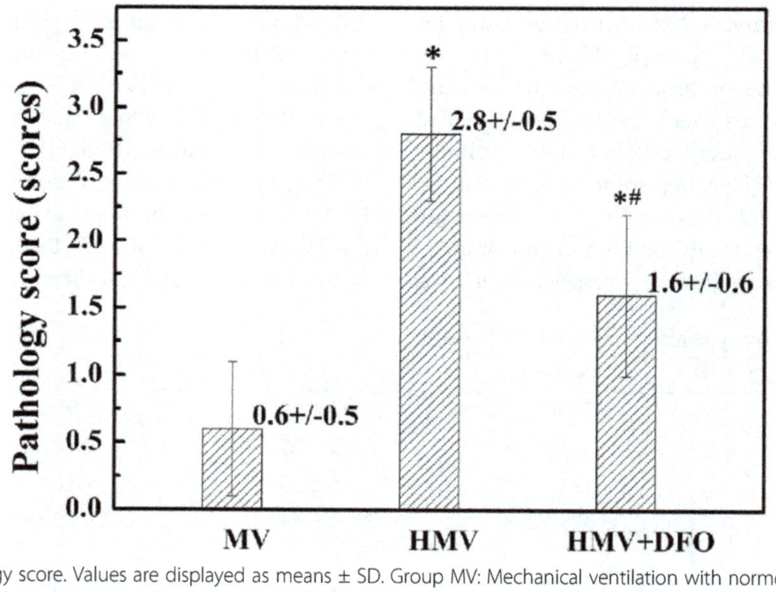

Fig. 2 Lung tissue pathology score. Values are displayed as means ± SD. Group MV: Mechanical ventilation with normoxia group; Group HMV: Mechanical ventilation with hyperoxia group; Group HMV + DFO: Mechanical ventilation with hyperoxia+DFO group. After mechanical ventilation with hyperoxia for 4 h, the pathological score of the lung tissues increased significantly as compared with the MV group ($P = 0.000$). After DFO treatment, the pathological score of the lung tissues decreased significantly as compared with the HMV group ($P = 0.001$), and it increased significantly as compared with the MV group ($P = 0.015$)

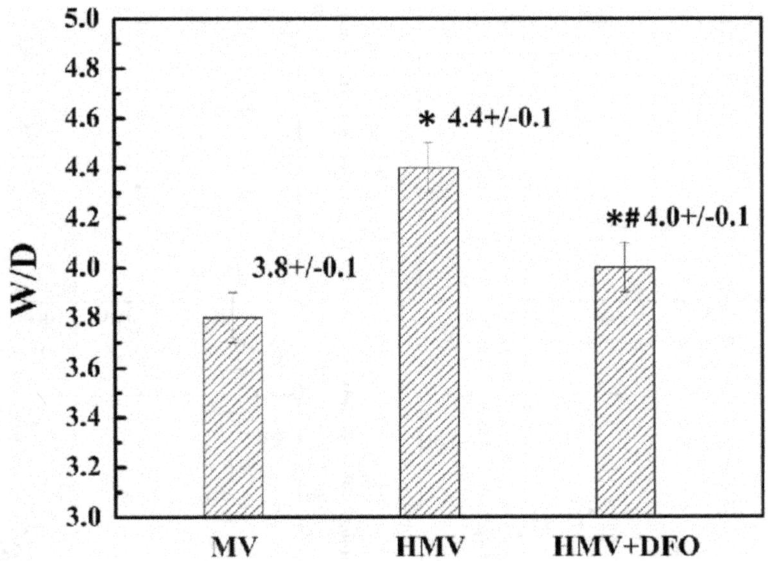

Fig. 3 Lung W/D ratio. Values are displayed as means ± SD. Group MV: Mechanical ventilation with normoxia group; Group HMV: Mechanical ventilation with hyperoxia group; Group HMV + DFO: Mechanical ventilation with hyperoxia+DFO group. After mechanical ventilation with hyperoxia for 4 h, the W/D ratio of the lung tissues increased significantly as compared with the MV group ($P = 0.000$). After DFO treatment, the W/D ratio of the lung tissues decreased significantly as compared with the HMV group ($P = 0.000$), and it increased significantly as compared with the MV group ($P = 0.000$)

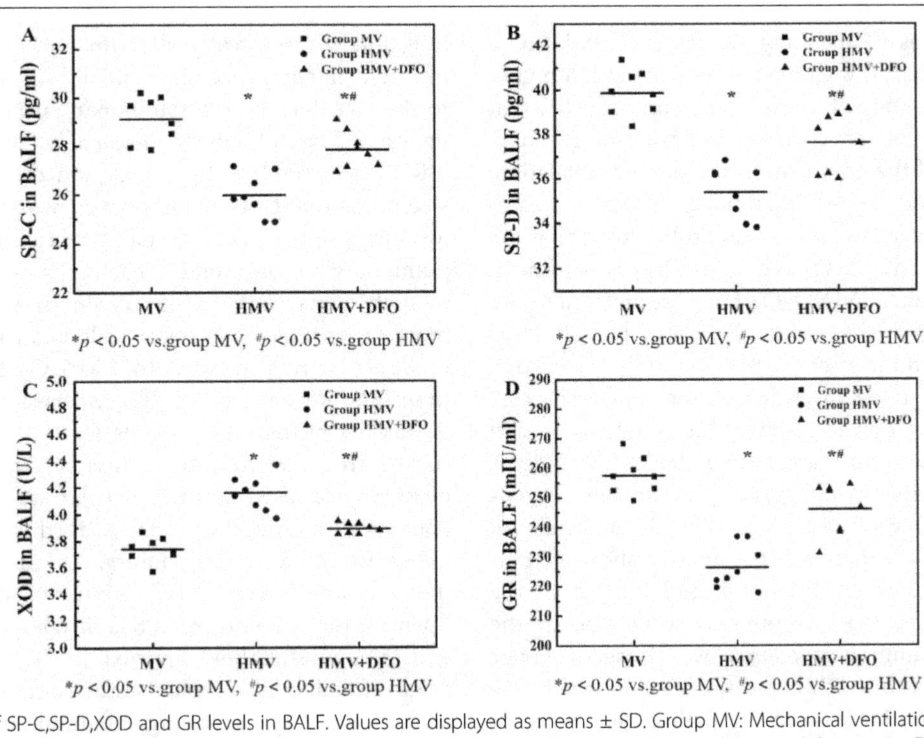

Fig. 4 Changes of SP-C,SP-D,XOD and GR levels in BALF. Values are displayed as means ± SD. Group MV: Mechanical ventilation with normoxia group; Group HMV: Mechanical ventilation with hyperoxia group; Group HMV + DFO: Mechanical ventilation with hyperoxia+DFO group; **a** shows the comparison of SP-C concentration in BALF between the three groups; **b** shows the comparison of SP-D concentration in BALF between the three groups; **c** shows the comparison of XOD concentration in BALF; **d** shows the comparison of GR concentration in BALF

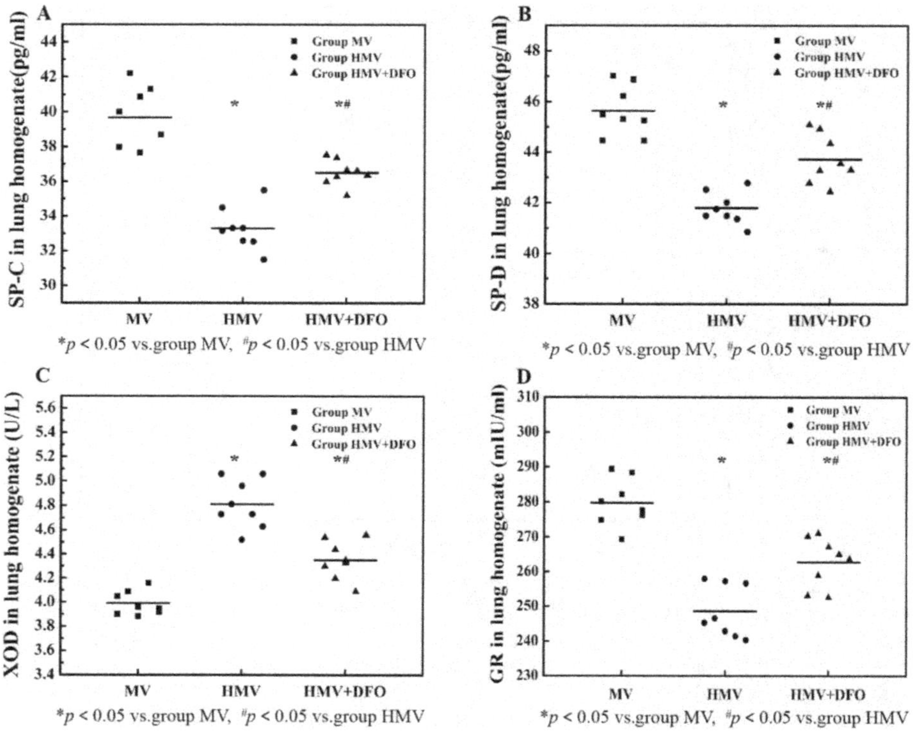

Fig. 5 Changes of SP-C,SP-D,XOD and GR levels in lung tissue homogenate.Values are displayed as means ± SD. Group MV: Mechanical ventilation with normoxia group; Group HMV: Mechanical ventilation with hyperoxia group; Group HMV + DFO: Mechanical ventilation with hyperoxia+DFO group; **a** shows the comparison of SP-C concentration in the lung tissue homogenate between the three groups; **b** shows the comparison of SP-D concentration in the lung tissue homogenate between the three groups; **c** shows the comparison of XOD concentration in the lung tissue homogenate; **d** shows the comparison of GR concentration in the lung tissue homogenate

pathological scores of the lung tissues at 2 and 4 h of mechanical ventilation with hyperoxia were much higher than those of the control group. Ferguson reported that PaO_2/FiO_2 ratio was an accurate indicator of the oxygenation status of the organism under oxygen inhalation. A PaO_2/FiO_2 ratio below 300 mmHg usually indicates respiratory insufficiency [27]. It should be noted that the relation between PaO_2/FiO_2 ratio and FiO_2 is nonlinear, factors that influence PaO_2/FiO_2 ratio are not only arise from the change of FiO_2, but also from the effect of intrapulmonary shunt affected by FiO_2 [28]. Therefore, using PaO_2/FiO_2 alone to evaluate lung injury has certain limitations in our experiment. It should be noted that high FiO_2 may cause absorptive atelectasis, and the atelectasis formation would possibly cause the oxygenation impairment. W/D ratio is an objective indicator of water content of the lung tissues. If it is above 4, pulmonary edema is usually indicated; and the higher the ratio, the more severity the pulmonary edema. In the present study, pulmonary edema was observed after mechanical ventilation with hyperoxia for 4 h, which was accompanied by an increase in the pathological score of the lung tissues. This further indicated that short-term mechanical ventilation with hyperoxia would induce injury of the lung tissues in rats. After DFO treatment, the lung injury was greatly alleviated, while the PaO_2/FiO_2 ratio did not improve substantially. This may be related to the fact that the intrapulmonary arteriovenous shunting caused by pulmonary edema affected PaO_2.

ROS generated by hyperoxia and the resulting excessive oxidative stress are important working mechanisms for lung injury [29, 30]. Early research indicated that pulmonary vascular endothelial cells are more sensitive to high concentrations of oxygen, and damage to pulmonary vascular endothelial cells is an important cause of death in rats exposed to 100% O_2 for a prolonged time [31]. Recent studies [32, 33] have shown that AEC II was the primary target cells for ROS. When the lung tissues are in an oxidative stress status, a large amount of ROS is released into the alveolar spaces, inducing the apoptosis of AECII, which is further related to the hyperoxia-induced lung injury. In case of hyperoxia-induced lung injury, AECII is injured, which further influences the secretion of PS. PS, composed of 10% SP and 90% phospholipid approximately, fulfills the functions of reducing alveolar surface tension, maintaining alveolar stability, inhibiting inflammatory response and enhancing the phagocytic function of alveolar macrophages. When the content of SP changes, it may cause pulmonary insufficiency and atelectasis [34]. SP-C is a hydrophobic glycoprotein secreted by AECII, which promotes the absorption of phospholipid and its distribution to the air-liquid interface of the lung. This will further reduce alveolar surface tension and ensure alveolar integrity and its normal biological role [35]. Sano et al. showed that SP-D knockout mice suffered from alveolar structural abnormalities, metabolic impairment of PS and host defense deficiency. SP-D deficiency could cause pulmonary injury to a certain degree [36]. In the present study, after mechanical ventilation with hyperoxia for 4 h, inhalation of hyperoxic gases led to alveolar injury of rats. It was thus inferred that the AECII structure was damaged. As the release of SP-C and SP-D from AECII was inhibited, the concentrations of SP-C and SP-D in the lung tissue homogenate and BALF decreased significantly. Moreover, as the concentrations of SP-C and SP-D changed, the composition of PS in AECII was altered. As a result, PS failed to perform the functions of reducing alveolar surface tension and maintaining alveolar volume, which further induced structural and functional abnormalities of the lung tissues. Thus the vicious cycle began, aggravating pulmonary edema and promoting lung injury. A significant increase in the concentrations of SP-C and SP-D was noted after DFO treatment, indicating an alleviation of pulmonary edema and lung injury and also a protective effect of DFO against the lung injury caused by hyperoxia.

XOD and GR are key enzymes in the oxidant-antioxidant system [37, 38]. Under normal conditions, XOD is inactive, and its activity increases when tissues are in an oxidative stress status. The active form of XOD can catalyze oxidation of xanthine, producing a large amount of ROS and mediating the peroxidation tissue injury. In the oxidative response, GR can clear excessive ROS by maintaining the content of reduced GSH, thus alleviating peroxidation tissue injury. Therefore, an increase in the activity of XOD and a decrease in the activity of GR usually suggest an increase in the ROS level and hence intense oxidative stress. In the present study, the XOD concentration increased and GR concentration decreased after mechanical ventilation with hyperoxia. This indicated ROS production-clearing imbalance and disorder of the oxidant-antioxidant enzyme system after mechanical ventilation with hyperoxia for 4 h, which further contributed to the lung injury.

DFO has proven to inhibit lipid peroxidation by reducing ROS generation [39]. Hybertson et al. found through animal experiments [17, 40] that DFO cleared excessive ROS by inhibiting XOD activity, reducing ROS production and increasing GSH content, which finally alleviated oxidative injury of the cells. GSH can protect lung tissues from hyperoxia-induced injury and GSH level reflects the activity of GR to a certain extent. In response to oxidative stress, GR activity is enhanced, and the content of reduced GSH increases as well, thus propelling ROS clearing and exerting an antioxidant effect. We found that (1) after DFO treatment, the XOD concentration decreased dramatically, suggesting that DFO alleviated the hyperoxia-induced lung injury by inhibiting XOD activity; (2) a significant increase in GR concentration after DFO treatment indicated that DFO might exert a protective effect for the lungs by enhancing GR activity and increasing the content of reduced GSH; (3) given a generally low ROS level, the injury to AECII was mild, and the reduction in the concentrations of SP-C and SP-D was redressed significantly by DFO, which finally alleviated pulmonary edema.

In the course of the experiment, the lack of positive end-expiratory pressure (PEEP) or lung recruitment maneuver applied and other related protective lung ventilation strategies for mechanically ventilated rats may affect our observations of lung tissue damage, which is one of the limitations of our experiment. In further researches, it is necessary to solve the above problems and take relevant measures (such as the application of PEEP to avoid or prevent the occurrence of atelectasis, thereby reducing the deviation of the experimental results.

Conclusions

Taken together, mechanical ventilation with hyperoxia for 4 h caused oxidative injury and a dramatic reduction in the concentrations of SP-C and SP-D in the lung tissue homogenate and BALF. This further led to respiratory impairment and pulmonary edema. DFO could alleviate the lung injury induced by mechanical ventilation with hyperoxia, exerting a protective effect for the lungs. Its working mechanism might be related to a reduction in XOD activity, an increase in the SP-C concentration and GR activity and alleviation of injury to AECII.

Abbreviations

FiO_2: Fraction of inspired oxygen; PS: Pulmonary Surfactant; AECII: Alveolar epithelial type II cells; SPs: Surfactant Proteins; DFO: Deferoxamine; ROS: Reactive Oxygen Species; XOD: Xanthine Oxidase; GSH: Glutathione; GR: Glutathion Reductase; HR: Heart Rate; PBS: Phosphate-buffered Saline; BALF: Bronchoalveolar Lavage Fluid; ELISA: Enzyme Linked ImmunoSorbent Assay; PEEP: Positive end-expiratory pressure

Acknowledgements

Not applicable.

Authors' contributions

WXX and SXL have contributed to study design and implementation, data collection and original draft of the manuscript writing; LYL helped to design the study, interpret of the results and revise the manuscript for important intellectual content; LCL, CSH and WJJ helped to execution the study; XZY helped to analyze the data and revise the manuscript. All authors read and approved the final manuscript. We would like to thank the Laboratory of Pharmacology, Gansu University of Traditional Chinese Medicine for their assistance with the study. This work was supported by Department of Anesthesiology, First Hospital of Lanzhou University.

Author details
[1]Department of Anesthesiology, First Hospital of Lanzhou University, Lanzhou 730000, People's Republic of China. [2]Department of Anesthesiology, The University of Hong Kong, Hong Kong 999077, People's Republic of China. [3]Department of Anesthesiology, Affiliated Hospital of Guangdong Medical University, Zhanjiang 524000, People's Republic of China.

References

1. Eastwood G, Bellomo R, Bailey M, et al. Arterial oxygen tension and mortality in mechanically ventilated patients. Intensive Care Med. 2012;38: 91–8. https://doi.org/10.1007/s00134-011-2419-6.
2. Suzuki S, Eastwood GM, Peck L, et al. Current oxygen management in mechanically ventilated patients: a prospective observational cohort study. J Crit Care. 2013;28:647–54. https://doi.org/10.1016/j.jcrc.2013.03.010.
3. de Graaff AE, Dongelmans DA, Binnekade JM, et al. Clinicians' response to hyperoxia in ventilated patients in a Dutch ICU depends on the level of FiO2. Intensive Care Med. 2011;37:46–51. https://doi.org/10.1007/s00134-010-2025-z.
4. Suzuki S, Mihara Y, Hikasa Y, et al. Current ventilator and oxygen management during general anesthesia: a multicenter, cross-sectional observational study. Anesthesiology. 2018;129:67–76. https://doi.org/10.1097/ALN.0000000000002181.
5. Munshi L, Ferguson ND. Evolving issues in oxygen therapy in acute care medicine. JAMA. 2020. https://doi.org/10.1001/jama.2019.22029.
6. Damiani E, Donati A, Girardis M. Oxygen in the critically ill: friend or foe? Curr Opin Anaesthesiol. 2018;31(2):129–35. https://doi.org/10.1097/ACO.0000000000000559.
7. Asfar P, Schortgen F, Boisramé-Helms J, et al. Hyperoxia and hypertonic saline in patients with septic shock (HYPERS2S): a two-by-two factorial, multicentre, randomised, clinical trial. Lancet Respir Med. 2017;5:180–90. https://doi.org/10.1016/S2213-2600(17)30046-2.
8. Mackle D, Bellomo R, Bailey M, et al. Conservative oxygen therapy during mechanical ventilation in the ICU. N Engl J Med. 2019. https://doi.org/10.1056/NEJMoa1903297.
9. Dias-Freitas F, Metelo-Coimbra C, Roncon-Albuquerque R Jr, et al. Molecular mechanisms underlying hyperoxia acute lung injury. Respir Med. 2016;119: 23–8. https://doi.org/10.1016/j.rmed.2016.08.010.
10. Sabaté S, Mazo V, Canet J. Predicting postoperative pulmonary complications: implications for outcomes and costs. Curr Opin Anaesthesiol. 2014;27:201–9. https://doi.org/10.1097/ACO.0000000000000045.
11. Barkauskas CE, Cronce MJ, Rackley CR, et al. Type 2 alveolar cells are stem cells in adult lung. J Clin Invest. 2013;123:3025–36. https://doi.org/10.1172/JCI68782.
12. Chroneos ZC, Sever-Chroneos Z, Shepherd VL. Pulmonary surfactant: an immunological perspective. Cell Physiol Biochem. 2010;25:13–26. https://doi.org/10.1159/000272047.
13. Tantawy AA, Adly AA, Ebeid FSE, et al. Surfactant protein D as a marker for pulmonary complications in pediatric patients with sickle cell disease: Relation to lung function tests. Pediatr Pulmonol. 2019;54:610–9. https://doi.org/10.1002/ppul.24257
14. Du J, Abdel-Razek O, Shi Q, et al. Surfactant protein D attenuates acute lung and kidney injuries in pneumonia-induced sepsis through modulating apoptosis, inflammation and NF-κB signaling. Sci Rep. 2018;8:15393. https://doi.org/10.1038/s41598-018-33828-7.
15. Jin Y, Peng LQ, Zhao AL. Hyperoxia induces the apoptosis of alveolar epithelial cells and changes of pulmonary surfactant proteins. Eur Rev Med Pharmacol Sci. 2018;22:492–7. https://doi.org/10.26355/eurrev_201801_14200.
16. Basaran UN, Ayvaz S, Aksu B, et al. Desferrioxamine reduces oxidative stress in the lung contusion. Sci World J. 2013;2013:376959. https://doi.org/10.1155/2013/376959.
17. Hybertson BM, Connelly KG, Buser RT, et al. Ferritin and desferrioxamine attenuate xanthine oxidase-dependent leak in isolated perfused rat lungs. Inflammation. 2002;26:153–9. https://doi.org/10.1023/a:1016511611435.
18. Kletkiewicz H, Nowakowska A, Siejka A, et al. Deferoxamine prevents cerebral glutathione and vitamin E depletions in asphyxiated neonatal rats: role of body temperature. Int J Hyperth. 2016;32:211–20. https://doi.org/10.3109/02656736.2015.1125955.
19. Britt RD Jr, Velten M, Locy ML, et al. The thioredoxin reductase-1 inhibitor aurothioglucose attenuates lung injury and improves survival in a murine model of acute respiratory distress syndrome. Antioxid Redox Signal. 2014; 20:2681–91. https://doi.org/10.1089/ars.2013.5332.
20. Kim SJ, Jung HJ, Hyun DH, et al. Glutathione reductase plays an anti-apoptotic role against oxidative stress in human hepatoma cells. Biochimie. 2010;92:927–32. https://doi.org/10.1016/j.biochi.2010.03.007.
21. Wolthuis EK, Choi G, Dessing MC, et al. Mechanical ventilation with lower tidal volumes and positive end-expiratory pressure prevents pulmonary inflammation in patients without preexisting lung injury [J]. Anesthesiology. 2008;108(1):46–54. https://doi.org/10.1097/01.anes.0000296068.80921.10.
22. Ozdemir R, Demirtas G, Parlakpinar H, et al. Dexpanthenol therapy reduces lung damage in a hyperoxic lung injury in neonatal rats. J Matern Fetal Neonatal Med. 2016;29:1801–7. https://doi.org/10.3109/14767058.2015.1064104.
23. Fukuhara K, Nakashima T, Abe M, et al. Suplatast tosilate protects the lung against hyperoxic lung injury by scavenging hydroxyl radicals. Free Radic Biol Med. 2017;106:1–9. https://doi.org/10.1016/j.freeradbiomed.2017.02.014.
24. Jaffal K, Six S, Zerimech F, et al. Relationship between hyperoxemia and ventilator associated pneumonia. Ann Transl Med. 2017;5:453–7. https://doi.org/10.21037/atm.2017.10.15.
25. Kawamura T, Wakabayashi N, Shigemura N, et al. Hydrogen gas reduces hyperoxic lung injury via the Nrf2 pathway in vivo. Am J Physiol Lung Cell Mol Physiol. 2013;304:L646–56. https://doi.org/10.1152/ajplung.00164.2012.
26. Damiani E, Adrario E, Girardis M, et al. Arterial hyperoxia and mortality in critically ill patients: a systematic review and meta-analysis. Crit Care. 2014; 18:711–26. https://doi.org/10.1186/s13054-014-0711-x.
27. Ferguson ND, Fan E, Camporota L, et al. The Berlin definition of ARDS: an expanded rationale, justification, and supplementary material. Intensive Care Med. 2012;38:1573–82. https://doi.org/10.1007/s00134-012-2682-1.
28. Aboab J, Louis B, Jonson B, et al. Relation between PaO_2/FiO_2 ratio and FiO_2: a mathematical description. Intensive Care Med. 2006;32(10):1494–7. https://doi.org/10.1007/s00134-006-0337-9.
29. Brueckl C, Kaestle S, Kerem A, et al. Hyperoxia-induced reactive oxygen species formation in pulmonary capillary endothelial cells in situ[J]. Am J Respir Cell Mol Biol. 2006;34(4):453–63. https://doi.org/10.1165/rcmb.2005-0223OC.
30. Veith AC, Bou AB, Jiang W, et al. Mice lacking the cytochrome P450 1B1 gene are less susceptible to hyperoxic lung injury than wild type. Toxicol Sci. 2018;165:462–74. https://doi.org/10.1093/toxsci/kfy154.
31. Crapo JD, Barry BE, Foscue HA, et al. Structural and biochemical changes in rat lungs occurring during exposures to lethal and adaptive doses of oxygen[J]. Am Rev Respir Dis. 1980;122(1):123–43. https://doi.org/10.1164/arrd.1980.122.1.123.
32. Lee HS, Kim CK. Effect of recombinant IL-10 on cultured fetal rat alveolar type II cells exposed to 65%-hyperoxia. Respir Res. 2011;12:68–82. https://doi.org/10.1186/1465-9921-12-68.
33. Kim MJ, Ryu JC, Kwon Y, et al. Dual oxidase 2 in lung epithelia is essential for hyperoxia-induced acute lung injury in mice. Antioxid Redox Signal. 2014;21:1803–18. https://doi.org/10.1089/ars.2013.5677.
34. Pace PW, Yao LJ, Wilson JX, et al. The effects of hyperoxia exposure on lung function and pulmonary surfactant in a rat model of acute lung injury. Exp Lung Res. 2009;35:380–98. https://doi.org/10.1080/01902140902745166.
35. Jin H, Ciechanowicz AK, Kaplan AR, et al. Surfactant protein C dampens inflammation by decreasing JAK/STAT activation during lung repair. Am J Physiol Lung Cell Mol Physiol. 2018;314:L882–92. https://doi.org/10.1152/ajplung.00418.2017.
36. Sano H, Kuroki Y. The lung collectins, SP-A and SP-D, modulate pulmonary innate immunity. Mol Immunol. 2005;42:279–87. https://doi.org/10.1016/j.molimm.2004.07.014.
37. Wang B, Yang RN, Zhu YR, et al. Involvement of xanthine oxidase and paraoxonase 1 in the process of oxidative stress in nonalcoholic fatty liver disease. Mol Med Rep. 2017;15:387–95. https://doi.org/10.3892/mmr.2016.6025.
38. Zhu Z, Du S, Du Y, et al. Glutathione reductase mediates drug resistance in glioblastoma cells by regulating redox homeostasis. J Neurochem. 2018;144: 93–104. https://doi.org/10.1111/jnc.14250.
39. Vlahakos D, Arkadopoulos N, Kostopanagiotou G, et al. Deferoxamine attenuates lipid peroxidation, blocks interleukin-6 production, ameliorates sepsis inflammatory response syndrome, and confers renoprotection after acute hepatic ischemia in pigs. Artif Organs. 2012;36:400–8. https://doi.org/10.1111/j.1525-1594.2011.01385.x.
40. Molina-Jijón E, Zarco-Márquez G, Medina-Campos ON, et al. Deferoxamine pretreatment prevents Cr(VI)-induced nephrotoxicity and oxidant stress: role of Cr(VI) chelation. Toxicology. 2012;291:93–101. https://doi.org/10.1016/j.tox.2011.11.003.

9

Inhibition of adenosine A1 receptors abolished the nutritional ketosis-evoked delay in the onset of isoflurane-induced anesthesia in wistar albino glaxo rijswijk rats

Zsolt Kovács[1], Brigitta Brunner[1,2], Dominic P. D'Agostino[3,4] and Csilla Ari[5*]

Abstract

Background: It has been demonstrated that administration of exogenous ketone supplement ketone salt (KS) and ketone ester (KE) increased blood ketone level and delayed the onset of isoflurane-induced anesthesia in different rodent models, such as Wistar Albino Glaxo Rijswijk (WAG/Rij) rats. The modulatory effect of adenosinergic system may have a role in the ketone supplementation-evoked effects on isoflurane-generated anesthesia. Thus, we investigated whether adenosine receptor antagonists can modulate the effect of exogenous ketone supplements on the onset of akinesia induced by isoflurane.

Methods: To investigate the effect of exogenous ketone supplements on anesthetic induction we used ketone supplement KE, KS, KEKS (1:1 mix of KE and KS), KSMCT and KEMCT (1:1 mix of KS and KE with medium chain triglyceride/MCT oil, respectively) in WAG/Rij rats. Animals were fed with standard diet (SD), which was supplemented by oral gavage of different ketone supplements (2.5 g/kg/day) for 1 week. After 7 days, isoflurane (3%) was administered for 5 min and the time until onset of isoflurane-induced anesthesia (time until immobility; light phase of anesthesia: loss of consciousness without movement) was measured. Changes in levels of blood β-hydroxybutyrate (βHB), blood glucose and body weight of animals were also recorded. To investigate the putative effects of adenosine receptors on ketone supplements-evoked influence on isoflurane-induced anesthesia we used a specific adenosine A1 receptor antagonist DPCPX (intraperitoneally/i.p. 0.2 mg/kg) and a selective adenosine A2A receptor antagonist SCH 58261 (i.p. 0.5 mg/kg) alone as well as in combination with KEKS.

Results: Significant increases were demonstrated in both blood βHB levels and the number of seconds required before isoflurane-induced anesthesia (immobility) after the final treatment by all exogenous ketone supplements. Moreover, this effect of exogenous ketone supplements positively correlated with blood βHB levels. It was also demonstrated that DPCPX completely abolished the effect of KEKS on isoflurane-induced anesthesia (time until immobility), but not SCH 58261.

Conclusions: These findings strengthen our previous suggestion that exogenous ketone supplements may modulate the isoflurane-induced onset of anesthesia (immobility), likely through A1Rs.

Keywords: Isoflurane, Anesthesia, Exogenous ketone supplements, Ketosis, Adenosine receptors

* Correspondence: csari2000@yahoo.com
[5]Department of Psychology, Hyperbaric Neuroscience Research Laboratory, University of South Florida, 4202 E. Fowler Ave, PCD 3127, Tampa, FL 33620, USA

Background

It has been demonstrated that exogenous ketone (ketogenic) supplements, such as ketone ester (KE), not only increase the level of ketone bodies (e.g., β-hydroxybutyrate/βHB) [1–5], but also maintain blood levels of ketone bodies in both animals and humans [2, 3, 6]. Ketone bodies, such as βHB, enter into the brain through blood-brain barrier and provide fuel to brain cells [7, 8] improving cell energy metabolism (e.g., enhance mitochondrial ATP synthesis) [9]. Moreover, ketone supplement-induced ketosis can suppress neuronal excitability [7, 10, 11], modulate functions of ion channels and neurotransmitter systems (e.g., increase GABA and adenosine levels) [7, 12–14] and influence inflammatory processes (e.g., decrease the concentration and expression of proinflammatory cytokines) [15]. It was suggested that these effects of ketosis may have therapeutic potential in the treatment of several central nervous system (CNS) diseases, such as Alzheimer's disease, Parkinson's disease, epilepsy and psychiatric disorders (e.g., anxiety, schizophrenia and depression) [1, 3, 8, 16]. It was also demonstrated that exogenous ketone supplements, such as KE and ketone salt (KS) are relatively well-tolerated without (or with minimal) adverse effects [1, 2, 6, 16, 17]. However, exact mechanism(s) of action of exogenous ketone supplement-generated ketosis on CNS diseases and other pathophysiological and physiological processes are largely unknown.

It was suggested that ketosis may modulate sleep and sleep-like effects [18–22]. Indeed, it has been demonstrated recently that nutritional ketosis (evoked by exogenous ketone supplements, such as KE) delayed the onset of inhalational anesthetics isoflurane (1-chloro-2,2, 2-trifluoroethyl difluoromethyl ether)- induced anesthesia (immobility) [23] (light phase of anesthesia: loss of consciousness without movement, which was defined as 'immobility') [24]. Nevertheless, mechanism of action of ketosis-induced changes in isoflurane-evoked anesthesia remains unknown. It was suggested that changes, for example, in functioning of different ion channels (e.g., K_{ATP} channels), neurotransmitter systems (e.g., GABAergic and adenosinergic system) and mitochondria (e.g., mitochondrial respiration) may have a role in ketone supplement-evoked effects on isoflurane-generated anesthesia [19, 23, 25–27]. However, it has also been demonstrated that ketosis (evoked by exogenous ketone supplements) [1, 2, 4, 5] may increase adenosine level in the brain [14] and adenosine may have a role not only in the sleep [28], but also the generation of sleep-like effects [29, 30]. Therefore, in this study, we examined the effect of ketone supplement KE, KS and their mix (KEKS), as well as mix of KS and KE with medium chain triglyceride (MCT) oil (KSMCT and KEMCT, respectively) on isoflurane-induced onset of anesthesia (latency to immobility). Animals (Wistar Albino Glaxo Rijswijk/WAG/Rij rats) were fed with standard diet (SD) and were gavaged with different ketogenic supplements for 1 week (2.5 g/kg/day). After the last supplement gavage we recorded the time until onset of immobility (under 3% isoflurane). In the second part of the study, the potential role of adenosine receptors in the nutritional ketosis-evoked effects on isoflurane-induced onset of anesthesia (immobility) was investigated. We used a specific adenosine A1 receptor (A1R) antagonist DPCPX (1,3-dipropyl-8-cyclopentylxanthine) (intraperitoneally/i.p. 0.2 mg/kg) and a selective adenosine A2A receptor (A2AR) antagonist SCH 58261 (7-(2-phenylethyl)-5-amino-2-(2-furyl)-pyrazolo-[4,3-e]-1,2,4-triazolo[1,5-c]pyrimidine) (i.p. 0.5 mg/kg) alone as well as in combination with KEKS (2.5 g/kg/day, gavage).

This study is the continuation of our previous study on genetically absence epileptic WAG/Rij rat strain (a well-investigated model of human absence epilepsy) [31], in which it was demonstrated that exogenous ketone supplements (such as KE) delayed the onset of isoflurane-induced anesthesia (increased the time required before immobility) [23]. These effects may be clinically relevant because administration of exogenous ketone supplements-induced ketosis are more and more widely used as a metabolic therapy in the treatment of different CNS diseases, such as epilepsy or other seizure disorders [2, 8, 32–35]. Consequently, in order to implement a safe and successful anesthesia, potential effects of ketosis on the latency to anesthesia might need to be considered when epileptic patients are undergoing anesthetic procedures. For this reason, this study was performed on WAG/Rij rats, to better understand the ketone supplement-evoked effects on isoflurane-generated onset of anesthesia and its mechanism of action under epileptic condition.

In this study we hypothesized that adenosine receptor inhibition may modulate the exogenous ketone supplement-evoked delay in the latency to onset of immobility.

Methods

Animals

Animal treatments were carried out according to the Hungarian Act of Animal Care and Experimentation (1998, XXVIII, section 243), European Communities Council Directive 24 November 1986 (86/609/EEC) and EU Directive 2010/63/EU to use and treat animals in experimental laboratories. The experimental design was approved by the Animal Care and Experimentation Committee of the Eötvös Loránd University (Savaria University Centre) and National Scientific Ethical Committee on Animal Experimentation (Hungary) under license number VA/ÉBNTF02/85–8/2016.

Male WAG/Rij rats ($n = 80$; 6 months old, 315–332 g; breeding colony of WAG/Rij rats at Eötvös Loránd University, Savaria University Centre, Szombathely,

Hungary) were kept in groups of 3–4 under standard laboratory conditions (12:12 h light-dark cycle, light was on from 08.00 AM to 08.00 PM; free access to food and water; air-conditioned room at 22 ± 2 °C). Rats were fed with standard rodent chow diet (SD), and received oral (intragastric) gavage of either water (control) or different ketone supplements (KE, KS, KSMCT, KEKS or KEMCT). The animals were euthanized after the last treatment and data collection by using isoflurane. All efforts were made to minimize pain and suffering and to reduce the number of animals used.

Treatment groups and detection of immobility

Both KE (1,3-butanediol – acetoacetate diester) and KS (Na^+/K^+ – βHB mineral salt) were developed by D'Agostino et al. [2] (University of South Florida/USF, United States) in collaboration with Savind, Inc. (Urbana, IL, United States). Ketone salt was mixed into a 50% solution (375 mg/g pure βHB and 125 mg/g of Na^+/K^+ in a 1:1 ratio). Medium chain triglyceride (MCT) oil (pharmaceutical grade; approximately 60% caprylic triglyceride and 40% capric triglyceride) was purchased from Now Foods (Bloomingdale, IL, United States).

We demonstrated previously the tolerability and effectiveness of exogenous ketone supplements KE, KS, KSMCT (mix of KS and MCT oil in a 1:1 ratio), KEKS (mix of KE and KS in a 1:1 ratio) and KEMCT (mix of KE and MCT oil in a 1:1 ratio) given by intragastric gavage (ad libitum access to normal rat chow + 2.5 g/kg body weight supplements by gavage once/day in WAG/Rij rats) [1, 4, 32, 36]. Mix of ketone supplements (KSMCT, KEKS, and KEMCT) was carried out at the Eötvös Loránd University (Savaria University Centre, HUNGARY). These types and dose of ketone supplements introduced by oral gavage once per day for 7 days effectively induced and maintained ketosis in our previous studies [1, 32, 36] without causing side effects. Therefore, in the first phase of this study, 2.5 g/kg/day dosage of ketone supplements (KE, KS, KSMCT, KEKS and KEMCT) was administered daily by gavage for 7 days. In the second phase of the study, to investigate the putative adenosinergic mechanism of action of ketone supplements on isoflurane-evoked anesthesia (latency to immobility), we also used a specific A1R antagonist DPCPX and a selective A2AR antagonist SCH 58261, which drugs were dissolved in 10% dimethyl sulfoxide (DMSO). All drugs were purchased from Sigma-Aldrich Inc. (Hungary, Budapest). In order to minimize the putative adverse effects of drugs and to induce antagonism of A1Rs and A2ARs without changes in absence epileptic activity we used previously tested and effective i.p. dose of DPCPX and SCH 58261 (0.2 mg/kg DPCPX and 0.5 mg/kg SCH 58261) alone as well as in combination with KEKS (2.5 g/kg/day, gavage) [32, 37, 38]. Moreover, it was demonstrated previously that 10% of DMSO alone has no effect on absence epileptic activity (spike-wave discharges, SWDs) in WAG/Rij rats [39] and on sleep architecture in rats [40].

Oral gavage is a relatively stressful administration method, which may affect the sensitivity of animals to anesthetics [41]. Thus, to familiarize the animals to the methods, the 7 days gavage treatment was preceded by i.p. injection of 0.5 ml saline/100 g body weight and (30 min later) by water gavage for 5 days (adaptation period). Following adaptation period, rats were randomly assigned into 10 groups with 8 animals in each group. All of the rats were injected i.p. by 0.5 ml saline/100 g body weight/every day 30 min before gavage. After the i.p. injection, water (2.5 g/kg body weight/day, group 1; SD, control group) or exogenous ketone supplements (KE, KS, KSMCT, KEKS or KEMCT: 2.5 g/kg body weight/day; group 2–6, respectively) were administered by gavage for 7 days. One hour after the 7th treatments, anesthesia was induced in an air tight anesthesia chamber with isoflurane (3% isoflurane gas mixed with air for 5 min). Time from chamber closure until immobility (loss of consciousness without movement) was measured and analyzed by a blinded observer similar to previously [23]. To test the putative effect of DPCPX and SCH 58261 alone on isoflurane-induced anesthesia (latency to immobility), animals were i.p. injected and gavaged similar to group 1, but on the 7th treatment (water gavage) day, i.p. injections contained 0.2 mg/kg DPCPX (group 7) or 0.5 mg/kg SCH 58261 (group 8) in 0.5 ml 10% DMSO solution/100 g body weight. Based on results on group 2–6, the most effective ketone supplement (KEKS) was chosen for investigation of the putative mechanism of action. Therefore, animals (group 9 and group 10) were i.p. injected by saline and gavaged for 7 days by KEKS similar to described above, but on the 7th treatment (KEKS gavage) day, the i.p. injections contained 0.2 mg/kg DPCPX (group 9) or 0.5 mg/kg SCH 58261 (group 10) in 0.5 ml 10% DMSO solution/100 g body weight. After administration of i.p. DPCPX (group 7) and SCH 58261 (group 8) alone as well as combined administration of KEKS with i.p. DPCPX (group 9) or SCH 58261 (group 10), anesthesia was induced and immobility was measured similar to group 1–6 on the 7th treatment days.

Each rat was used only in one of the treatment groups and was euthanized with isoflurane after the 7th treatment and data collection.

Measurement of blood βHB and glucose levels as well as body weight

Blood was taken from the tail vein of rats. βHB levels were measured by a commercially available glucose and ketone monitoring system (Precision Xtra™, Abbott Laboratories, Abbott Park, IL, USA) [1, 23, 32]. Total blood ketone levels (D-βHB + L-βHB + acetoacetate + acetone) would be higher than we measured because this instrument only measures blood levels of D-βHB. Baseline βHB and glucose levels were measured on the last (5th) day of the adaptation period (group 1–6). Levels of βHB and glucose were measured again after the last (7th) day of water (group 1, control) and ketone supplementation (gavage; group 2–6) on awake animals, approximately 10 min after the detection of isoflurane-induced anesthesia (immobility) [23].

Body weight of rats were measured before (on last/5th day of the adaptation period) and after (on last/7th day of gavage) the treatments (group 1–6).

Statistics

All data were presented as the mean ± standard error of the mean (S.E.M.). We compared the latency of isoflurane-induced anesthesia (immobility) in control group (SD; group 1; gavaged by water for 7 days) and treated groups (gavaged by different exogenous ketone supplements for 7 days: group 2–6; i.p. injected by DPCPX or SCH 58261 alone on 7th treatment days: group 7, and group 8; administration of KEKS in combination with i.p. DPCPX or SCH 58261 on 7th treatment days: group 9, and group 10). Moreover, baseline (last/5th day of the adaptation period; group 1–6), control (SD; group 1; 7th day) and ketone supplements-induced (group 2–6; 7th day) blood glucose and βHB levels as well as body weight (before treatment and after treatment: group 1–6) were also compared. Data analysis was performed using GraphPad Prism version 6.0a using a two-way ANOVA with Tukey's multiple comparisons test. Pearson correlation was calculated for blood βHB and anesthesia latency as individual data points and as group means [23]. Results were considered significant when $p < 0.05$.

Results

Effects of exogenous ketone supplements on blood βHB and glucose levels and body weight

A significant increase in blood βHB levels was demonstrated after the final (7th) treatment by all exogenous ketone supplements (KE, KS, KSMCT, KEKS and KEMCT; group 2–6), compared to both control (SD; $p < 0.01$ for KS; $p < 0.001$ for KSMCT; $p < 0.0001$ for KE, KEKS and KEMCT) and baseline ($p < 0.001$ for KS; $p < 0.0001$ for KE, KSMCT, KEKS and KEMCT) levels (Fig. 1a; Table 1).

After the 7th treatment day, changes in glucose levels and body weight of animals were not detected (Fig. 1b and c; Table 1 and Table 2).

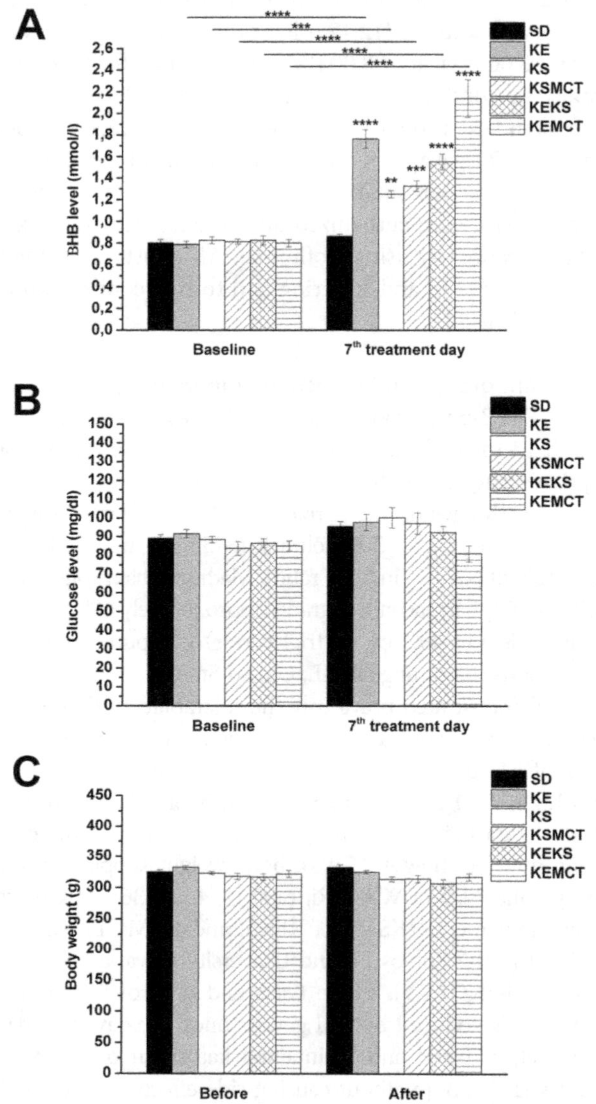

Fig. 1 Ketone supplements-evoked changes in blood βHB and glucose levels as well as body weight. Blood βHB levels were significantly elevated in all groups (group 2–6) gavaged by ketone supplements (KE, KS, KSMCT, KEKS and KEMCT) for 7 days, compared to both control (standard diet/SD, gavaged with water for 7 days) and to their baseline (**a**). After different treatments, glucose level (**b**) and body weight (**c**) of animals did not change compared to both control (SD) and to their baseline. Abbreviations: After, after the treatments; Before, before the treatments; KE, ketone ester; KEKS, mix of KE and KS in a 1:1 ratio; KEMCT, mix of KE and medium chain triglyceride (MCT) oil in a 1:1 ratio; KS, ketone salt; KSMCT, mix of KS and MCT oil in a 1:1 ratio; SD, standard diet/control; **$p < 0.01$; ***$p < 0.001$; ****$p < 0.0001$

Effect of exogenous ketone supplements on isoflurane-induced anesthesia: delay in the latency to onset of immobility

Treatments by all exogenous ketone supplements (KE, KS, KSMCT, KEKS and KEMCT; group 2–6) caused a significant increase in the number of seconds required before anesthetic induction (the time until immobility), compared to control (SD; $p < 0.05$ for KSMCT; $p < 0.001$ for KS; $p < 0.0001$ for KE, KEKS and KEMCT) (Fig. 2a; Table 3) on the 7th day of treatment.

Exogenous ketone supplement-induced delay in isoflurane-generated anesthesia (increase in latency to immobility) positively correlated with blood βHB levels when individual data points ($R^2 = 0.2933$) or the group

Table 1 Effect of ketone supplements on blood βHB and glucose levels on the 7th day of gavage

Treatments (2.5 g/kg/day; Fig. 1a)	Blood βHB level			
	Baseline	7th treatment day		
	mmol/l (mean ± S.E.M.)	mmol/l (mean ± S.E.M.)	Compared to baseline (significance level/q-value)	Compared to control (significance level/q-value)
SD (control; group 1)	0.80 ± 0.037	0.86 ± 0.018	–/0.945	–
KE (group 2)	0.79 ± 0.029	1.76 ± 0.087	****/14.550	****/13.610
KS (group 3)	0.83 ± 0.031	1.25 ± 0.033	***/6.805	**/5.860
KSMCT (group 4)	0.81 ± 0.023	1.33 ± 0.049	****/7.939	***/6.994
KEKS (group 5)	0.83 ± 0.041	1.55 ± 0.073	****/11.340	****/10.400
KEMCT (group 6)	0.80 ± 0.033	2.14 ± 0.172	****/20.230	****/19.280
	Blood glucose level			
Treatments (2.5 g/kg/day; Fig. 1b)	Baseline	7th treatment day		
	mg/dl (mean ± S.E.M.)	mg/dl (mean ± S.E.M.)	Compared to baseline (significance level/q-value)	Compared to control (significance level/q-value)
SD (control; group 1)	89.00 ± 1.937	95.38 ± 2.672	–/1.764	–
KE (group 2)	91.50 ± 2.284	97.63 ± 4.342	–/2.386	–/0.623
KS (group 3)	88.38 ± 1.772	100.13 ± 5.482	–/3.078	–/1.314
KSMCT (group 4)	83.63 ± 3.600	97.00 ± 5.745	–/2.213	–/0.449
KEKS (group 5)	86.38 ± 2.398	92.13 ± 3.388	–/0.865	–/0.899
KEMCT (group 6)	85.00 ± 2.659	80.88 ± 4.286	–/2.248	–/4.011

Abbreviations: KE, ketone ester; KEKS, mix of KE and KS in a 1:1 ratio; KEMCT, mix of KE and medium chain triglyceride (MCT) oil in a 1:1 ratio; KS, ketone salt; KSMCT, mix of KS and MCT oil in a 1:1 ratio; SD, standard diet/control; ** $p < 0.01$; *** $p < 0.001$; **** $p < 0.0001$

means were considered ($R^2 = 0.5553$) (Fig. 2b and c, respectively).

Effect of A1R and A2AR inhibition on KEKS-evoked increase in latency to immobility

Administration of i.p. DPCPX (0.2 mg/kg; group 7) and SCH 58261 (0.5 mg/kg; group 8) alone (without KEKS administration) did not cause significant changes in the number of seconds required before isoflurane-induced anesthesia (latency to immobility), compared to control (SD; Fig. 3; Table 3) on the 7th day of gavage. It was demonstrated that i.p. 0.2 mg/kg DPCPX completely abolished the effect of KEKS on latency to immobility (group 9) (Fig. 3), whereas i.p. 0.5 mg/kg SCH 58261 (group 10) was ineffective on the KEKS-induced effect (Fig. 3; Table 3). After combined administration of KEKS with SCH 58261 on the 7th day of gavage, latency to immobility significantly increased, compared to control (SD; Fig. 3; Table 3) and both the rate of this increase and its significance level ($p < 0.0001$) was similar to results, which were recorded after gavage of KEKS alone (group 5) (Fig. 3; Table 3).

Table 2 Effect of ketone supplements on body weight

Treatments (2.5 g/kg/day; Fig. 1)	Body weight		
	Before the treatments	After the treatments	
	Gram (mean ± S.E.M.)	Gram (mean ± S.E.M.)	Compared to 'Before the treatments' (significance level/q-value)
SD (control, group 1)	325.0 ± 3.134	331.8 ± 4.427	–/1.464
KE (group 2)	331.9 ± 2.496	324.9 ± 2.608	–/0.027
KS (group 3)	323.1 ± 2.394	313.5 ± 3.942	–/2.495
KSMCT (group 4)	318.0 ± 5.119	314.0 ± 5.719	–/2.386
KEKS (group 5)	316.9 ± 5.377	306.6 ± 6.434	–/3.986
KEMCT (group 6)	321.8 ± 5.502	316.8 ± 5.640	–/1.790

Abbreviations: KE, ketone ester; KEKS, mix of KE and KS in a 1:1 ratio; KEMCT, mix of KE and medium chain triglyceride (MCT) oil in a 1:1 ratio; KS, ketone salt; KSMCT, mix of KS and MCT oil in a 1:1 ratio; SD, standard diet/control

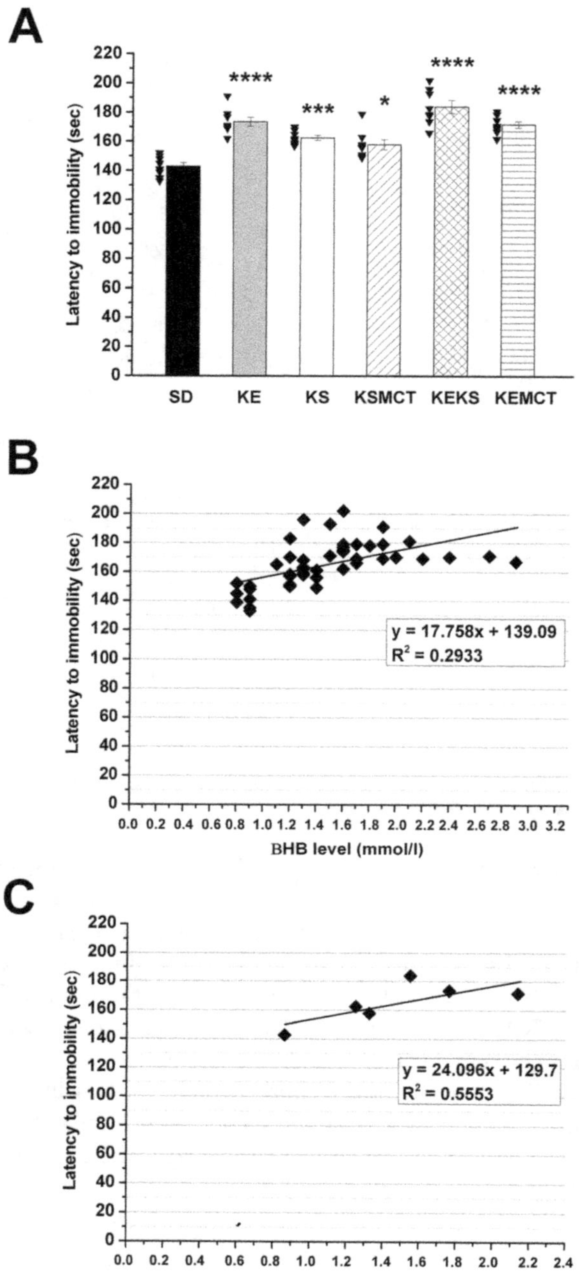

Fig. 2 Effect of ketone supplements on isoflurane-induced anesthesia (latency to immobility). Gavage by exogenous ketone supplements (KE, KS, KSMCT, KEKS and KEMCT; group 2–6) significantly increased the latency to anesthetic induction (the time until immobility), compared to control (SD) on the 7th day of gavage (**a**; the raw data was plotted as filled black triangles to the left of the columns). There was a positive correlation between latency to immobility and blood βHB levels when all data point (**b**; $R^2 = 0.2933$) or the group means (**c**; $R^2 = 0.5553$) were considered. Abbreviations: KE, ketone ester; KEKS, mix of KE and KS in a 1:1 ratio; KEMCT, mix of KE and medium chain triglyceride (MCT) oil in a 1:1 ratio; KS, ketone salt; KSMCT, mix of KS and MCT oil in a 1:1 ratio; SD, standard diet/control; *$p < 0.05$; ***$p < 0.001$; ****$p < 0.0001$

Discussion

In this study we demonstrated that inhibition of A1Rs completely abolished the KEKS-evoked delay in isoflurane-induced anesthesia (immobility) in WAG/Rij rats. Moreover, we extended our previous results showing that not only gavage of KE and KS [23], but also KSMCT, KEKS and KEMCT are able to increase both the blood level of βHB (ketosis) and number of seconds required before induction of anesthesia (immobility).

Although isoflurane has been used in patients for nearly 50 years [19], its mechanism of action remains largely unknown. In spite of that both behavioral and physiological differences in functioning of sleep and general anesthetics-induced sleep-like state were demonstrated (e.g., general anesthesia is not able to appear spontaneously), it was suggested that several brain areas, such as cerebral cortex and the hypothalamic nucleus ventrolateral preoptic area may participate in both processes [42–44]. It was hypothesized, that anesthetics, such as isoflurane may induce anesthesia through common endogenous arousal neural circuitry/sleep pathways [44, 45].

Administration of exogenous ketone supplements by gavage and subsequent metabolism [17, 46, 47] increases levels of ketone bodies in the blood stream (nutritional ketosis) [1, 2, 4, 32]. Ketone bodies, such as βHB may enter into the brain through blood brain barrier and modulate different physiological and pathophysiological processes, such as sleep or seizures [7, 8, 12]. As ketosis (βHB) increases adenosine level [14] in the brain tissue and adenosine has a role in the sleep generation [28, 29], enhanced level of βHB generated by ketone supplements may modulate naturally occurring sleep. Indeed, exogenous ketone supplement-generated ketosis may evoke a decrease in total sleep time through ventrolateral preoptic area [20, 21, 44]. Moreover, it has been demonstrated that level and metabolism of both ketone bodies [7, 18, 48], as well as adenosine and expression of adenosine receptors [49] are regionally different in the brain, which strengthen the modulatory role of ketone bodies and adenosine in processes such as sleep and sleep-like states. Ketosis-evoked increase in extracellular adenosine levels may change neuronal activity in different brain areas [22, 49] implicated in sleep/sleep-like effects by its receptors. Increased level of adenosine was demonstrated during waking whereas adenosine concentration decreased during sleep in the brain [50]. Adenosine agonists induced sleep/electroencephalographic slow-wave activity, but adenosine receptor antagonists (e.g., a non-selective antagonist of adenosine receptors caffeine) reversed effects of adenosine on the sleep [51]. Moreover, adenosine accumulates under, for example, sleep deprivation and may have a role in the anesthetic action of isoflurane [28, 44]: theophylline (a non-selective antagonist of adenosine receptors) reversed the cerebral

Table 3 Effect of ketone supplements, DPCPX, and SCH 58261 alone as well as ketone supplement KEKS in combination with DPCPX or SCH 58261 on latency to immobility on the 7th day of gavage

Treatments (2.5 g/kg/day; Figs. 2a and 3)	Latency to immobility Sec (mean ± S.E.M.)	Compared to control (significance level/q-value)
SD (control, group 1)	142.88 ± 2.474	–
KE (group 2)	173.50 ± 3.105	****/10.220
KS (group 3)	162.50 ± 1.679	***/6.548
KSMCT (group 4)	157.88 ± 3.446	*/5.005
KEKS (group 5)	183.88 ± 4.299	****/13.680
KEMCT (group 6)	171.75 ± 2.226	****/9.634
DPCPX (group 7)	146.25 ± 4.443	–/0.765
SCH 58261 (group 8)	141.63 ± 4.935	–/0.283
KEKS + DPCPX (group 9)	138.13 ± 4.202	–/1.177
KEKS + SCH 58261 (group 10)	187.13 ± 5.531	****/12.290

Abbreviations: DPCPX (DP), 1,3-dipropyl-8-cyclopentylxanthine (a specific adenosine A1 receptor/A1R antagonist); KE, ketone ester; KEKS, mix of KE and KS in a 1:1 ratio; KEMCT, mix of KE and medium chain triglyceride (MCT) oil in a 1:1 ratio; KS, ketone salt; KSMCT, mix of KS and MCT oil in a 1:1 ratio; SCH (SC), SCH 58261, 7-(2-phenylethyl)-5-amino-2-(2-furyl)-pyrazolo-[4,3-e]-1,2,4-triazolo[1,5-c] pyrimidine (a selective adenosine A2A receptor/A2AR antagonist); SD, standard diet/control; *$p < 0.05$; ***$p < 0.001$; ****$p < 0.0001$

effects of isoflurane in dogs (e.g., EEG has been changed from a sleep pattern to an awake pattern) [30] and caffeine accelerated emergence from isoflurane-evoked anesthesia in humans [52]. Moreover, enhanced activity of A1Rs (e.g., by an A1R agonist N-sulfophenyl adenosine) may cause increase in anesthesia recovery time [53]

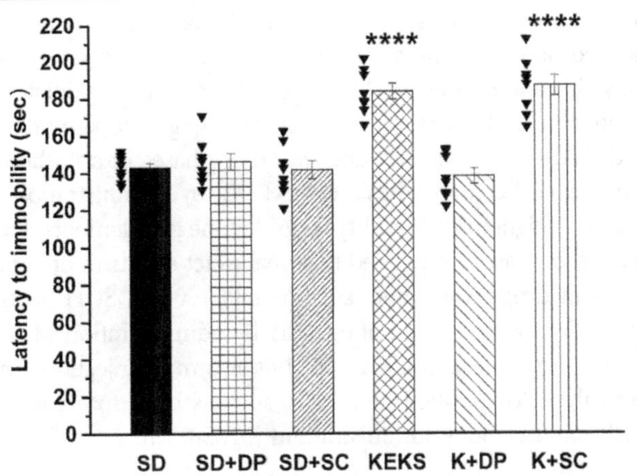

Fig. 3 Influence of A1R antagonist DPCPX and A2AR antagonist SCH 58261 on KEKS-generated changes in isoflurane-evoked anesthesia (latency to immobility). Administration of DPCPX (i.p. 0.2 mg/kg; SD + DP; group 7) and SCH 58261 (i.p. 0.5 mg/kg; SD + SC; group 8) alone did not modulate the latency to immobility, compared to control (SD; the raw data was plotted as filled black triangles to the left of the columns). Combined administration of DPCPX (i.p. 0.2 mg/kg) with KEKS (K + DP; group 9) completely abolished the effect of KEKS on latency to immobility, whereas SCH 58261 (i.p. 0.5 mg/kg) was ineffective on the KEKS-induced influence (K + SC; group 10); Abbreviations: DP (DPCPX), 1,3-dipropyl-8-cyclopentylxanthine (a specific adenosine A1 receptor/A1R antagonist); KEKS, mix of KE and KS in a 1:1 ratio; SC (SCH 58261), 7-(2-phenylethyl)-5-amino-2-(2-furyl)-pyrazolo-[4,3-e]-1,2,4-triazolo[1,5-c] pyrimidine (a selective adenosine A2A receptor/A2AR antagonist); SD, standard diet/control; ****$p < 0.0001$

and isoflurane may activate A1Rs [54]. It has been demonstrated that receptors of adenosine, such as inhibitory A1Rs and excitatory A2ARs are expressed brain areas implicated in the generation of sleep and sleep-like effects, such as ventrolateral/lateral preoptic area and basal forebrain [29]. Thus, adenosine may be a link between the anesthetic actions of isoflurane and sleep regulation as an endogenous sleep factor.

It was also demonstrated that inhibition or disinhibition by A1Rs (e.g., in wake-promoting neurons of basal forebrain or sleep-active neurons of ventrolateral preoptic area, respectively) may induce sleep [29, 55, 56]. Nevertheless, A1Rs may also promote wakefulness by inhibition of sleep-active neurons in lateral preoptic area [57] and in ventrolateral preoptic area [58]. Consequently, we can hypothesize that adenosinergic system may modulate the influence of exogenous ketone supplements, such as KEKS, on the onset of isoflurane-induced anesthesia (immobility) by inhibition of sleep active neurons (possibly by ketosis and, as a consequence, through increase in adenosine level as well as its A1Rs) [14, 23], which processes lead to delay in the anesthetic effects of isoflurane. Indeed, although the A1R antagonist DPCPX alone did not change the isoflurane-generated anesthetic effect (immobility), combined administration of DPCPX with KEKS completely abolished the KEKS-evoked increase in latency to immobility under isoflurane anesthesia (Fig. 3). Moreover, adenosine receptors may also modulate anesthesia recovery time [52, 53]. Thus, it is possible that exogenous ketone supplements not only delay the onset of isoflurane-induced anesthesia (immobility) [23] (Fig. 2a and 3), but also modulate the time required for recovery from anesthesia. However, further studies are needed to determine the exact effect and mechanism(s) of action of exogenous ketone supplements (ketosis) on isoflurane-generated anesthetic effects.

As it was demonstrated, not only A1Rs but also A2ARs are implicated in sleep generation, and A2ARs are considered more important in sleep regulation [29]: increased activity of A2ARs, for example, in ventrolateral/lateral preoptic area may induce sleep through sleep-active/promoting neurons [57, 59]. It has been demonstrated that A1Rs are abundantly expressed in the brain whereas A2AR expression is week in most of brain areas such as ventrolateral preoptic area [29, 49, 60]. Thus, as it was demonstrated, effects of adenosine on both sleep [29, 55–58] and processes of anesthesia may be brain region- and receptor-dependent. In addition, our knowledge relating to the exact role of adenosinergic system in modulation of both isoflurane-evoked anesthesia and connections between brain areas implicated in processes of anesthesia is far from complete. Consequently, it is possible that A1Rs are predominant whereas A2ARs are secondary (if any) in adenosine-evoked influences on anesthesia at least at this level of isoflurane-generated anesthesia (loss of consciousness without movement: immobility) in WAG/Rij rats. Indeed, our results suggest that A2ARs have no effect on isoflurane-generated anesthesia (immobility): neither isoflurane-induced anesthesia (latency to immobility) nor the effect of exogenous ketone supplement KEKS on isoflurane-induced anesthesia (latency to immobility) were modulated by the A2AR antagonist SCH 58261 (Fig. 3). Nevertheless, it cannot be excluded that this physiologically effective dose of A2AR antagonist SCH 58261 (0.5 mg/kg) may not have been adequate to investigate its influence on isoflurane-generated light phase of anesthesia (loss of consciousness without movement, immobility), but may modulate the later/deeper phase(s) of isoflurane-evoked anesthesia. However, more studies are needed to explain the exact role of adenosine and its receptors in isoflurane-induced anesthesia.

It has been demonstrated that gavage of exogenous ketone supplements, such as KSMCT for 7 days not only increases the number of seconds required before isoflurane-induced anesthetic induction (the time until immobility) (Fig. 2a) [23], but also generates decrease in both anxiety level on elevated plus maze [36] and absence epileptic activity [32] in WAG/Rij rats. These effects may be in correlation with enhanced level of βHB [23, 32, 36] (Fig. 2b and c). Moreover, it was showed that inhibition of A1Rs may abolish the anti-anesthetic (Fig. 3), antiepileptic [32] and anxiolytic [36] effects of exogenous ketone supplements, suggesting that adenosinergic system may modulate the ketone supplements (ketosis) induced influences in the CNS. Indeed, it was proposed that adenosinergic system (e.g., through A1Rs) has a role in the modulation of sleep and sleep-like effects [28–30], different types of epilepsies [61–63] and anxiety [64–66]. However, new studies are needed to reveal the likely (at least partly) common mechanism(s), as well as interactions of adenosine receptors and adenosine receptor-evoked changes (e.g., in ion channels, signal transduction, metabolic processes) in different brain areas involved in sleep/sleep-like effects, epilepsy and anxiety, by which ketone supplements could exert its above mentioned influences.

One limitation of our study is that we used the WAG/Rij rat strain exclusively to investigate the effect of ketone supplementation on isoflurane-induced anesthesia. In addition, during this study we narrowed our focus on the influence of ketone supplement-evoked effects to the adenosinergic system. Nevertheless, this WAG/Rij rat strain is extensively used for investigation of different drugs on CNS diseases [1, 67–71], and the present study further supports our previous experiments [23] on the role of the adenosinergic system. It has been suggested that the ketosis/βHB-evoked increase in adenosine levels [14] can modulate influence of ketone supplements not only on different CNS diseases [8, 32, 36], but also sleep and sleep-like effects [20, 21, 28–30] via adenosinergic system (likely through A1Rs). Consequently, we propose that the adenosinergic system may be one of main neurotransmitter systems by which ketone supplements can exert their influence on isoflurane-induced anesthesia. However, to get comprehensive view on influence of ketone supplements on isoflurane-evoked anesthesia more studies are needed on other animal strains and humans, on changes not only in adenosinergic, but also other neuromodulatory/neurotransmitter systems (such as cholinergic, dopaminergic, and GABAergic system), and on other phases of anesthesia/emergence from anesthesia [24, 53, 72] by administration of different/higher doses and types of ketone supplements. Further studies are also needed to reveal exact effects of different doses of drugs were used, such as DPCPX and SCH 58261, on isoflurane-generated anesthesia by administration of distinct methods (e.g., not only i.p., but also microinjections/microdialysis to specific brain areas, such as basal forebrain, as well as intravenous administration) [57, 58, 73].

Conclusion

The present study strengthened the putative clinical and surgical relevance of ketone supplements-evoked influences on sleep and sleep-like effects suggested by our previous results: exogenous ketone supplements may increase the resistance to the isoflurane-induced anesthetic influence by delaying the onset of anesthesia (immobility). Thus, monitoring of blood ketone levels in humans undergoing isoflurane and (theoretically) other inhalational anesthesia may be important and helpful for the anesthesiologists. Moreover, inhibitory effect of DPCPX on KEKS-evoked delay in isoflurane-generated anesthesia (immobility) suggests that the adenosinergic system, likely via A_1Rs, may modulate the exogenous ketone supplements-evoked anti-anesthetic influence. However, further studies are needed to reveal the exact mechanism(s) of action of exogenous ketone supplements (ketosis) on isoflurane-generated anesthesia not only in animals, but also in human subjects because ketone supplements used in normal and pathological conditions may modify the time needed for anesthesia.

Abbreviations

A_1R: Adenosine A_1 receptor; A2AR: Adenosine A2A receptor; CNS: Central nervous system; DMSO: Dimethyl sulfoxide; DPCPX: 1,3-dipropyl-8-cyclopentylxanthine; i.p.: intraperitoneal; K_{ATP} channels: ATP-sensitive potassium channels; KE (ketone ester): 1,3 butanediol-acetoacetate diester; KEKS: (mix of KE and KS); KEMCT: (mix of KE and MCT oil); KS: ketone salt; KSMCT: (mix of KS and MCT oil); MCT: medium chain triglyceride; SCH 58261: 7-(2-phenylethyl)-5-amino-2-(2-furyl)-pyrazolo-[4,3-e]-1,2,4-triazolo[1,5-c]pyrimidine; SD: Standard rodent chow diet; WAG/Rij: Wistar Albino Glaxo/Rijswijk; βHB: beta-hydroxybutyrate

Acknowledgements

Not Applicable.

Authors' contributions

All authors read and approved the final manuscript. ZK: design of experiments, acquisition, analysis, and interpretation of data, writing manuscript, BS: acquisition of data, DPD: revising manuscript, CA: analysis of data, writing manuscript.

Author details

[1]Savaria Department of Biology, ELTE Eötvös Loránd University, Savaria University Centre, Szombathely, Hungary. [2]Institute of Biology, University of Pécs, Pécs, Hungary. [3]Department of Molecular Pharmacology and Physiology, Laboratory of Metabolic Medicine, Morsani College of Medicine, University of South Florida, Tampa, FL, USA. [4]Institute for Human and Machine Cognition, Ocala, FL, USA. [5]Department of Psychology, Hyperbaric Neuroscience Research Laboratory, University of South Florida. 4202 E. Fowler Ave, PCD 3127, Tampa, FL 33620, USA.

References

1. Ari C, Kovács Z, Juhasz G, Murdun C, Goldhagen CR, Koutnik AM, Poff AM, Kesl SL, D'Agostino D. Exogenous ketone supplements reduce anxiety-related behavior in Sprague-Dawley and Wistar albino Glaxo/Rijswijk rats. Front Mol Neurosci. 2016;9:137.
2. D'Agostino DP, Pilla R, Held HE, Landon CS, Puchowicz M, Brunengraber H, Ari C, Arnold P, Dean JB. Therapeutic ketosis with ketone ester delays central nervous system oxygen toxicity seizures in rats. Am J Physiol Regul Integr Comp Physiol. 2013;304(10):829–36.
3. Hashim SA, VanItallie TB. Ketone body therapy: from the ketogenic diet to the oral administration of ketone ester. J Lipid Res. 2014;55(9):1818–26.
4. Kesl SL, Poff AM, Ward NP, Fiorelli TN, Ari C, Van Putten AJ, Sherwood JW, Arnold P, D'Agostino DP. Effects of exogenous ketone supplementation on blood ketone, glucose, triglyceride, and lipoprotein levels in Sprague-Dawley rats. Nutr Metab. (Lond.) 2016;13:9.
5. Kovács Z, D'Agostino DP, Diamond DM, Ari C. Exogenous ketone supplementation decreased the lipopolysaccharide-induced increase in absence epileptic activity in Wistar albino Glaxo Rijswijk rats. Front Mol Neurosci. 2019;12:45.
6. Stubbs BJ, Cox PJ, Evans RD, Santer P, Miller JJ, Faull OK, Magor-Elliott S, Hiyama S, Stirling M, Clarke K. On the metabolism of exogenous ketones in humans. Front Physiol. 2017;8:848.
7. Achanta LB, Rae CD. β-Hydroxybutyrate in the brain: one molecule, multiple mechanisms. Neurochem Res. 2017;42(1):35–49.
8. Kovács Z, D'Agostino DP, Diamond D, Kindy MS, Rogers C, Ari C. Therapeutic potential of exogenous ketone supplement induced ketosis in the treatment of psychiatric disorders: review of current literature. Front Psychiatry. 2019;10:363.
9. Sato K, Kashiwaya Y, Keon C, Tsuchiya N, King MT, Radda GK, Chance B, Clarke K, Veech RL. Insulin, ketone bodies, and mitochondrial energy transduction. FASEB J. 1995;9(8):651–8.
10. Juge N, Gray JA, Omote H, Miyaji T, Inoue T, Hara C, Uneyama H, Edwards RH, Nicoll RA, Moriyama Y. Metabolic control of vesicular glutamate transport and release. Neuron. 2010;68(1):99–112.
11. Simeone TA, Simeone KA, Rho JM. Ketone bodies as anti-seizure agents. Neurochem Res. 2017;42(7):2011–8.
12. Newman JC, Verdin E. Ketone bodies as signaling metabolites. Trends Endocrinol Metab. 2014;25(1):42–52.
13. McNally MA, Hartman AL. Ketone bodies in epilepsy. J Neurochem. 2012; 121(1):28–35.
14. Sharma AK, Rani E, Waheed A, Rajput SK. Pharmacoresistant epilepsy: a current update on non-conventional pharmacological and non-pharmacological interventions. J Epilepsy Res. 2015;5(1):1–8.
15. Youm YH, Nguyen KY, Grant RW, Goldberg EL, Bodogai M, Kim D, D'Agostino D, Planavsky N, Lupfer C, Kanneganti TD, Kang S, Horvath TL, Fahmy TM, Crawford PA, Biragyn A, Alnemri E, Dixit VD. The ketone metabolite β-hydroxybutyrate blocks NLRP3 inflammasome-mediated inflammatory disease. Nat Med. 2015;21(3):263–9.
16. Newport MT, VanItallie TB, Kashiwaya Y, King MT, Veech RL. A new way to produce hyperketonemia: use of ketone ester in a case of Alzheimer's disease. Alzheimers Dement. 2015;11(1):99–103.
17. Clarke K, Tchabanenko K, Pawlosky R, Carter E, Todd King M, Musa-Veloso K, Ho M, Roberts A, Robertson J, Vanitallie TB, Veech RL. Kinetics, safety and tolerability of (R)-3-hydroxybutyl (R)-3-hydroxybutyrate in healthy adult subjects. Regul Toxicol Pharmacol. 2012;63(3):401–8.
18. Allen CN. Circadian rhythms, diet, and neuronal excitability. Epilepsia. 2008; 49(Suppl 8):124–6.
19. Constantinides C, Murphy K. Molecular and integrative physiological effects of isoflurane anesthesia: the paradigm of cardiovascular studies in rodents using magnetic resonance imaging. Front Cardiovasc Med. 2016;3:23.
20. Hallböök T, Ji S, Maudsley S, Martin B. The effects of the ketogenic diet on behavior and cognition. Epilepsy Res. 2012;100(3):304–9.
21. Hallböök T, Lundgren J, Rosén I. Ketogenic diet improves sleep quality in children with therapy-resistant epilepsy. Epilepsia. 2007;48(1):59–65.
22. Masino SA, Kawamura M, Wasser CD, Pomeroy LT, Ruskin DN. Adenosine, ketogenic diet and epilepsy: the emerging therapeutic relationship between metabolism and brain activity. Curr Neuropharmacol. 2009;7(3):257–68.
23. Ari C, Kovács Z, Murdun C, Koutnik AP, Goldhagen CR, Rogers C, Diamond D, D'Agostino DP. Nutritional ketosis delays the onset of isoflurane induced anesthesia. BMC Anesthesiol. 2018;18(1):85.
24. Hanusch C, Hoeger S, Beck GC. Anaesthesia of small rodents during magnetic resonance imaging. Methods. 2007;43(1):68–78.
25. Joksovic PM, Weiergräber M, Lee W, Struck H, Schneider T, Todorovic SM. Isoflurane-sensitive presynaptic R-type calcium channels contribute to inhibitory synaptic transmission in the rat thalamus. J Neurosci. 2009;29(5): 1434–45.
26. Kofke WA, Hawkins RA, Davis DW, Biebuyck JF. Comparison of the effects of volatile anesthetics on brain glucose metabolism in rats. Anesthesiology. 1987;66(6):810–3.
27. Rogawski MA, Löscher W, Rho JM. Mechanisms of action of antiseizure drugs and the ketogenic diet. Cold Spring Harb Perspect Med. 2016;6(5), pii: a022780.
28. Porkka-Heiskanen T, Strecker RE, Thakkar M, Bjorkum AA, Greene RW, McCarley RW. Adenosine: a mediator of the sleep-inducing effects of prolonged wakefulness. Science. 1997;276(5316):1265–8.
29. Huang ZL, Urade Y, Hayaishi O. The role of adenosine in the regulation of sleep. Curr Top Med Chem. 2011;11(8):1047–57.
30. Roald OK, Forsman M, Steen PA. Partial reversal of the cerebral effects of isoflurane in the dog by theophylline. Acta Anaesthesiol Scand. 1990;34(7): 548–51.
31. Coenen AM, Van Luijtelaar EL. Genetic animal models for absence epilepsy: a review of the WAG/Rij strain of rats. Behav Genet. 2003;33(6):635–55.
32. Kovács Z, D'Agostino DP, Dobolyi A, Ari C. Adenosine A1 receptor antagonism abolished the anti-seizure effects of exogenous ketone supplementation in Wistar albino Glaxo Rijswijk rats. Front Mol Neurosci. 2017;10:235.
33. Lee E, Kang HC, Kim HD. Ketogenic diet for children with epilepsy: a practical meal plan in a hospital. Clin Nutr Res. 2016;5(1):60–3.
34. Rho JM. How does the ketogenic diet induce anti-seizure effects? Neurosci Lett. 2017;637:4–10.
35. Yudkoff M, Daikhin Y, Melø TM, Nissim I, Sonnewald U, Nissim I. The ketogenic diet and brain metabolism of amino acids: relationship to the anticonvulsant effect. Annu Rev Nutr. 2007;27:415–30.

36. Kovács Z, D'Agostino DP, Ari C. Anxiolytic effect of exogenous ketone supplementation is abolished by adenosine A1 receptor inhibition in Wistar albino Glaxo/Rijswijk rats. Front Behav Neurosci. 2018;12:29.
37. Dubroqua S, Yee BK, Singer P. Sensorimotor gating is disrupted by acute but not chronic systemic exposure to caffeine in mice. Psychopharmacology. 2014;231(21):4087–98.
38. Fontinha BM, Delgado-García JM, Madroñal N, Ribeiro JA, Sebastião AM, Gruart A. Adenosine a(2A) receptor modulation of hippocampal CA3-CA1 synapse plasticity during associative learning in behaving mice. Neuropsychopharmacology. 2009;34(7):1865–74.
39. Kovács Z, Czurkó A, Kékesi KA, Juhász G. The effect of intraperitoneally administered dimethyl sulfoxide on absence-like epileptic activity of freely moving WAG/Rij rats. J Neurosci Methods. 2011;197(1):133–6.
40. Cavas M, Beltrán D, Navarro JF. Behavioural effects of dimethyl sulfoxide (DMSO): changes in sleep architecture in rats. Toxicol Lett. 2005;157(3):221–32.
41. Wang L, Holland L, Fong R, Khokhar S, Fox AP, Xie Z. A pilot study showing that repeated exposure to stress produces alterations in subsequent responses to anesthetics in rats. PLoS One. 2019;14(3):e0214093.
42. Moore JT, Chen J, Han B, Meng QC, Veasey SC, Beck SG, Kelz MB. Direct activation of sleep-promoting VLPO neurons by volatile anesthetics contributes to anesthetic hypnosis. Curr Biol. 2012;22(21):2008–16.
43. Saper CB, Chou TC, Scammell TE. The sleep switch: hypothalamic control of sleep and wakefulness. Trends Neurosci. 2001;24(12):726–31.
44. Tung A, Mendelson WB. Anesthesia and sleep. Sleep Med Rev. 2004;8(3): 213–25.
45. Nelson LE, Guo TZ, Lu J, Saper CB, Franks NP, Maze M. The sedative component of anesthesia is mediated by GABA(a) receptors in an endogenous sleep pathway. Nat Neurosci. 2002;5(10):979–84.
46. Schönfeld P, Wojtczak L. Short- and medium-chain fatty acids in energy metabolism: the cellular perspective. J Lipid Res. 2016;57(6):943–54.
47. Tate RL, Mehlman MA, Tobin RB. Metabolic fate of 1,3-butanediol in the rat: conversion to -hydroxybutyrate. J Nutr. 1971;101(12):1719–26.
48. Hawkins RA, Biebuyck JF. Ketone bodies are selectively used by individual brain regions. Science. 1979;205(4403):325–7.
49. Kovács Z, Juhász G, Palkovits M, Dobolyi A, Kékesi KA. Area, age and gender dependence of the nucleoside system in the brain: a review of current literature. Curr Top Med Chem. 2011;11(8):1012–33.
50. Porkka-Heiskanen T, Strecker RE, McCarley RW. Brain site-specificity of extracellular adenosine concentration changes during sleep deprivation and spontaneous sleep: an in vivo microdialysis study. Neuroscience. 2000;99(3): 507–17.
51. Schwierin B, Borbély AA, Tobler I. Effects of N6-cyclopentyladenosine and caffeine on sleep regulation in the rat. Eur J Pharmacol. 1996;300(3):163–71.
52. Fong R, Wang L, Zacny JP, Khokhar S, Apfelbaum JL, Fox AP, Xie Z. Caffeine accelerates emergence from isoflurane anesthesia in humans: a randomized, double-blind, crossover study. Anesthesiology. 2018;129(5):912–20.
53. Gettys GC, Liu F, Kimlin E, Baghdoyan HA, Lydic R. Adenosine a(1) receptors in mouse pontine reticular formation depress breathing, increase anesthesia recovery time, and decrease acetylcholine release. Anesthesiology. 2013; 118(2):327–36.
54. Tas PW, Eisemann C, Roewer N. The volatile anesthetic isoflurane suppresses spontaneous calcium oscillations in vitro in rat hippocampal neurons by activation of adenosine A1 receptors. Neurosci Lett. 2003;338(3):229–32.
55. Blanco-Centurion C, Xu M, Murillo-Rodriguez E, Gerashchenko D, Shiromani AM, Salin-Pascual RJ, Hof PR, Shiromani PJ. Adenosine and sleep homeostasis in the basal forebrain. J Neurosci. 2006;26(31):8092–100.
56. Morairty S, Rainnie D, McCarley R, Greene R. Disinhibition of ventrolateral preoptic area sleep-active neurons by adenosine: a new mechanism for sleep promotion. Neuroscience. 2004;123(2):451–7.
57. Methippara MM, Kumar S, Alam MN, Szymusiak R, McGinty D. Effects on sleep of microdialysis of adenosine A1 and A2a receptor analogs into the lateral preoptic area of rats. Am J Physiol Regul Integr Comp Physiol. 2005; 289(6):1715–23.
58. Zhang J, Yin D, Wu F, Zhang G, Jiang C, Li Z, Wang L, Wang K. Microinjection of adenosine into the hypothalamic ventrolateral preoptic area enhances wakefulness via the A1 receptor in rats. Neurochem Res. 2013;38(8):1616–23.
59. Scammell TE, Gerashchenko DY, Mochizuki T, McCarthy MT, Estabrooke IV, Sears CA, Saper CB, Urade Y, Hayaishi O. An adenosine A2a agonist increases sleep and induces Fos in ventrolateral preoptic neurons. Neuroscience. 2001;107(4):653–63.
60. Fredholm BB, IJzerman AP, Jacobson KA, Klotz KN, Linden J. International Union of Pharmacology. XXV. Nomenclature and classification of adenosine receptors. Pharmacol Rev. 2001;53(4):527–52.
61. D'Alimonte I, D'Auro M, Citraro R, Biagioni F, Jiang S, Nargi E, Buccella S, Di Iorio P, Giuliani P, Ballerini P, Caciagli F, Russo E, De Sarro G, Ciccarelli R. Altered distribution and function of A2A adenosine receptors in the brain of WAG/Rij rats with genetic absence epilepsy, before and after appearance of the disease. Eur J Neurosci. 2009;30(6):1023–35.
62. Masino SA, Li T, Theofilas P, Sandau US, Ruskin DN, Fredholm BB, Geiger JD, Aronica E, Boison D. A ketogenic diet suppresses seizures in mice through adenosine A1 receptors. J Clin Invest. 2011;121(7):2679–83.
63. Kovács Z, Kékesi KA, Juhász G, Dobolyi A. The antiepileptic potential of nucleosides. Curr Med Chem. 2014;21(6):788–821.
64. Klein E, Zohar J, Geraci MF, Murphy DL, Uhde TW. Anxiogenic effects of m-CPP in patients with panic disorder: comparison to caffeine's anxiogenic effects. Biol Psychiatry. 1991;30(10):973–84.
65. Johansson B, Halldner L, Dunwiddie TV, Masino SA, Poelchen W, Giménez-Llort L, Escorihuela RM, Fernández-Teruel A, Wiesenfeld-Hallin Z, Xu XJ, Hårdemark A, Betsholtz C, Herlenius E, Fredholm BB. Hyperalgesia, anxiety, and decreased hypoxic neuroprotection in mice lacking the adenosine A1 receptor. Proc Natl Acad Sci U S A. 2001;98(16):9407–12.
66. Giménez-Llort L, Fernández-Teruel A, Escorihuela RM, Fredholm BB, Tobeña A, Pekny M, Johansson B. Mice lacking the adenosine A1 receptor are anxious and aggressive, but are normal learners with reduced muscle strength and survival rate. Eur J Neurosci. 2002;16(3):547–50.
67. Sarkisova K, van Luijtelaar G. The WAG/Rij strain: a genetic animal model of absence epilepsy with comorbidity of depression. Prog Neuro-Psychopharmacol Biol Psychiatry. 2011;35(4):854–76.
68. Kovács Z, Kékesi KA, Szilágyi N, Abrahám I, Székács D, Király N, Papp E, Császár I, Szego E, Barabás K, Péterfy H, Erdei A, Bártfai T, Juhász G. Facilitation of spike-wave discharge activity by lipopolysaccharides in Wistar albino Glaxo/Rijswijk rats. Neuroscience. 2006;140(2):731–42.
69. Kovács Z, Czurkó A, Kékesi KA, Juhász G. Neonatal tricyclic antidepressant clomipramine treatment reduces the spike-wave discharge activity of the adult WAG/Rij rat. Brain Res Bull. 2012;89(3–4):102–7.
70. Kovács Z, Kékesi KA, Dobolyi Á, Lakatos R, Juhász G. Absence epileptic activity changing effects of non-adenosine nucleoside inosine, guanosine and uridine in Wistar albino Glaxo Rijswijk rats. Neuroscience. 2015;300:593–608.
71. Citraro R, Iannone M, Leo A, De Caro C, Nesci V, Tallarico M, Abdalla K, Palma E, Arturi F, De Sarro G, Constanti A, Russo E. Evaluation of the effects of liraglutide on the development of epilepsy and behavioural alterations in two animal models of epileptogenesis. Brain Res Bull. 2019;153:133–42.
72. Kelz MB, García PS, Mashour GA, Solt K. Escape from oblivion: neural mechanisms of emergence from general anesthesia. Anesth Analg. 2019; 128(4):726–36.
73. Tung A, Herrera S, Szafran MJ, Kasza K, Mendelson WB. Effect of sleep deprivation on righting reflex in the rat is partially reversed by administration of adenosine A1 and A2 receptor antagonists. Anesthesiology. 2005;102(6):1158–64.

10

A small dose of dezocine suppresses remifentanil-induced cough in general anesthesia induction

Rui Ma[1†], Yu Wei[1†] and Zifeng Xu[1,2*]

Abstract

Background: The aim of this prospective randomized controlled study was to evaluate whether pretreatment with a small dose of dezocine could prevent remifentanil-induced cough in general anesthesia induction.

Trial design: a prospective, randomized, controlled study.

Methods: A total of 210 patients receiving elective operative hysteroscopy from December 2018 to April 2019 were enrolled in the present study. They were randomly equally separated into dezocine group ($n = 105$) and control group ($n = 105$). Patients were intravenously pre-administrated with dezocine 0.03 mg/kg (diluted to 5 mL) or the same volume of normal saline 1 min prior to remifentanil infusion. One minute later, intravenous injection of propofol 1.5 mg/kg and cisatracurium 0.1 mg/kg were given to all patients for induction of general anesthesia. The counts of coughs occurred during the anesthesia induction period were recorded and the severity of cough was scaled.

Results: There were 7 cases of mild cough in dezocine group and 18 cases of mild cough, 12 cases of moderate cough and 4 cases of severe cough in control group. The incidence rate of cough was significantly lower and the severity of cough was obviously relieved in dezocine group compared to control group (6.67% vs. 32.38%, $P < 0.001$). The two groups were not significantly different in heart rate and mean arterial pressure before the induction, before and after the intubation, and in operating time and postoperative visual analog scale pain scores.

Conclusion: This study recommends the efficacy and safety of a pretreatment with a small dose of dezocine in reducing remifentanil-induced cough during general anesthesia.

Keywords: Opioids, Cough, General anesthesia, Dezocine, Remifentanil

* Correspondence: ZiFengXu_ipm@163.com
†Rui Ma and Yu Wei contributed equally to this work.
[1]Department of Anesthesiology, international Peace Maternal and Child Health Hospital, School of Medicine, Shanghai Key Laboratory of Embryo Original Disease, Shanghai Municipal Key Clinical Specialty, Shanghai Jiao Tong University, Huashan Rd. 1961, Shanghai 200030, China
[2]Shanghai Key Laboratory of Embryo Original Diseases, Shanghai, China

Background

Opioids are conventionally used as adjunct drugs for induction of general anesthesia [1]. Application of opioids such as fentanyl [2] and sufentanil [3] often elicits cough during induction of general anesthesia. This adverse effect may lead to increased intracranial pressure and intraocular pressure and is extraordinarily dangerous for patients with diseases such as cerebral aneurysm, open eye injury and airway [4]. Remifentanil is a fentanyl congener characterized by short onset and short action time, and has been widely applied for induction of general anesthesia [5]. Remifentanil shows an antitussive effect on brainstem μ-opioid receptors [6]; however, some studies reported it also causes coughing just like fentanyl with a incidence rate varies from 26 to 57% during general anesthesia [7–10].

There is a growing interest in suitable agents and methods to prevent remifentanil-induced cough. For instance, Kim et al. suggests that elongating injection time over than 60 s could inhibit remifentanil-cough during anesthesia in children [7]. Limited maximal infusion rate appears to alleviate remifentanil-induced cough as well [11]. Moreover, there is evidence that pretreatment of several agents such as dexamethasone [12], ketamine or their combination [13] and propofol [14] has been reported to be useful for suppressing cough provoked by remifentanil. Dezocine is a mixed agonist-antagonist opioid analgesic [15]. It was initially identified as a full agonist of κ-receptor and partial agonist/antagonist of μ-receptor [15]. Later study suggested it is a κ-receptor antagonist [15, 16]. Increasing studies have demonstrated that dezocine administration is effective and feasible in preventing the occurrence of sufentanil-induced cough during the induction of general anesthesia [17, 18]. Nevertheless, few studies are focused on the effect of dezocine on remifentanil-induced cough.

Our study pretreated the patients undergoing elective hysteroscopic surgery with a small dose of dezocine prior to remifentanil infusion with a view to investigating whether dezocine pretreatment is a reliable strategy to relieve the incidence and severity of remifentanil-induced cough. This prospective randomized controlled trial would provide some useful clues for further development of anesthesia management.

Methods

Study design

This study was approved by the National science and technology ethics committee (approval number: 2017–101) and registered in the Chinese Clinical Trial Register (registration number: ChiCTR2000032035). A total of 210 patients with ASA physical status I-II who received elective hysteroscopic surgery in our hospital from December 2018 to April 2019 were enrolled in this study. Exclusion criteria were: known hypersensitivity to the drugs used in this study; body mass index > 30 kg/m^2; a history of hypertension; severe arrhythmias; chronic bronchitis, asthma, or other respiratory diseases; increased intraocular pressure, intrathoracic pressure or intracranial pressure before surgery. Written informed consent was obtained from each participant.

The incidence of remifentanil (1.5 μg/kg)-induced cough in control group was around 30% in our early study (unpublished). We hypothesized that the incidence rate of cough in dezocine group was lower than 10%. Based on $\alpha = 0.05$ (two-sided) and power = 0.95 ($\beta = 0.05$), a medium effect size (Cohen's $f = 0.25$), the estimated sample size was 104. Taking the dropout into account, the sample size was set at 105 in each group.

The 210 patients were randomly and equally divided into two groups: dezocine group and control group by a computer-generated allocation program.

Anesthesia and monitoring

In brief, all patients of the two groups were fasted for 8 h. Peripheral venous access was established using a 20-gauge cannula on the dorsal hand in the operating room. Heart rate (HR) and blood pressure were monitored. Two minutes prior to induction of general anesthesia, patients of the dezocine group received intravenous infusion of dezocine 0.03 mg/kg (diluted to 5 mL), while patients of the control group received an injection of 5 mL normal saline.

One minute later, remifentanil 1.5 μg/kg (1 mg remifentanil diluted with normal saline in a 50 mL syringe; Yichang Humanwell Pharmaceutical Co., LTD, Yichang, Hubei Province, China) was administrated to all patients of the two groups by a syringe pump at a rate of 600 mL/h, followed by intravenous injection of propofol 1.5 mg/kg and cisatracurium 0.1 mg/kg (Hengrui Pharmacutical Co., LTD, Shanghai, China) 1 min later to induce general anesthesia. Endotracheal intubation was then conducted and the patients were ventilated mechanically.

HR and mean arterial pressure (MAP) before the anesthesia induction, immediately before and 1 min after intubation were recorded. Side effects such as vomiting [19], hypoxemia ($SpO_2 < 90\%$) [20] or other intended effects during the induction period were also recorded. The number of coughs of the two groups was recorded and the severity of cough was defined as follows: mild, 1–2; moderate, 3–4; severe, 5 or more [21, 22]. In addition, operative time and visual analog scale (VAS) pain score 30 mins and 60 mins postoperatively were recorded and analyzed as well.

Statistical analysis

The primary endpoint was the incidence of cough in different groups. All statistical analyses were done by SPSS

Table 1 Demographic characteristics of patients in two groups

Group	Control group	Dezocine group	*P*
n	105	105	
Age (year)	41.99 ± 10.43	42.61 ± 11.26	0.680
Body weight (kg)	58.82 ± 7.92	59.50 ± 9.93	0.586
ASA class (I/II)	78/27	74/31	0.644

Data represent mean ± SD or numbers. Difference between groups were compared by students' t test or chi-square test

software 22.0 (IBM, Chicago, IL, USA). Categorical data, such as ASA and incidence of cough were expressed as number (percentage) and compared between groups by Chi-square test or Wilcoxon rank-sum test. Continuous data, including age and body weight were expressed as mean ± standard deviation and compared by Students' t test. Repeated continuous variables, including HR, MAP were analyzed by repeated measure ANOVA with Bonferroni correction. $P < 0.05$ was defined as significance level.

Results

Demographic characteristics

Total 210 ASA I and II patients were included in this study. They were randomly assigned to dozocine group ($n = 105$) or control group ($n = 105$). The age range of patients in dozocine group was 25–73 years and body weight range was 43–80 kg. The age range and body weight of patients in control group were 22–75 years and 42–89 kg, respectively. There was no significant difference between the two groups in age (41.99 ± 10.43 years vs. 42.61 ± 11.26 years, $P = 0.680$), body weight (58.82 ± 7.92 kg vs.59.50 ± 9.93 kg, $P = 0.586$) and ASA class ($P = 0.644$) (Table 1).

Hysteroscopic surgery was successful in all patients. Intraoperative oxygen saturation (SpO_2) of each patient was 100%. Adverse effects such as nausea and vomiting were not observed in any patient. HR and MAP were not significantly different between the two groups before the anesthesia induction, before intubation and 1 min after intubation ($P > 0.05$, Table 2). Moreover, both the two groups had significantly decreased HR and MAP before intubation and 1 min after intubation compared to those before the anesthesia induction ($P < 0.05$, Table 2).

Incidence and severity of cough, operating time and VAS pain score

As shown in Table 3, mild cough was observed in 7 patients of dozocine group, with an incidence of 6.67%. Control group had 34 patients with cough (32.38%), including 18 patients with mild cough, 12 patients with moderate cough and 4 patients with severe cough. The patients in dozocine group had a significantly lower incidence of cough and improved severity of cough in comparison with those in control group ($P < 0.001$). Additionally, there were no significant differences in operating time, 30-min and 60-min postoperative VAS pain scores ($P > 0.05$, Table 4).

Discussion

Our study enrolled a total of 210 patients scheduled for hysteroscopic surgery who were equally randomized into dozocine group and control group. Patients in these two groups had similar age and body weight. The patients in the dozocine group received a small dose of dezocine prior to remifentanil administration, while patients in control group were given the same volume of normal saline. A pre-emptive administration of dezocine decreased the incidence of cough from 32.38 to 6.67% and relieved the severity of cough. These findings suggest that pretreatment with dezocine could effectively prohibit remifentanil-induced cough during general anesthesia induction in patients undergoing operative hysteroscopy.

Hysteroscopy is an established endoscopic surgical procedure in obstetrics and gynecology practice for diagnosis and management of endometrial problems, with advantages of fewer complications, shorter recovery time and lower costs [23, 24]. However, pain is the most common complication of hysteroscopy because of several procedures such as cervical dilatation, uterine distension and peritoneal irritation [25]. Application of appropriate anesthetic agents for maximal anesthetic effect is a critical issue for hysteroscopy [26]. Remifentanil is a short-acting anilidopiperidine opioid with unique pharmacokinetic characteristics, facilitating fast and efficient analgesia. It is metabolized by esterases independently of hepatic and renal functions, and was therefore eliminated at a more rapid speed than other anilidopiperidine opioids [27]. Remifentanil alone or in combination with

Table 2 Observations of MAP and HR

Variable	Group	Before induction	1 min before intubation	1 min after intubation
(mmHg)	Control group	85.64 ± 8.32	70.26 ± 7.47*	69.79 ± 6.19*
	Dezocine group	88.03 ± 14.91	70.06 ± 8.24*	70.07 ± 7.94*
HR (beats/min)	Control group	81.77 ± 13.04	60.86 ± 8.04*	60.28 ± 7.81*
	Dezocine group	79.58 ± 13.71	60.89 ± 7.55*	60.19 ± 6.69*

Difference between groups at same time point was compared by Student's t test. Difference among different time points in the same group was compared by repeated measure ANOVA. *$P < 0.05$ vs. before anesthesia induction. MAP, mean arterial pressure; HR, heart rate

Table 3 Incidence and severity of cough in two groups

Group	N	None (N/%)	Mild cough (N/%)	Moderate cough (N/%)	Severe cough (N/%)	Cough (N/%)	P
Control group	105	71(67.62%)	18(17.31%)	12(11.43%)	4(3.81%)	34(32.38%)	< 0.001
Dezocine group	105	98(93.33%)	7(6.67%)	0	0	7(6.67%)	

adjunct agents has been widely utilized for general anesthesia in hysteroscopy [28]. In the present study, similarly, intravenous infusion of remifentanil 1.5 μg/kg in synergy with propofol 1.5 mg/kg and cisatracurium 0.1 mg/kg 1 min later were used for the induction of general anesthesia in all patients. Cough is often elicited by remifentanil infusion and is a causative factor of undesirable conditions including elevated intracranial, intra-ocular and intra-abdominal pressure [29]. In the present study, the incidence of remifentanil-induced cough without any pretreatment was 32.38% (34/105). Previous studies showed an incidence range of 26–57% during general anesthesia [7, 9–11]. The variance may be possibly attributed to different doses, effect-site concentrations and infusion speeds used in different studies.

The exact mechanisms behind opioid-induced cough remain elusive. One possible mechanism is that opioids cause suppression of central sympathetic outflow and strengthening of the vagus nerve, thus resulting in cough [30]. Pulmonary chemoreflex mediated by irritant receptors or vagal C-fiber receptors close to pulmonary vessels, opioid-induced histamine release from lung mast cells and tracheal smooth muscle constriction may be responsible for occurrence of cough [31]. Control of opioid-induced cough is of paramount clinical significance. Dezocine is a mixed agonist-antagonist opioid and its inhibitory action on opioid-induced cough has been proved in prior studies [17, 32]. In our study, the incidence of remifentanil-induced cough was 32.38% (18 cases of mild cough, 12 cases of moderate cough and 4 cases of severe cough) in the patients pre-administrated with normal saline, and was 6.67% (7 cases of mild cough) in the patients pre-administrated with dezocine. This result revealed that pre-administration of dezocine was effective in suppressing remifentanil-induced cough during general anesthesia induction. In a previous study, no patient pretreated with infusion of dezocine 0.1 mg/kg reports sufentanil-induced cough, in contrast the control patients had a cough incidence of 31.9% [17]. Although dezocine 0.1 mg/kg seems to exert a more potent suppressive effect, higher HR and blood pressure are detected in the patients receiving a pre-emptive infusion of dezocine compared to the control patients in their study. In the current study, 0.03 mg/kg dezocine, a third of an analgesic dose of dezocine was selected. Patients in the dozocine group and the control group were not significantly different in HR and MAP before the anesthesia induction, prior to intubation and 1 min after intubation, and in operating time, 30-min and 60-min postoperative VAS pain scores. These observations indicated that pre-administration of dezocine 0.03 mg/kg does not affect hemodynamics, operating time and postoperative pain of patients. Postoperative analgesia demands a larger dose of dezocine.

Dezocine was thought to be a κ opioid receptor agonist, but recent data suggest it could be a κ opioid receptor antagonist [16]. The cough suppression by dezocine may be due to κ receptors antagonism or decreased norepinephrine and serotonin reuptake [33]. Xu et al. speculated that dezocine may reduce fentanyl-induced cough by antagonizing fentanyl-activated μ receptors via activating κ receptors [34]. Our study did not unveil the exact mechanisms underlying the suppression on remifentanil-induced cough by dezocine. More in-depth studies are necessary to decipher the exact mechanisms. Cough suppressing effect of different doses of dezocine was not explored in the present study. These limitations should be addressed in future studies.

Table 4 Operative duration and postoperative VAS pain scores of two groups

Group	Operative time (min)	30-min postoperative VAS pain scores	60-min postoperative VAS pain scores
Group C	20.4 ± 3.5	2.83 ± 1.33	3.81 ± 1.12
Group D	19.8 ± 4.3	2.65 ± 0.97	3.79 ± 1.11

VAS Visual analog scale

Conclusion

Our study showed that premedication of a low dose of dezocine was capable of effectively and safely repressing remifentanil-induced cough during general anesthesia in the patients receiving operative hysteroscopy. This study offers more insights concerning alternative regimens to prevent remifentanil-induced cough.

Abbreviations

HR: Heart rate; MAP: Mean arterial pressure; VAS: Visual analog scale

Acknowledgements

Not applicable.

Authors' contributions

RM designed the project and wrote the manuscript; YW performed the data analysis; ZX collected the data and revised this paper. All authors read and approved the final manuscript.

References

1. Egan TD. Are opioids indispensable for general anaesthesia? Br J Anaesth. 2019;122(6):e127–e35.
2. Lin CS, Sun WZ, Chan WH, Lin CJ, Yeh HM, Mok MS. Intravenous lidocaine and ephedrine, but not propofol, suppress fentanyl-induced cough. Can J Anaesth. 2004;51(7):654–9.
3. An LJ, Gui B, Su Z, Zhang Y, Liu HL. Magnesium sulfate inhibits sufentanil-induced cough during anesthetic induction. Int J Clin Exp Med. 2015;8(8): 13864–8.
4. Sun S, Huang SQ. Effects of pretreatment with a small dose of dexmedetomidine on sufentanil-induced cough during anesthetic induction. J Anesth. 2013;27(1):25–8.
5. Yu Z, Zhang P, Wang H, Zhang L, Wei W, Fang W, Mu X. Effects of dexmedetomidine versus remifentanil on mothers and neonates during cesarean section under general anesthesia. Biomed Pap Med Fac Univ Palacky Olomouc Czech Repub. 2019. https://doi.org/10.5507/bp.2019.055.
6. Nasra J, Belvisi MG. Modulation of sensory nerve function and the cough reflex: understanding disease pathogenesis. Pharmacol Ther. 2009;124(3): 354–75.
7. Kim DH, Yoo JY, Moon BK, Yoon BH, Kim JY. The effect of injection speed on remifentanil-induced cough in children. Korean J Anesthesiol. 2014;67(3): 171–4.
8. Min SK, Kim DH, Cho HB, Moon BK, Kim JY. Limited maximal flow rate of target-controlled remifentanil infusion and induced cough. Anaesthesia. 2012;67(2):145–8.
9. Cho HB, Kwak HJ, Park SY, Kim JY. Comparison of the incidence and severity of cough after alfentanil and remifentanil injection. Acta Anaesthesiol Scand. 2010;54(6):717–20.
10. Shen JC, Xu JG, Zhou ZQ, Liu HJ, Yang JJ. Effect of equivalent doses of fentanyl, sufentanil, and remifentanil on the incidence and severity of cough in patients undergoing abdominal surgery: a prospective, randomized, double-blind study. Curr Ther Res Clin Exp. 2008;69(6):480–7.
11. Min S, Kim D, Cho H, Moon B, Kim J. Limited maximal flow rate of target-controlled remifentanil infusion and induced cough. Anaesthesia. 2012;67(2): 145–8.
12. Yu MS, Kim JY, Kim HY. Intravenous dexamethasone pretreatment reduces remifentanil induced cough. Korean J Anesthesiol. 2011;60(6):403–7.
13. Honarmand A, Safavi M, Khalighinejad F. A comparison of the effect of pretreatment with intravenous dexamethasone, intravenous ketamine, and their combination, for suppression of remifentanil-induced cough: a randomized, double-blind, placebo-controlled clinical trial. Adv Biomed Res. 2013;2:60.
14. Kim JY, Lee SY, Kim DH, Park SK, Min SK. Effect-site concentration of propofol for reduction of remifentanil-induced cough. Anaesthesia. 2010; 65(7):697–703.
15. Liu R, Huang XP, Yeliseev A, Xi J, Roth BL. Novel molecular targets of dezocine and their clinical implications. Anesthesiology. 2014;120(3):714–23.
16. Gharagozlou P, Hashemi E, DeLorey TM, Clark JD, Lameh J. Pharmacological profiles of opioid ligands at kappa opioid receptors. BMC Pharmacol. 2006;6:3.
17. Liu XS, Xu GH, Shen QY, Zhao Q, Cheng XQ, Zhang J, Gu EW. Dezocine prevents sufentanil-induced cough during general anesthesia induction: a randomized controlled trial. Pharmacol Rep. 2015;67(1):52–5.
18. Soleimani A, Kiabi FH, Habibi MR, Emami Zeydi A, Assarroudi A, Sharifi H. Intravenous dezocine for suppressing fentanyl-induced cough during general anesthesia induction: a potentially effective and clinically feasible method. J Anaesthesiol Clin Pharmacol. 2017;33(4):556–7.
19. Shinpo K, Hirai Y, Maezawa H, Totsuka Y, Funahashi M. The role of area postrema neurons expressing H-channels in the induction mechanism of nausea and vomiting. Physiol Behav. 2012;107(1):98–103.
20. Roze H, Lafargue M, Ouattara A. Case scenario: management of intraoperative hypoxemia during one-lung ventilation. Anesthesiology. 2011; 114(1):167–74.
21. Phua WT, Teh BT, Jong W, Lee TL, Tweed WA. Tussive effect of a fentanyl bolus. Can J Anaesth. 1991;38(3):330–4.
22. Saleh AJ, Zhang L, Hadi SM, Ouyang W. A priming dose of intravenous ketamine-dexmedetomidine suppresses fentanyl-induced coughing: a double-blind, randomized, controlled study. Ups J Med Sci. 2014;119(4):333–7.
23. Centini G, Troia L, Lazzeri L, Petraglia F, Luisi S. Modern operative hysteroscopy. Minerva Ginecol. 2016;68(2):126–32.
24. Ma T, Readman E, Hicks L, Porter J, Cameron M, Ellett L, McIlwaine K, Manwaring J, Maher P. Is outpatient hysteroscopy the new gold standard? Results from an 11 year prospective observational study. Aust N Z J Obstet Gynaecol. 2017;57(1):74–80.
25. Ahmad G, O'Flynn H, Attarbashi S, Duffy JM, Watson A. Pain relief for outpatient hysteroscopy. Cochrane Database Syst Rev. 2010;11:CD007710.
26. Munro MG. Anesthesia and analgesia for office-based uterine procedures. In: *Hysteroscopy*. Berlin: Springer; 2018. p. 19–32.
27. Beers R, Camporesi E. Remifentanil update: clinical science and utility. CNS Drugs. 2004;18(15):1085–104.
28. Gazi M, Abitagaoglu S, Turan G, Koksal C, Akgun FN, Ari DE. Evaluation of the effects of dexmedetomidine and remifentanil on pain with the analgesia nociception index in the perioperative period in hysteroscopies under general anesthesia. A randomized prospective study. Saudi Med J. 2018;39(10):1017–22.
29. Kim JY, Chae YJ, Kim JS, Park YJ, Min SK. A target-controlled infusion regimen for reducing remifentanil-induced coughs. Korean J Anesthesiol. 2012;63(1):30–5.
30. Agarwal A, Azim A, Ambesh S, Bose N, Dhiraj S, Sahu D, Singh U. Salbutamol, beclomethasone or sodium chromoglycate suppress coughing induced by iv fentanyl. Can J Anaesth. 2003;50(3):297–300.
31. Zhang J, Miao S, Tu Q, Shi M, Zou L, Liu S, Wang G. Effect of butorphanol on opioid-induced cough: a meta-analysis of randomized controlled trials. Drug Des Devel Ther. 2018;12:3263–8.
32. Shuying L, Ping L, Juan N, Dong L. Different interventions in preventing opioid-induced cough: a meta-analysis. J Clin Anesth. 2016;34:440–7.
33. Jiang WX, Huang JM, Zhang JM, Li HN, Lu X, Zhang J, Lv ZT. Effect of dezocine administration in the prevention of fentanyl-induced cough during general anesthesia induction: a systematic review and meta-analysis of randomized controlled trials. Int J Clin Exp Med. 2017;10(12):15866–77.
34. Xu YJ, Zhu Y, Wang SL, Ren Y, Miao CH. Dezocine attenuates fentanyl-induced cough in a dose-dependent manner-a randomized controlled trial. Int J Clin Exp Med. 2015;8(4):6091–6.

11

Comparison of supreme laryngeal mask airway versus endotracheal intubation for airway management during general anesthesia for cesarean section

Wei Yu Yao[1], Shi Yang Li[1], Yong Jin Yuan[2], Hon Sen Tan[3], Nian-Lin R. Han[4], Rehena Sultana[5], Pryseley N. Assam[6], Alex Tiong-Heng Sia[3,7] and Ban Leong Sng[3,7*]

Abstract

Background: The obstetric airway is a significant cause of maternal morbidity and mortality. Endotracheal intubation is considered the standard of care but the laryngeal mask airway (LMA) has gained acceptance as a rescue airway and has been incorporated into the obstetric airway management guidelines. In this randomized controlled equivalence trial, we compared the Supreme LMA (SLMA) with endotracheal intubation (ETT) in managing the obstetric airway during cesarean section.

Methods: Parturients who underwent elective cesarean section under general anesthesia were randomized to receive either an SLMA or ETT as their airway device. Our primary outcome was first-attempt insertion success. Successful insertion was defined as adequate bilateral air entry with auscultation and the presence of end-tidal carbon dioxide on the capnogram. The first-attempt insertion success rate was compared using the Chi-Square test. Secondary outcomes included time-to-ventilation, seal pressure, ventilation/hemodynamic parameters, occurrence of clinical aspiration, fetal outcomes, and maternal side effects associated with the airway device.

Results: We recruited 920 parturients (460 SLMA, 460 ETT) who underwent elective cesarean section under general anesthesia. Patient characteristics were similar between the groups. First attempt success was similar (Odds Ratio--$OR_{SLMA/ETT}$: 1.00 (95%CI: 0.25, 4.02), $p = 1.0000$). SLMA was associated with reduced time to effective ventilation (Mean Difference--MD -22.96; 95%CI: − 23.71, − 22.21 s) compared to ETT group ($p < 0.0001$). Ventilation parameters, maternal and fetal outcomes were similar between the groups, and there was no aspiration.

Conclusions: SLMA could be an alternative airway management technique for a carefully selected low-risk obstetric population, with similar insertion success rates, reduced time to ventilation and less hemodynamic changes compared with ETT. Our findings are consistent with the airway guidelines in recommending the second-line use of LMA in the management of the obstetric airway.

Keywords: Laryngeal mask airway, Obstetric, Cesarean section, General anesthesia

* Correspondence: sng.ban.leong@singhealth.com.sg
[3]Department of Women's Anaesthesia, KK Women's and Children's Hospital, 100 Bukit Timah Road, Singapore, Singapore
[7]Anaesthesiology and Perioperative Sciences Academic Clinical Program, Duke-NUS Medical School, 8 College Road, Singapore, Singapore

Background

Airway complications are one of the main causes of anesthetic-related obstetric adverse events in developed countries, with the incidence of failed intubation estimated to be around 0.4% [1–5]. Obstetric airway management is complex, due to the unique challenges posed by the physiological changes of pregnancy, including reduced oncotic pressure, oxytocin-related water retention, and Valsalva maneuver during labor leading to mucosal capillary engorgement and edema. This is often confounded by inadequate fasting time, urgency of cesarean section requiring general anesthesia, and the need to balance the potential conflicting needs of the mother and fetus [6–8].

The introduction of second-generation supraglottic airway devices (SAD) such as the Proseal Laryngeal Mask Airway (LMA) and Supreme LMA (SLMA) with a double-lumen specifically designed to physically separate the respiratory and alimentary tract, reduces the risk of aspiration [8–12] and has changed obstetric airway management. The first Difficult Airway Society (DAS) guideline for managing an unanticipated difficult intubation published in 2004 incorporated the LMA as a second-line rescue device, though obstetric patients were specifically excluded [13]. Subsequently, the important role of the LMA in obstetric difficult airway management was recognized in the first obstetric-specific guideline jointly released by Obstetric Anaesthetists' Association (OAA) and DAS [14]. In addition, the OAA-DAS guideline recommends an active decision process that takes into consideration the maternal risk of proceeding without endotracheal intubation versus the fetal risk of delayed surgery. The guideline also drew attention to the traditional notion that general anesthesia for cesarean section is unacceptable without endotracheal intubation, due to concerns of increased risk of pulmonary aspiration.

The practice of rapid sequence induction (RSI) and ETT as the standard of care for obstetric airway management originated from concerns of pulmonary aspiration of gastric contents following general anesthesia [15]. Current obstetric anesthesia practice is associated with a low but significant incidence of pulmonary aspiration of about 0.1% [3]. The increasing use of neuraxial anesthesia, aspiration prophylaxis, stricter adherence to fasting guidelines, and airway control via RSI and ETT for general anesthesia are factors that may enhance the margin of safety in this respect. However, rising rates of obesity and other risk factors for pulmonary aspiration may necessitate endotracheal intubation as standard of care.

Recently, the efficacy and safety of LMA use in selected patients undergoing cesarean section under general anesthesia has been demonstrated in several prospective and retrospective cohort studies [12, 16–18]. However, to date, there are no randomized controlled trials comparing airway outcomes of the LMA compared to ETT in cesarean section. This prospective, randomized controlled trial aims to evaluate the first insertion attempt success rate of the SLMA compared to ETT in elective cesarean section under general anesthesia.

Methods

This study was approved by the Institutional Review Board (approval obtained on 25th October 2012) at the Quanzhou Women's and Children's Hospital, Fujian Province, China, and registered at http://www.clinicaltrials.gov (NCT01858467). At the time of the study, the majority of cesarean sections at Quanzhou Women's and Children's Hospital were performed under general anesthesia largely due to patients' request, with routine airway management using the SLMA in both elective and urgent cases [18]. The hospital cesarean section rate is 35% and the SLMA technique for general anesthesia is used in about 2000 deliveries annually, with endotracheal intubation employed as an alternative airway management.

We recruited parturients with singleton pregnancies aged 18 to 50 years old who are healthy or with well-controlled medical conditions (American Society of Anesthesiology; ASA 2) undergoing elective cesarean section under general anesthesia at Quanzhou Women's and Children's Hospital, China between May 2013 and July 2014. Written informed consent was obtained from every participant. Our exclusion criteria included parturients with body mass index (BMI) $\geq 35\,kg/m^2$, anticipated difficult airway (modified Mallampati grade 4, or known upper respiratory tract or neck pathology) or self-reported gastro-esophageal reflux disease. All parturients were fasted for a minimum of 6 h. Once enrolled in the study, the parturients were randomized into 2 groups and allocation concealed using sealed opaque envelopes prepared by a statistician not involved in the study recruitment. The 2 groups were (1) SLMA group; and (2) ETT group. The parturients and independent assessors were blinded to the assigned group, but the investigators managing the airway were not blinded.

The induction of anesthesia and airway device insertion reflects the clinical standard at our study center [18]. As per our institutional standard, all parturients received premedication with intravenous ranitidine, following which electrocardiography, pulse oximetry, capnography and non-invasive blood pressure measurements were started. Following preoxygenation for three minutes, RSI was performed with cricoid pressure applied by a trained anesthetic nurse. Anesthesia was induced with intravenous propofol (2-3 mg/kg) and 100 mg succinylcholine. After the airway device was inserted, rocuronium (0.5 mg/kg) was used to maintain muscle relaxation and fentanyl (100mcg) was administered for intraoperative analgesia after the fetus was delivered. All cases regardless of assigned study groups were induced in similar fashion.

The SLMA size was chosen based on manufacturer's recommendations, however, a more appropriate size could be selected based on parturient's weight, BMI, and mouth opening at the discretion of the investigators. ETTs of intraluminal diameters between 6.5 to 7.0 mm were used, chosen at the investigators' discretion. Three investigators (Yao, Li, and Yuan), each with more than five years of experience in the use of both SLMA and ETT as well as difficult airway management in general anesthesia, managed the airway for all parturients enrolled in this study.

In the SLMA group, SLMA insertion using the recommended single-handed rotational technique was performed with the maintenance of cricoid pressure. Subsequently, a manometer was used to inflate the cuff to 60 cmH_2O, and we recorded the volume of air required to achieve this pressure. Next, the ability to ventilate was confirmed as evidenced by the presence of auscultation of bilateral air entry and carbon dioxide trace on capnography, after which cricoid pressure was released. Following successful SLMA placement, a pre-mounted #14 gastric tube was advanced through the gastric drainage channel, and confirmed adequate placement by: (1) aspiration of gastric fluid; or (2) injection of air into the orogastric tube and auscultating a "swoosh" over the epigastrium. We recorded the number of attempts needed for successful placement, and suctioning of the orogastric tube was performed before commencement of the surgery. Finally, SLMA seal pressure was determined by recording the peak airway pressure after closing the adjustable pressure-limiting valve while maintaining a fresh gas flowrate of 3 L/min into the closed circuit.

If required, the use of additional maneuvers such as chin lift, head extension, jaw thrust, or SLMA repositioning were permitted to maintain a patent airway. Failure to achieve successful SLMA placement (1) after 2 attempts, (2) within one minute, or (3) before desaturation occurred (oxygen saturation < 92%), would result in securing of the airway via direct laryngoscopy and endotracheal intubation. Cesarean section would commence if the following were met: (1) presence of a square-wave capnogram; (2) SLMA cuff pressure of 60cmH_2O; (3) SLMA bite block positioned between the incisors; (4) successful orogastric tube placement and suctioning performed; and (5) recorded SLMA seal pressure was ≥20cmH_2O.

In the ETT group, oral endotracheal intubation via direct laryngoscopy was performed using a Macintosh blade (size 3–4 based on anesthesiologist's preference). The ETT cuff was inflated to 25 cmH_2O using a manometer, and we recorded the volume of air needed to achieve this pressure. Following confirmation of the ability to ventilate, as evidenced by the auscultation of bilateral air entry and carbon dioxide trace on capnography, cricoid pressure was released. A #14 orogastric tube was then inserted, and the position confirmed, as above.

For all parturients irrespective of assigned group, successful placement of the airway device was confirmed by auscultation of bilateral breath sounds and the capnographic presence of end-tidal carbon dioxide. We defined an insertion attempt as the insertion and complete removal of the airway device, and recorded the number of attempts required. We also measured the time to effective airway placement, which we defined as the duration from when the device was picked up till the first carbon dioxide waveform was seen.

Intraoperative anesthesia management reflects the clinical practice at the study center [18]. Maintenance of general anesthesia was achieved with 1.5 to 2.0% sevoflurane in a 50% mix of nitrous oxide and oxygen, with all parturients positioned in left lateral tilt using a wedge. During anesthesia, complications including the loss of airway, inadequate oxygenation or ventilation, and bleeding into the airway device were recorded. Parturients were ventilated with a tidal volume of 6 to 10 mL/kg at 10 to 16 breaths/min, targeting an end-tidal carbon dioxide concentration of 30 to 40 mmHg. The presence of clinical signs of aspiration, including perioperative hypoxemia, lung auscultation revealing wheezing or crepitations, and postoperative dyspnea would trigger investigation of the parturient with bronchoscopy or chest X-rays.

The obstetricians were advised to reduce fundal pressure during delivery regardless of the device used. Upon completion of surgery, reversal of muscle paralysis followed by suctioning and removal of the orogastric tube were performed. After achieving adequate spontaneous respiration and consciousness (defined as when parturient was able to follow instructions to open her eyes and mouth), the airway devices were removed and inspected for blood. An independent assessor recorded the incidence of sore throat and hoarseness before discharge from the post-anesthesia care unit.

Our primary outcome was the first-insertion attempt success rate of the airway devices. Secondary anesthetic outcomes included:

1. time to effective ventilation; airway device seal pressure;
2. ventilation parameters (tidal volume, respiratory rate, peak ventilation pressure) to maintain effective oxygenation and ventilation, which we defined as $SpO_2 \geq 92\%$ and end-tidal carbon dioxide concentration of < 50 mmHg, achieved via inspired oxygen concentration ≤ 0.5, respiratory rate of 10 to 16

breaths/min, and tidal volume of 6 to 10 mL/kg; and
3. hemodynamic parameters including heart rate and blood pressure for 6 min after induction.

We also recorded the amount and pH of gastric aspirate; as well as the incidence of regurgitation (presence of clear/bile-stained fluid during surgery or removal of the airway device); incidence of aspiration (bile-stained fluid noted in the lung via bronchoscopy or suggestive radiographical signs), and the pH of SLMA laryngeal surface and ETT cuff. Apart from neonatal weight, the obstetric outcomes recorded included neonatal Apgar scores at 1 and 5 min and umbilical cord venous pH. Maternal satisfaction (question asked, "how would you rate your overall satisfaction with your anesthetic care from 0 to 100%") was assessed one day after surgery by an independent assessor.

Statistical analysis

The primary outcome measure of first-attempt success rate of SLMA insertion and secondary outcomes, namely incidence of regurgitation, aspiration, blood staining of the airway devices and voice hoarseness were treated as categorical data, with categories *"yes"* or *"no"*. All demographic, anesthetic and clinical categorical variables were summarized as frequency with the corresponding proportion; and continuous variables were expressed as mean (standard deviation (SD)) or median [interquartile range (IQR)], whichever applicable with respect to two study groups SLMA and ETT. Difference in outcomes between ETT and SLMA were represented as odds ratio (OR) and mean difference or median difference, whichever applicable, with 95% confidence interval for categorical and continuous data respectively. Difference in categorical and continuous variables between SLMA and ETT were tested using Chi-Square test and Student's t-test or Mann-Whitney U test, whichever applicable, respectively. Significance level was set at p-value < 0.05 and all tests were two-sided. Data analysis was generated using SAS 9.3 software (SAS Institute Inc., Cary, NC, USA).

We performed a sample size calculation based on our previous experience estimate of 98% in first attempt insertion success rate of SLMA insertion [18]. An equivalence boundary of 0.034 i.e. (96.3, 99.7%) as the maximum difference between maximum likelihood estimates of the true proportions in the first attempt insertion success rate in SLMA and ETT use was considered as clinical equivalence. A sample size of 916 parturients (458 per group) would achieve 80% power with the above-mentioned equivalence limits, based on a one-sided test with a significance level of 2.5% and retrospective estimate in the first attempt success rate of 98%. We aimed to recruit a total of 920 parturients in this study.

Results

We screened 998 parturients between May 2013 and July 2014. There were 49 parturients who did not give consent and 29 parturients did not meet the recruitment criteria. A total of 920 parturients were randomized (460 assigned to each group) and there was no withdrawal or dropout (Fig. 1 consort diagram).

We summarized the demographic and clinical characteristics of the parturients in Table 1. There were no significant differences in maternal age, weight, height, ASA scores, Mallampati scores and fetal gestational age. There was no significant difference in duration from the time of anesthesia to delivery, and the overall duration of surgery.

The anesthesia outcomes are presented in Table 2. The primary outcome first attempt success was similar in in both groups: SLMA 456/460 (99.1%), ETT 456/460 (99.1%), with OR of 1.00 (95%CI: 0.25, 4.02; $p = 1.0000$) when SLMA was compared with respect to ETT. We found there was a statistically significant reduction in time to effective ventilation (defined as the duration from when the device was picked up to appearance of first end-tidal carbon dioxide waveform) with MD of − 22.96 (95%CI: − 23.71, − 22.21; $p < 0.0001$) in SLMA insertion compared to ETT. There was a significant difference in seal pressure obtained (MD: -0.77; 95%CI: − 1.25, − 0.30; $p = 0.0014$). The rest of the ventilation parameters were similar between the groups, in terms of lowest tidal volume, lowest respiratory rate, highest peak airway pressure, seal minus highest peak airway pressure and lowest SpO_2 achieved. We did not observe hypoxemia, laryngospasm or bronchospasm intra-operatively. Although the baseline heart rate and systolic blood pressure were similar, we found that SLMA insertion was associated with less hemodynamic alterations compared to endotracheal intubation, with lower heart rate and systolic blood pressure during the airway insertion period.

Maternal and fetal outcomes are summarized in Table 3. There were no significant mean differences in fetal weight, or median differences in APGAR scores at 1 and 5 min, and umbilical venous cord pH. The volume of gastric aspirate was similar between the groups, but the SLMA group had a lower pH with MD of − 0.06 (95%CI: − 0.11, − 0.02) compared to the ETT group ($p = 0.0309$). More importantly, the pH of the SLMA laryngeal surface was similar to that of the ETT cuff, suggesting the absence of gastric contents in the airway (− 0.001; 95%CI: − 0.004, 0.002 for both ETT and SLMA groups, $p = 0.5613$). There was no clinical suggestion of pulmonary aspiration.

There was a low incidence of airway complications in this study. Odds of blood on SLMA was lower compared to ETT insertion with OR of 0.76 (95%CI: 0.46, 1.27; $p = 0.2999$). The incidence of sore throat was similar (OR

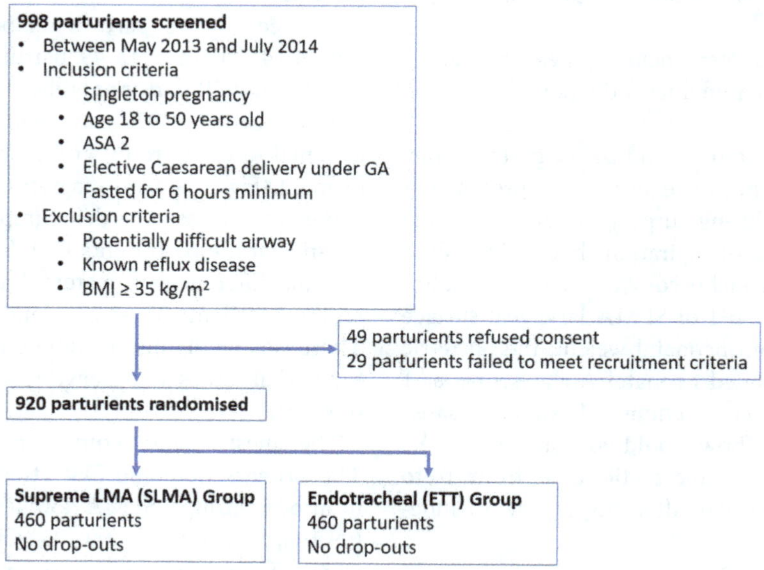

Fig. 1 Consort diagram. 998 parturients who were planned for elective cesarean section in Quanzhou Women's and Children's Hospital were screened between May 2013 and July 2014. Inclusion criteria: singleton pregnancy, aged 18 to 50 years old, ASA 2, and fasted for at least 6 h. Parturients with potentially difficult airway, known reflux disease, or with BMI ≥ 35 kg/m^2 were excluded. 49 parturients refused consent, and 29 did not meet the recruitment criteria. The remaining 920 parturients were randomized by opaque envelope to obtain 460 in each group. There were no dropouts or withdrawal

0.59; 95%CI: 0.26, 1.37, $p = 0.2146$), and there was no voice hoarseness reported in both groups. Patient satisfaction scores were also similar between the groups (MD 0.86; 95%CI: – 0.14, 1.86; $p = 0.0931$).

Discussion

This large prospective randomized controlled trial involving parturients receiving general anesthesia for cesarean section showed similar first attempt insertion success rates in both SLMA and ETT groups. However, SLMA use was associated with a significant reduction in the time to effective ventilation and less hemodynamic fluctuation in the immediate period after airway insertion. The respiratory, airway, and fetal outcomes were similar between both groups. No evidence of pulmonary aspiration was detected, and the incidence of complications were low in both groups (blood on the airway device, sore throat, voice hoarseness). Maternal satisfaction was also similar.

The first attempt SLMA insertion success rate of 99.1% is comparable to rates previously reported in LMA studies in obstetric general anesthesia (97.7 to 98.0%) [12, 17–19]. The high success rate could be

Table 1 Baseline patient demographics and clinical characteristics of participants receiving SLMA or ETT while undergoing cesarean section under general anesthesia

Characteristics	SLMA ($n = 460$)	ETT ($n = 460$)	*p*-value
Age (years), mean (SD)	28.4 (4.1)	28.4 (4.0)	0.9869
Weight (kg), mean (SD)	65.6 (6.5)	65.0 (6.5)	0.1230
Height (cm), mean (SD)	158.9 (5.0)	158.1 (4.7)	**0.0130**
BMI (kg/m^2), mean (SD)	26.0 (2.27)	26.0 (2.33)	0.9875
Mallampati, n (%)			0.8644
Mallampati 1	183 (39.8)	177 (38.5)	
Mallampati 2	244 (53.0)	252 (54.8)	
Mallampati 3	33 (7.2)	31 (6.7)	
Gestational age (weeks), mean (SD)	38.1 (1.2)	38.3 (1.2)	0.7422
Duration from anesthesia to delivery (min), mean (SD)	12.0 (7.9)	12.5 (7.9)	0.3307
Duration of surgery (min), mean (SD)	33.1 (10.5)	32.1 (10.1)	0.1524

Categorical values are compared using Chi-Square test and continuous variables are compared using two-sample Student's t-test. *P*-values of 0.05 or less are considered significant

Table 2 Anesthetic outcomes of participants receiving either SLMA or ETT while undergoing cesarean section under general anesthesia

Characteristics	SLMA (n = 460)	ETT (n = 460)	Mean Difference / Odds ratio (95%CI)	p-value
Number of insertion attempts, n (%)				
First attempt	456 (99.1)	456 (99.1)	Reference	–
Second attempt or more	4 (0.9)	4 (0.9)	1.00 (0.25, 4.02)	1.0000
Time to effective ventilation (s), mean (SD)	16.1 (3.9)	39.1 (7.2)	-22.96 (−23.71, −22.21)	**< 0.0001**
Seal pressure (cmH_2O), mean (SD)	27.1 (3.8)	27.9 (3.6)	-0.77 (−1.25, −0.30)	**0.0014**
Lowest tidal volume (ml), mean (SD)	430.9 (39.2)	429.2 (39.3)	1.76 (−3.32, 6.84)	0.4965
Lowest respiratory rate (breaths /min), median (IQR)	12 (12.0, 12.0)	12 (12.0, 12.0)	0.00 (0.00, 0.00)	0.7957
Highest peak airway pressure (cmH_2O), mean (SD)	16.8 (3.4)	17.0 (3.6)	−0.14 (−0.59, 0.31)	0.5320
Seal pressure minus highest peak airway pressure (cmH_2O), mean (SD)	10.3 (4.2)	10.9 (4.3)	−0.63 (−1.18, – 0.08)	**0.0250**
Lowest SpO2 (%), median (IQR)	99.0 (97.0, 99.0)	98.5 (97.0, 99.0)	0.50 (0.00, 0.00)	0.2109
Baseline systolic blood pressure (mmHg), mean (SD)	116.8 (8.6)	116.8 (11.2)	−0.002 (−1.297, 1.292)	0.9974
Systolic blood pressure 2 min after induction (mmHg), mean (SD)	114.0 (11.1)	133.9 (18.2)	−19.96 (−21.91, – 18.01)	**< 0.0001**
Systolic blood pressure 5 min after induction (mmHg), mean (SD)	103.7 (10.4)	111.2 (13.3)	−7.51 (−9.06, −5.97)	**< 0.0001**
Baseline heart rate (beats /min), mean (SD)	84.4 (10.3)	85.5 (10.1)	−1.04 (−2.36, 0.28)	0.1210
Heart rate 2 min after induction (beats /min), mean (SD)	93.6 (12.9)	105.4 (11.7)	−11.75 (– 13.34, – 10.16)	**< 0.0001**
Heart rate 5 min after induction (beats /min), mean (SD)	88.0 (13.3)	92.9 (11.9)	−4.87 (−6.5, −3.24)	**< 0.0001**

Difference between the two categories are expressed as mean difference or median difference and odds ratio with 95% confidence interval for continuous and categorical values, respectively. Categorical values are compared using Chi-Square test and continuous variables are compared using two-sample Student's t-test or Wilcoxon test. *P*-values of 0.05 or less are considered significant

attributed to adherence of the manufacturers' recommended technique, insertion by experienced anesthetists, and the routine use of SLMA at the study site for cesarean section under general anesthesia. Of note, we achieved a high SLMA insertion success rate despite maintenance of cricoid pressure, which could impede the LMA insertion into the post-cricoid hypopharyngeal space. This issue could have been attenuated by the relative rigidity of the SLMA. The high success rate of SLMA insertion in obstetrics further strengthens our hypothesis that the use of second-generation LMAs such as the SLMA is suitable in selected parturients, and this is consistent with the OAA-DAS recommendations for use in difficult and failed intubation.

Table 3 Fetal and maternal outcomes of participants receiving either SLMA or ETT while undergoing cesarean section under general anesthesia

Characteristics	SLMA (n = 460)	ETT (n = 460)	Mean Difference / Odds ratio (95%CI)	p-value
Fetal weight (g), mean (SD)	3150.7 (457.9)	3137.8 (417.0)	12.83 (−43.84, 69.49)	0.6570
APGAR score 1 min, median (IQR)	10.0 (9.0, 10.0)	10.0 (9.0, 10.0)	0.00 (0.00, 0.00)	0.9517
APGAR score 5 min, median (IQR)	10.0 (10.0, 10.0)	10.0 (10.0, 10.0)	0.00 (0.00, 0.00)	0.7208
Umbilical venous cord pH, median (IQR)	7.3 (7.3, 7.3)	7.3 (7.3, 7.3)	0.00 (0.00, 0.001)	0.2298
Presence of blood on airway device, n (%)	28 (6.1)	36 (7.8)	0.76 (0.46, 1.27)	0.2999
Incidence of sore throat, n (%)	9 (2.0)	15 (3.3)	0.59 (0.26, 1.37)	0.2146
Incidence of voice hoarseness, n (%)	0 (0.0)	0 (0.0)	–	NA
Patient satisfaction (%), mean (SD)	85.4 (7.6)	84.5 (7.9)	0.86 (−0.14, 1.86)	0.0931
Volume of gastric aspirate (ml), mean (SD)	17.3 (13.4)	17.6 (16.3)	−0.28 (−2.21, 1.65)	0.7756
pH of gastric aspirate, mean (SD)	3.5 (1.4)	3.7 (1.6)	−0.06 (– 0.11, – 0.02)	**0.0309**
pH of SLMA laryngeal surface / ETT cuff, mean (SD)	7.0 (0.2)	7.0 (0.2)	−0.001 (– 0.004, 0.002)	0.5613

Difference between the two categories are expressed as mean difference or median difference and odds ratio with 95% confidence interval for continuous and categorical values, respectively. Categorical values are compared using Chi-Square test and continuous variables are compared using two-sample Student's t-test or Wilcoxon test. *P*-values of 0.05 or less are considered significant

Parturients are considered to be at higher risk for gastric regurgitation and pulmonary aspiration. The risk could be exacerbated especially with concomitant obesity, labor pain or opioid analgesia administration. Although this study was not powered to investigate the risk of pulmonary aspiration, we did not detect any clinical evidence of regurgitation or aspiration, including no significant acidification of SLMA laryngeal surface to reflect gastric pH, which is a surrogate indication of the presence of gastric contents in the trachea [20]. The lack of clinical aspiration is possibly due to: (1) the ability of the double-lumen system of second-generation LMAs to facilitate gastric tube insertion and attenuation of intra-gastric fluid volume; (2) a better pharyngeal seal that prevents stomach insufflation and gastric fluid at the hypopharynx from entering the airway; (3) performance of rapid sequence induction and cricoid pressure; (4) careful patient selection with exclusion of parturients at risk of gastric regurgitation; and (5) adherence to the minimum recommended fasting time. We also requested the obstetricians to reduce fundal pressure for all cases, though the benefit of this in terms of aspiration risk is uncertain.

Our results concurred with previous studies evaluating the role of supraglottic airway devices in parturients receiving general anesthesia for cesarean section. The prospective study using the Classic™ LMA in 1067 parturients undergoing elective cesarean section by Han et al. in 2001 detected no aspiration or regurgitation [19]. The use of the ProSeal LMA in 3000 parturients by Halaseh et al. reported a single event of gastric regurgitation after LMA insertion, but with no clinical evidence of aspiration [17]. More recently, our team demonstrated the safety of SLMA use for airway management in obstetric general anesthesia, in a cohort study involving 700 low-risk parturients undergoing elective and urgent cesarean section [12], followed by a higher-risk 584 women requiring emergent Category 2 or 3 cesarean section, of which 38.4% were in active labor [18]. Both studies reported a high first attempt success rate of SLMA insertion of 98% and no clinical evidence of regurgitation or aspiration.

There are several limitations in our study. Our participants were carefully selected to reduce the risk of gastric regurgitation and our study was not powered to detect such rare events. By extension, we are also unable to extrapolate our findings to parturients who are at a higher risk of pulmonary aspiration. Based on a previous study by Halaseh et al., with a baseline risk of aspiration of 1: 1000, at least 3000 cases are required based on a cohort study [17]. This would make the study feasibility difficult given the large numbers. The cesarean section rate is 35% in our institution and the SLMA technique for general anesthesia is used in 2000 deliveries annually. Since we have adopted the SLMA in airway management of selected parturients, we have not noted any adverse events (aspiration). However, the current practice of endotracheal intubation for cesarean section should still be advocated as pulmonary aspiration is one of the main concerns with SLMA use in obstetrics, for which our study was not powered to detect. We noted that the familiarity with the use of SLMA in general anesthesia for cesarean section and less familiarity with endotracheal intubation could have led to faster time to ventilation and high insertion success rate with SLMA in this study center. Thus, these findings may not be applicable to other centers. Also, cricoid pressure was applied by the anesthetic nurses, who were briefed on the study and the need for consistency. They applied cricoid pressure according to routine hospital practice, but cricoid pressure was not directly measured. Although the obstetricians were not blinded, they were instructed to reduce fundal pressure uniformly for all cases. Lastly, there is no reliable method to blind the anesthesiologists who performed the airway management in this study. Hence, outcome measures including the primary outcome could be influenced by the experience and familiarity with the airway devices used.

The faster speed to establish a secure airway and the reduced risk of hemodynamic fluctuations renders potential justification for future studies on the effectiveness of second-generation LMAs in the obstetric population especially in difficult obstetric airway management. Higher-risk obstetric parturients with medical conditions such as preeclampsia and cardiac disease could benefit from reduced hemodynamic alterations associated with SLMA use [21, 22]. Furthermore, during emergency airway management, a shorter time to ventilation could reduce potential hypoxia [8, 23].

Conclusion

We found that in parturients undergoing elective cesarean section under general anesthesia, the SLMA group has similar high first attempt success rate, while potentially reducing the time taken to achieve effective ventilation and less hemodynamic changes, as compared to ETT group. However, there is still limited information of the safety of SLMA use, especially pertaining to pulmonary aspiration risk. Given the higher incidence of difficult and failed intubation in obstetrics, our findings support the current DAS-OAA guidelines in recommending the use of second-generation LMAs as a second-line airway device, in place of persistent attempts at endotracheal intubation.

Abbreviations

ASA: American Society of Anesthesiology; BMI: Body mass index; CI: Confidence interval; DAS: Difficult Airway Society; ETT: Endotracheal intubation; IQR: Interquartile range; LMA: Laryngeal mask airway; MD: Mean difference; OAA: Obstetric Anaesthetists' Association; OR: Odds ratio; RSI: Rapid sequence induction; SAD: Supraglottic airway devices; SD: Standard deviation; SLMA: Supreme laryngeal mask airway

Acknowledgements
The authors would like to acknowledge the staff of Quanzhou Women's and Children's Hospital for their help in patient care for this study.

Authors' contributions
BLS: study design, data collection, data analysis, revising the article critically for important intellectual content and final approval of the version to be submitted. WYY: data collection, patient recruitment and final approval of the version to be submitted. SYL: study design, data collection, patient recruitment and final approval of the version to be submitted. YJY: data collection, patient recruitment and final approval of the version to be submitted. HST: data analysis, revising the article and final approval of the version to be submitted. NLH: data analysis, revising the article and final approval of the version to be submitted. RS: data analysis, revising the article and final approval of the version to be submitted. PNA: data analysis, revising the article and final approval of the version to be submitted. ATS: study design, data analysis, revising the article critically for important intellectual content and final approval of the version to be submitted. All authors read and approved the final manuscript.

Author details
[1]Department of Anesthesiology and Perioperative Medicine, Quanzhou Macare Women's Hospital, Quanzhou, Fujian Province, China. [2]Department of Anesthesiology, Qinghai University Affiliated Hospital, Xining, Qinghai Province, China. [3]Department of Women's Anaesthesia, KK Women's and Children's Hospital, 100 Bukit Timah Road, Singapore, Singapore. [4]Division of Clinical Support Services, KK Women's and Children's Hospital, 100 Bukit Timah Road, Singapore, Singapore. [5]Center for Quantitative Medicine, Duke-NUS Medical School, 8 College Road, Singapore, Singapore. [6]Singapore Clinical Research Institute, 31 Biopolis Way, Singapore, Singapore. [7]Anaesthesiology and Perioperative Sciences Academic Clinical Program, Duke-NUS Medical School, 8 College Road, Singapore, Singapore.

References

1. Barnardo PD, Jenkins JG. Failed tracheal intubation in obstetrics: a 6-year review in a UK region. Anaesthesia. 2000;55:690–4.
2. Hawthorne L, Wilson R, Lyons G, Dresner M. Failed intubation revisited: 17-yr experience in a teaching maternity unit. Br J Anaesth. 1996;76:680–4.
3. McDonnell NJ, Paech MJ, Clavisi OM, Scott KL, Group AT. Difficult and failed intubation in obstetric anaesthesia: an observational study of airway management and complications associated with general anaesthesia for caesarean section. Int J Obstet Anesth. 2008;17:292–7.
4. Quinn AC, Milne D, Columb M, Gorton H, Knight M. Failed tracheal intubation in obstetric anaesthesia: 2 yr national case-control study in the UK. Br J Anaesth. 2013;110:74–80.
5. Rahman K, Jenkins JG. Failed tracheal intubation in obstetrics: no more frequent but still managed badly. Anaesthesia. 2005;60:168–71.
6. Harmer M. Difficult and failed intubation in obstetrics. Int J Obstet Anesth. 1997;6:25–31.
7. McKeen DM, George RB, O'Connell CM, Allen VM, Yazer M, Wilson M, Phu TC. Difficult and failed intubation: incident rates and maternal, obstetrical, and anesthetic predictors. Can J Anaesth. 2011;58:514–24.
8. Mushambi MC, Kinsella SM. Obstetric Anaesthetists' Association/difficult airway society difficult and failed tracheal intubation guidelines--the way forward for the obstetric airway. Br J Anaesth. 2015;115:815–8.
9. Bercker S, Schmidbauer W, Volk T, Bogusch G, Bubser HP, Hensel M, Kerner T. A comparison of seal in seven supraglottic airway devices using a cadaver model of elevated esophageal pressure. Anesth Analg. 2008;106: 445–8.
10. Keller C, Brimacombe J, Kleinsasser A, Loeckinger A. Does the ProSeal laryngeal mask airway prevent aspiration of regurgitated fluid? Anesth Analg. 2000;91:1017–20.
11. Lim Y, Goel S, Brimacombe JR. The ProSeal laryngeal mask airway is an effective alternative to laryngoscope-guided tracheal intubation for gynaecological laparoscopy. Anaesth Intensive Care. 2007;35:52–6.
12. Yao WY, Li SY, Sng BL, Lim Y, Sia AT. The LMA supreme in 700 parturients undergoing cesarean delivery: an observational study. Can J Anaesth. 2012; 59:648–54.
13. Henderson JJ, Popat MT, Latto IP, Pearce AC. Difficult airway S. difficult airway society guidelines for management of the unanticipated difficult intubation. Anaesthesia. 2004;59:675–94.
14. Mushambi MC, Kinsella SM, Popat M, Swales H, Ramaswamy KK, Winton AL, Quinn AC, Obstetric Anaesthetists. Association; difficult airway society. Obstetric Anaesthetists' Association and difficult airway society guidelines for the management of difficult and failed tracheal intubation in obstetrics. Anaesthesia. 2015;70:1286–306.
15. Mendelson CL. The aspiration of stomach contents into the lungs during obstetric anesthesia. Am J Obstet Gynecol. 1946;52:191–205.
16. Geng ZY, Wang DX. Laryngeal mask airway for cesarean delivery: a 5-year retrospective cohort study. Chin Med J. 2017;130:404–8.
17. Halaseh BK, Sukkar ZF, Hassan LH, Sia AT, Bushnaq WA, Adarbeh H. The use of ProSeal laryngeal mask airway in caesarean section--experience in 3000 cases. Anaesth Intensive Care. 2010;38:1023–8.
18. Li SY, Yao WY, Yuan YJ, Tay WS, Han NLR, Sultana R, Assam PN, Sia AT, Sng BL. Supreme™ laryngeal mask airway use in general anesthesia for category 2 and 3 cesarean delivery: a prospective cohort study. BMC Anesthesiol. 2017;17.
19. Han TH, Brimacombe J, Lee EJ, Yang HS. The laryngeal mask airway is effective (and probably safe) in selected healthy parturients for elective cesarean section: a prospective study of 1067 cases. Can J Anaesth. 2001;48: 1117–21.
20. Hagberg CA, Vartazarian TN, Chelly JE, Ovassapian A. The incidence of gastroesophageal reflux and tracheal aspiration detected with pH electrodes is similar with the laryngeal mask airway and esophageal tracheal Combitube--a pilot study. Can J Anaesth. 2004;51:243–9.
21. Benhamou D, Chassard D, Mercier FJ, Bouvier-Colle MH. The seventh report of the confidential enquiries into maternal deaths in the United Kingdom: comparison with French data. Ann Fr Anesth Reanim. 2009;28:38–43.
22. Gogarten W. Preeclampsia and anaesthesia. Curr Opin Anaesthesiol. 2009;22: 347–51.
23. Cook TM, Kelly FE. Time to abandon the 'vintage' laryngeal mask airway and adopt second-generation supraglottic airway devices as first choice. Br J Anaesth. 2015;115:497–9.

12

Oral mosapride can provide additional anti-emetic efficacy following total joint arthroplasty under general anesthesia

Jinwei Xie[1], Yingchun Cai[1,2], Jun Ma[1], Qiang Huang[1] and Fuxing Pei[1*]

Abstract

Background: We sought to determine (1) whether the addition of prophylactic oral mosapride to a protocol including dexamethasone and ondansetron further reduces postoperative nausea and vomiting (PONV) compared with ondansetron alone or the combination of both; (2) whether preemptive application of oral mosapride provides additional clinical benefits for bowel function and appetite, thus improving functional recovery.

Methods: We randomized 240 patients undergoing total hip and knee arthroplasty to receive placebo (Control, $n = 80$), dexamethasone (10 mg) before anesthesia induction (Dexa, $n = 82$), or dexamethasone (10 mg) before anesthesia induction as well as oral mosapride (5 mg) before and after surgery (Mosa+Dexa, $n = 78$). Patients were assessed at 0–6, 6–12, 12–24, and 24–48 h postoperatively. Primary outcomes were incidence and severity of PONV as well as complete response. Secondary outcomes were appetite, time until first defecation and ambulation, patient satisfaction score, and length of hospital stay.

Results: Mosa+Dexa patients showed significantly lower incidence of nausea at 6–12 h (3.8%) and over the entire evaluation period (6.4%), as well as a higher rate of complete response (89.7%) than other patients. Mosa+Dexa patients required less time to achieve first defecation and ambulation, they were hospitalized for shorter time, and they were more satisfied with clinical care.

Conclusion: Addition of oral mosapride further reduced incidence of PONV, especially postoperative nausea, during 6–12 h postoperatively. Moreover, preemptive application of oral mosapride can further improve appetite, bowel function, ambulation and length of hospital stay.

Keywords: PONV, Total joint arthroplasty, General anesthesia, Bowel function

* Correspondence: peifuxinghuaxi@126.com
[1]Department of Orthopaedic Surgery, National Clinical Research Center for Geriatrics, West China Hospital, Sichuan University, No. 37 Guoxue Road, Chengdu, Sichuan Province 610041, People's Republic of China

Background

Total hip and knee arthroplasty remain one of the most commonly performed major orthopedic procedures; the number of procedures in most countries has increased rapidly over the past decades [1, 2]. Postoperative nausea and vomiting (PONV) are one of the most common and distressing complications after surgery, especially when the surgery is performed under general anesthesia: PONV occurs in 25–30% of all patients, and the rate can reach 80% among at-risk patients without prophylactic intervention [3, 4]. PONV can lead to dehydration, hypertension and other postoperative morbidities, which may prolong hospital stay and increase risk of readmission, raising healthcare costs [5]. This was a paradox in the circumstance that surgeons and healthcare providers have been shifting their focus from the surgical technique to perioperative management in order to improve patients' psychological and functional recovery [6].

Several prophylactic interventions have been reported to prevent and treat PONV, e.g. 5-HT_3 receptor antagonists, NK-1 receptor antagonists, corticosteroids, butyrophenone and antihistamines [7]. While these measures can be effective, PONV remains a persistent problem [8, 9]. One reason for this persistence is the gap between implementation and our goal of a "PONV-free hospital". We previously found that PONV occurred in up to 48.8% of patients undergoing total joint arthroplasty under general anesthesia at our medical center (unpublished data). Another reason for this persistence is that anti-PONV measures can be associated with adverse effects. For example, use of the 5-HT_3 receptor antagonist ondansetron can aggravate the postoperative constipation that occurs in up to 65% of total joint arthroplasty patients [10]. We have shown that low-dose dexamethasone can reduce the incidence of PONV following total hip and knee arthroplasty [11, 12], but it can be contraindicated in the presence of diabetes or gastrointestinal ulcers. Therefore, it's necessary and practical to search for other antiemetic protocol.

The major risk factor of PONV is use of opioids, which can stimulate the release of 5-HT and inhibit gastrointestinal peristalsis [13]]. Indeed, selective 5-HT_4 agonists can stimulate the gastrointestinal tract and promote motility [14]. The selective 5-HT_4 agonist mosapride can reduce vomiting caused by chemotherapy [15]. This inspired us to examine whether the anti-emetic effects of oral mosapride might offer clinical benefits for total joint arthroplasty patients.

Thus, we sought to determine in the present study (1) whether the addition of prophylactic oral mosapride to a protocol including dexamethasone and ondansetron can further reduce PONV compared with ondansetron alone or the combination of both; and (2) whether preemptive application of oral mosapride can provide additional clinical benefits for recovery of bowel function and appetite.

Methods

Study design

This prospective, randomized, clinical trial was performed on patients undergoing primary total hip or knee arthroplasty between November 2017 and December 2018. Institutional review board approval (2012–268) was obtained before the enrollment of patients. All patients provided written informed consent and research authorization before surgery. The study was conducted in compliance with the recommendations of the CONSORT Statement and the Declaration of Helsinki. The study protocol was registered at the Chinese Clinical Trial Registry (ChiCTR1800015896).

Participants

Eligible patients included those at least 18 years old who were at risk of PONV (at least 1 score of Apfel), and scheduled for primary total hip or knee arthroplasty for end-stage joint diseases such as osteoarthritis, development dysplasia of hip, and osteonecrosis of the femoral head. Exclusion criteria included a history of intolerance of any drugs used in the current study, administration of another antiemetic drug or systemic steroid within 24 h before surgery, allergy to experimental drugs or history of adverse reactions, diabetes with poor blood glucose control, history of steroid or immunosuppressive drug use within the previous 6 months, history of cardiac disease such as heart failure, heart block, ventricular arrhythmia or severe impairment of bowel motility, renal function or hepatic function.

Randomization and treatment

Patients in this double-blind study were randomly allocated into three groups using a computer-generated randomization list in a 1: 1: 1 ratio. A random allocation sequence concealed in opaque sealed envelopes only opened before surgery. The control group received 2 ml of normal saline during anesthesia induction, followed by oral placebo at 3 h before surgery and three times per day after surgery. The Dexa group received 10 mg of dexamethasone (in 2 ml) during anesthesia induction, as well as oral placebo at 3 h before surgery and three times per day after surgery. The Mosa+Dexa group received 10 mg of dexamethasone (in 2 ml) during anesthesia induction, as well as 5 mg of oral Mosapride at 3 h before surgery and three times per day after surgery. Dexamethasone was administered intraoperatively by the anesthesiologist and oral drugs were given postoperatively by nurses who were not involved in the study. Patients, surgeons, data collectors and analysts were blinded to group allocation.

Anesthesia and perioperative pain management

All surgeries were performed under general anesthesia by the same surgeons; standard medial parapatellar arthrotomy was performed for total knee arthroplasty, and the posterolateral approach was used for total hip arthroplasty. A cemented posteriorly stabilized prosthesis was implanted in all total knee arthroplasty patients, and cementless acetabular and femoral components were implanted in total hip arthroplasty patients.

All patients received the same anesthetic regimen and multimodal pain management protocol. Cefuroxime (1.5 g) was given intravenously as prophylactic antibiotic prior to incision. Sufentanil (0.2 μg/kg) propofol (2 mg/kg), atracurium (1 mg/kg) and midazolam (2 mg) were used for anesthesia induction. Then sufentanil (0.1 μg/kg), atracurium (0.5 mg/kg) and sevoflurane (1–3%) were used to maintain anesthesia during surgery. After prosthesis insertion, propofol (4 mg per kg per h) and remifentanil (0.1 μg per kg per min) were used to maintain anesthesia. Anesthetic drugs were discontinued before wound closure. At the end of surgery, 8 mg ondansetron was administered intravenously to all patients.

After prosthesis insertion, a periarticular infiltration of 200 mg ropivacaine (100 mg per 10 ml) in 60 ml of normal saline was injected all around the capsule before closure. A dose of 40 mg of parecoxib was injected intravenously to manage pain. Postoperative pain control consisted of 50 mg of oral voltaren (Diclofenac Sodium Sustained Release Tablets) and 10 mg of oxycodone every 12 h. Breakthrough pain was recorded using a Visual Analgesic Scale (VAS) score that ranged from 0 (no pain) to 10 (most severe). If the VAS score was > 6, 50 mg of pethidine was given as an intramuscular injection when required, up to every 6 h. No nerve block or intravenous patient-controlled analgesia was utilized perioperatively.

Outcome measurements

The primary outcome variables were the incidence of PONV, severity of PONV and complete response. Secondary outcome variables included time until first defecation and ambulation, postoperative appetite score, patient satisfaction score and length of hospital stay. A blinded clinical investigator reviewed the diagnosis and medical histories of patients and prospectively collected demographic data and surgical information. The investigator also recorded all episodes of nausea and vomiting, severity of nausea, requirement for anti-emetic rescue, and complete response during four postoperative periods (0–6, 6–12, 12–24 and 24–48 h). Nausea was defined as a subjective unpleasant sensation associated with awareness of the urge to vomit, and vomiting was defined as the forceful expulsion of gastric contents from the mouth [16]. The incidence of nausea and vomiting was determined in each of the four periods and during the entire study by calculating the proportion of patients who experienced PONV. In order to avoid double counting, the patients experienced both nausea and vomiting would be counted as episode of vomiting. Following institutional guidelines, 10 mg of intramuscular metoclopramide was used as a first-line anti-emetic rescue treatment when patients experienced two or more episodes of PONV within 2 h. This was followed by 4 mg of intravenous ondansetron when two consecutive boluses of metoclopramide alone, delivered 30 min apart, were ineffective.

We used a standardized scoring algorithm to classify the severity of PONV on a 4-level scale during the 48-h observation period. Complete response was defined as no additional PONV or no requirement for anti-emetic rescue. Mild PONV described the occurrence of mild nausea or one episode of vomiting caused by exogenous stimulus (drinking or movement). Moderate PONV referred to when the patient vomited up to two times or experienced nausea that required anti-emetic rescue only once. Patients were classified as having severe PONV if they suffered more than two emetic episodes or required more than one dose of rescue anti-emetic [17, 18].

The same blinded investigator also recorded the time until first defecation, ambulation and length of hospital stay, and evaluated appetite score on postoperative days 0–2 as follows: 1 point, lower appetite than preoperatively; 2 points, same appetite as preoperatively; and 3 points, more appetite than preoperatively. The same investigator assessed patient satisfaction before discharge using a VAS score that ranged from 0 (extremely dissatisfied) to 10 (very satisfied). During the perioperative period, all the patients would be carefully evaluated for side effects and cardiac complications such as atrioventricular block, or QT interval prolongation with the use of electrocardiogram if necessary.

Statistical analysis

We performed a priori power analysis based on our preliminary results showing that PONV incidence was 49% in patients receiving ondansetron prophylaxis alone after total joint arthroplasty [unpublished data]. We calculated that 228 patients (76 in each arm) were required to detect a 50% reduction in PONV incidence at an alpha level of 0.05 and a power of 0.9 using a two-sided test. To allow for exclusions and dropouts, we aimed to enroll 246 patients.

Inter-group differences in categorical variables such as incidence of PONV or proportion of complete response were assessed for significance using the chi-square or Fisher's exact tests. When differences were significant, multiple comparisons between groups were performed using a Bonferroni-corrected post hoc test. Inter-group differences in continuous variables were assessed for significance using either one-way ANOVA, in the case of body mass index, length of hospital stay, time until first defecation or ambulation; or the Wilcoxon signed-rank test, in the case of appetite and patient satisfaction scores. When differences were significant, multiple comparisons between groups were performed using a post hoc Tukey test. Differences associated with $p < 0.05$ were considered statistically significant. All statistical analyses were conducted in SPSS 21.0 (IBM, Chicago, IL, USA).

Results

A total of 82 patients were initially allocated to each of the three groups. We excluded two patients from the control group and four from the Mosa+Dexa group because of incomplete data and spinal anesthesia. In the end, 240 patients (80 in the control group, 82 in the Dexa group and 78 in the Mosa+Dexa group) were included in the final analysis (Fig. 1). These groups showed no significant differences in clinical or demographic characteristics (Table 1).

Prophylactic use of concurrent dexamethasone and oral mosapride reduced the overall incidence and severity of PONV, and improved the overall complete response during the entire 48-h evaluation period. Across the entire evaluation period, incidence of postoperative nausea was lowest in the Mosa+Dexa group (6.4%), followed by the Dexa group (19.5%) and the control group (43.8%) ($p < 0.01$ for all, Table 2). Similarly, incidence of postoperative vomiting was lowest in the Mosa+Dexa group (3.9%), followed by the Dexa group (6.1%) and the control group (11.2%), although these differences were not significant ($p = 0.176$). The rate of complete response was significantly higher in the Mosa+Dexa group (89.7%) than in the Dexa group (74.4%, $p =$ 0.012) or control group (45%, $p < 0.001$). The rate of severe PONV was significantly lower in the Mosa+Dexa group (1.3%) than in the Dexa group (7.3%, $p = 0.062$) and control group (18.8%, $p < 0.001$).

Simultaneous application of mosapride and dexamethasone reduced the incidence of nausea mainly during the first 12 h (Tables 3 and 4): the incidence during 6–12 h was significantly lower in the Mosa+Dexa group (3.8%) than in the Dexa group (15.9%, $p < 0.016$) and control group (32.5%, $p < 0.016$). Moreover, all vomiting episodes occurred during the first 12 h in the Mosa+Dexa patients, while some vomiting incidents in other groups occurred later (Table 4). Nevertheless, the vomiting incidence during the first 12 h did not differ significantly among the three groups. Less patients in Mosa+Dexa group (2.6%) required rescue treatment for PONV when compared with Dexa group (9.8%, $p = 0.06$) and Control group (21.3%, $p < 0.001$, Table 5), as well as total dose of metoclopramide. No significances were detected among the three groups regarding the postoperative pain score and rescue requirement.

The preemptive use of mosapride also reduced the time until first defecation, which was significantly shorter in the Mosa+Dexa group (36.4 ± 18.3 h) than in the Dexa group (54.7 ± 15.8 h, $p < 0.001$) and control group (60.7 ± 24.6 h, $p < 0.001$; Table 6). Appetite score was significantly higher in the Mosa+Dexa group than in the control group on postoperative days 0 ($p = 0.019$), 1 ($p < 0.001$) and 2 ($p = 0.022$); and higher than in the Dexa group on postoperative day 1 ($p = 0.001$; Table 6).

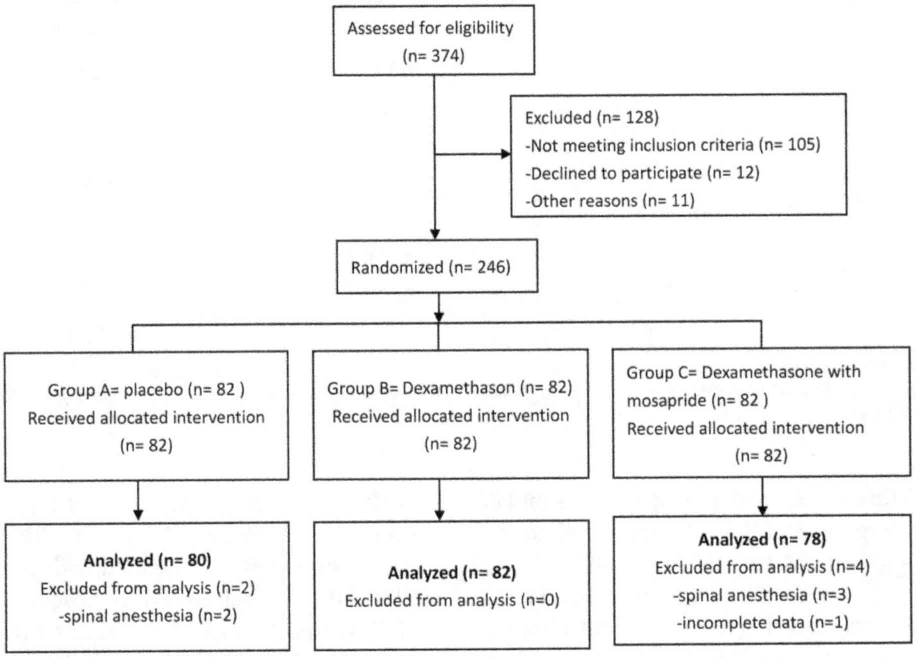

Fig. 1 A flow diagram shows the patients recruitment

Table 1 Baseline characteristics of all patients

	Control (*n* = 80)	Dexa (n = 82)	Mosa+Dexa (*n* = 78)	p
Age (years)	61.2 (8.9)	62.7 (11.8)	62.2 (12.5)	0.376
Female / Male	47 / 33	61 / 21	53 / 25	0.104
Height (m)	1.61 (0.07)	1.58 (0.07)	1.59 (0.06)	0.055
Weight (kg)	63.4 (13.5)	62.2 (9.0)	60.1 (8.7)	0.143
BMI (kg/m^2)	24.4 (4.6)	24.9 (3.4)	23.5 (3.0)	0.057
Smoking				0.266
Yes	33 (41.2%)	24 (29.3%)	26 (33.3%)	
No	47 (58.8%)	58 (70.7%)	52 (66.7%)	
History of PONV				0.856
Yes	10 (12.5%)	8 (9.8%)	10 (12.8%)	
No	70 (87.5%)	74 (91.2%)	68 (87.2%)	
History of motion sickness				0.994
Yes	27 (33.8%)	28 (34.1%)	33 (42.3%)	
No	53 (66.2%)	54 (65.9%)	45 (57.7%)	
ASA Score				0.806
2	56 (70%)	55 (67.1%)	56 (71.8%)	
3	24 (30%)	27 (32.9%)	22 (28.2%)	
Surgery				0.439
THA	36 (45%)	31 (37.8%)	37 (47.4%)	
TKA	44 (55%)	51 (62.2%)	41 (52.6%)	
Number of comorbidities				0.978
1	52 (65%)	52 (63.4%)	50 (64.1%)	
≥ 2	28 (35%)	30 (36.6%)	28 (35.9%)	
Operation time (min)	76.3 (21.6)	77.6 (20.1)	76.2 (27.8)	0.920
Anesthesia time (min)	125.5 (26.0)	127.1 (26.5)	120.1 (33.6)	0.280
PACU time (min)	70.3 (48.5)	80.9 (44.7)	76.1 (35.5)	0.300
Sufentanil (μg)	24.24 (2.92)	24.18 (2.59)	24.89 (3.17)	0.195
Remifentanil (mg)	0.58 (0.15)	0.62 (0.10)	0.62 (0.30)	0.329
Propofol (mg)	219.45 (109.40)	196.93 (79.12)	220.54 (178.85)	0.420
Midazolam (mg)	2.09 (0.51)	2.12 (0.41)	2.11 (0.48)	0.946
Atracurium (mg)	13.19 (1.91)	13.37 (2.60)	13.65 (2.18)	0.436
Sevoflurane (ml)	29.97 (6.71)	30.23 (5.47)	30.53 (11.11)	0.913
VAS pain score- rest	3.81 (1.98)	3.58 (1.55)	3.42 (1.26)	0.374

Data presented as mean (stand deviation) or number (percentage)
ASA American Society of Anesthesiologists; *BMI* body mass index; *Dexa* dexamethasone; *Mosa* mosapride; *THA* total hip arthroplasty; *TKA* total knee arthroplasty; *PACU*, post-anesthesia care unit

Patients in the Mosa+Dexa group began to ambulate 20.6 ± 5.9 h after surgery, significantly sooner than patients in the Dexa group (23.4 ± 5.8 h, $p = 0.005$) or control group (23.3 ± 4.6 h, $p = 0.008$). Patients in the Mosa+Dexa group were more satisfied with their hospital experience than patients in the control group ($p < 0.001$) and Dexa group ($p = 0.008$). Length of hospitalization was shorter in the Mosa+Dexa group than in the contrl group (4.9 ± 1.4 vs 5.6 ± 1.5 d, $p = 0.012$).

No adverse events associated with mosapride including prolonged QT syndrome were observed during the study or follow-up. A total of 5 patients (including 1 abdominal pain, 2 dry mouth, 2 insomnia) experienced side effects in control group, 5 patients (1 diarrhea, 1 dry

Table 2 Incidence of PONV during the first postoperative 48 h

	Control (n = 80)	Dexa (*n* = 82)	Mosa + Dexa (*n* = 78)	p*	p1†	p2†	p3†
Total	44 (55%)	21 (25.6%)	8 (10.3%)	< 0.001	**< 0.001**	**< 0.001**	**0.014**
Nausea	35 (43.8%)	16 (19.5%)	5 (6.4%)	< 0.001	**0.001**	**< 0.001**	**0.014**
Vomiting	9 (11.2%)	5 (6.1%)	3 (3.9%)	0.176	NA	NA	NA
Complete response	36 (45%)	61 (74.4%)	70 (89.7%)	< 0.001	**< 0.001**	**< 0.001**	**0.012**
Severe PONV	15 (18.8%)	6 (7.3%)	1 (1.3%)	0.001	0.030	**< 0.001**	0.062

Data presented as number of patients (percentage)
Dexa dexamethasone; *Mosa* mosapride; *PONV* postoperative nausea and vomiting
* Uncorrected *p* values (for the three-way comparison)
† Bonferroni-corrected *p* values: p1, Control vs Dexa; p2, Control vs. Mosa+Dexa; p3, Dexa vs. Mosa-Dexa. The corrected significance threshold was 0.016

mouth, 3 insomnia) in Dexa group and 6 (in abdominal pain, 2 dry mouth and 3 insomnia) in Mosa + Dexa group without significance ($p = 0.908$, Table 7).

Discussion

PONV remains a challenge in recovery after total joint arthroplasty surgery, because it creates anxiety in patients, lowers their appetite, delays ambulation and even disturbs water and electrolyte balance. This increases risk of postoperative complications and prolongs hospitalization and consensus guidelines have been formulated for the management of PONV [7]. Fifteen years have passed since the first international recommendations for the prophylaxis and treatment of PONV [19], and the incidence of PONV has fallen from approximately 80% to 20–30% [20], which is still relatively high. Our own work suggests that at least certain patient populations may show much higher incidence: we reported, for example, 48% incidence in patients who underwent total joint arthroplasty with general anesthesia [unpublished data]. Indeed, risk of PONV appears to be 11-fold higher when surgery is performed under general anesthesia than under regional anesthesia [21]. While modification of risk factors should be taken firstly according to the recommendation of latest consensus [7], some risk factors such as gender or history of smoking and PONV were non-modifiable. Moreover, in our country, total joint arthroplasty is performed under general anesthesia routinely, because of the different medical system. On the other hand, spinal anesthesia is conductive to early ambulation and postoperative anticoagulation following enhanced total joint arthroplasty. These considerations highlight the need to improve PONV prophylaxis and treatment.

In our current study, we compared a new multimodal PONV prophylaxis protocol with a traditional anti-emetic protocol involving ondansetron and/or dexamethasone. The latter two drugs are the most commonly used perioperatively to prevent PONV. Our results indicate that addition of the oral prokinetic drug mosapride can lead to lower PONV incidence and severity, especially postoperative nausea, during the first 12 h postoperatively than the use of ondansetron alone or in combination with dexamethasone, although the

Table 3 Timing of PONV events during the postoperative period

Time	Control (n = 80)	Dexa (n = 82)	Mosa+Dexa (n = 78)	p*	p1†	p2†	p3†
Nausea	35 (43.8%)	16 (19.5%)	5 (6.4%)	< 0.001	0.001	< 0.001	0.014
0–6 h	30 (37.5%)	14 (17.1%)	5 (6.4%)	< 0.001	0.003	< 0.001	0.037
6–12 h	26 (32.5%)	13 (15.9%)	3 (3.8%)	< 0.001	0.002	< 0.013	0.011
12–24 h	8 (10%)	3 (3.7%)	0	0.006	0.109	0.007	0.246
24–48 h	6 (7.5%)	1 (1.2%)	0	0.013	0.062	0.028	1.000
Vomiting	9 (11.2%)	5 (6.1%)	3 (3.9%)	0.176			
0–6 h	7 (23.8%)	4 (12.2%)	3 (3.8%)	0.380			
6–12 h	3 (12.5%)	2 (6.1%)	1 (1.3%)	0.610			
12–24 h	1 (1.3%)	1 (1.2%)	0	1.000			
24–48 h	1 (1.3%)	0	0	0.652			

Data presented as number of patients (percentage). Dexa, dexamethasone; Mosa, mosapride; PONV, postoperative nausea and vomiting
* Uncorrected values
† Bonferroni-corrected p values: p1, Control vs Dexa; p2, Control vs. Mosa+Dexa; p3, Dexa vs. Mosa-Dexa. The corrected significance threshold was 0.016

Table 4 Duration of PONV during the first postoperative 48 h

Duration	Control (n = 80)	Dexa (n = 82)	Mosa+Dexa (n = 78)	p*	p1†	p2†	p3†
< 6 h	18 (22.5%)	12 (14.6%)	7 (9.0%)	0.061			
6–12 h	8 (10.0%)	6 (7.3%)	1 (1.3%)	0.068			
12–24 h	8 (10.0%)	2 (2.4%)	0	0.004	0.046	0.007	0.497
> 24 h	10 (12.5%)	1 (1.2%)	0	< 0.001	0.004	0.001	1.000

Data presented as number of patients (percentage)
* Uncorrected values
† Bonferroni-corrected p values: p1, Control vs Dexa; p2, Control vs. Mosa+Dexa; p3, Dexa vs. Mosa-Dexa. The corrected significance threshold was 0.016

difference of severe PONV rate between Dexa + Mosa group and Dexa Group was not statistically significant ($p = 0.062$). Moreover, preemptive application of oral mosapride can improve appetite, bowel function, time until ambulation and length of hospital stay.

5-HT_3 receptor antagonists and corticosteroids are the anti-emetic drugs most commonly used perioperatively to prevent and treat PONV. These drugs act by antagonizing 5-HT_3 receptors both peripherally on vagal afferents and centrally in the area postrema. Dexamethasone is a synthetic glucocorticoid showing higher potency, greater bioavailability, and longer acting time than the most widely used antagonist, ondansetron [22–24]. Low-dose systemic dexamethasone can show good anti-emetic efficacy [25, 26], although the mechanism remains unclear. The drug may inhibit prostaglandin synthesis and endogenous opioid release, controlling pain and reducing the need for opioid drugs, which can help prevent PONV. The half-life of dexamethasone is about 36–72 h, much longer than the 4 h of ondansetron [22, 23]. Therefore, the combination of dexamethasone and ondansetron can be particularly effective at reducing PONV incidence during the first 12–48 h after surgery (Tables 3 and 4). We found that combining dexamethasone with ondansetron led to lower incidence of PONV and higher incidence of complete response than with ondansetron alone. Similarly, previous work showed that combining dexamethasone with ramosetron further reduced postoperative emesis and pain without increasing risk of wound complications [27]. Studies also have suggested that dexamethasone can help reduce postoperative pain and inflammatory responses [11, 12, 24, 27, 28], which we did not examine here. Future work should explore the full range of benefits offered by dexamethasone.

Here we investigated additional clinical benefits of the anti-emetic mosapride, a selective 5-HT_4 receptor agonist. Mosapride can promote the release of acetylcholine and stimulate the gastrointestinal tract to promote motility, thereby improving the gastrointestinal symptoms of patients with functional dyspepsia. Mosapride can inhibit emesis induced by selective serotonin reuptake inhibitors (SSRIs) in laboratory animals [14], probably by reversing the SSRI-induced delay in gastric emptying. We found in the present study that the preemptive use of oral mosapride can provide additional anti-emetic effects beyond dexamethasone and ondansetron in total joint arthroplasty patients. In fact, mosapride may antagonize the ability of 5-HT_3 receptor antagonists to reduce gastrointestinal motility, which may help reduce the risk of constipation that affects many total hip and knee arthroplasty patients [29]. Indeed, this motility-inducing effect may help explain why the patients in our Mosa+Dexa group showed better postoperative appetite and shorter times to first defecation and ambulation

Table 5 The requirement of rescue treatment and postoperative VAS pain score

	Control (n = 80)	Dexa (n = 82)	Mosa+Dexa (n = 78)	p*	p1†	p2†	p3†
Metoclopramide							
Number	17 (21.3%)	8 (9.8%)	2 (2.6%)	0.001	0.043	< 0.001	0.060
Mean dose (mg)	2.88 (40)	1.10 (20)	0.26 (10)	0.002	0.044	0.002	0.496
VAS-rest 24 h	2.66 ± 0.72	2.45 ± 0.91	2.59 ± 0.82	0.333			
VAS-rest 48 h	2.16 ± 0.99	2.03 ± 0.73	2.15 ± 0.71	0.551			
Pethidine							
Number	30 (37.5%)	19 (23.2%)	21 (26.9%)	0.116			
Mean dose (mg)	20 (100)	17.38 (50)	16.99 (100)	0.486			

Data presented as number of patients (percentage), mean (range) or mean ± standard deviation. *Dexa* dexamethasone; *Mosa* mosapride
* Uncorrected p values (for the three-way comparison)
† Bonferroni-corrected *p* values: p1, Control vs Dexa; p2, Control vs. Mosa+Dexa; p3, Dexa vs. Mosa-Dexa. The corrected significance threshold was 0.016

Table 6 Other clinical outcomes

	Control (n = 80)	Dexa (n = 82)	Mosa+Dexa (n = 78)	p*	p1[†]	p2[†]	p3[†]
Time to first defecation (h)	60.7 ± 24.6	54.7 ± 15.8	36.4 ± 18.3	< 0.001	0.136	< 0.001	< 0.001
Appetite on POD 0	2.26 ± 0.67	2.34 ± 0.65	2.55 ± 0.68	0.020	0.731	0.019	0.117
Appetite on POD 1	2.38 ± 0.62	2.41 ± 0.63	2.76 ± 0.51	< 0.001	0.905	< 0.001	0.001
Appetite on POD 2	2.63 ± 0.49	2.73 ± 0.45	2.82 ± 0.45	0.030	0.306	0.022	0.443
Time to first ambulation (h)	23.4 ± 5.8	23.3 ± 4.6	20.6 ± 5.9	0.002	0.976	0.005	0.008
Satisfaction	7.7 ± 1.1	8.7 ± 1.1	9.2 ± 0.9	< 0.001	< 0.001	< 0.001	0.008
Length of hospitalization (d)	5.6 ± 1.5	5.1 ± 1.5	4.9 ± 1.4	0.013	0.095	0.012	0.683

Data presented as mean ± standard deviation. Dexa, dexamethasone; Mosa, mosapride; POD, postoperative day
p1, Control vs Dexa; p2, Control vs. Mosa+Dexa; p3, Dexa vs. Mosa-Dexa. *p values with one-way ANOVA or Wilcoxon signed-rank test and [†]p values with Tukey post hoc test

than patients who did not receive mosapride. Although some patients in Mosa + Dexa group experienced digestive side effects such as abdominal pain or dry mouth, we could not conclude the correlation between mosapride and these side effects because of non-significant difference.

As far as we know, our study provides comprehensive evidence supporting the potential clinical benefit of prokinetic drugs following total joint arthroplasty, although the results need to be interpreted in light of the following limitations. First, patients receiving mosapride alone were not included. Therefore, we cannot make the conclusion that mosapride alone was effective at reducing PONV incidence after total joint arthroplasty. Although our results implicated no incidence of prolonged QT syndrome, more further works are needed to confirm and extend our results, especially the safety profile of mosapride, because another 5-HT_4 agonist that antagonizes 5-HT_3 activity and that can rapidly relieve nausea induced by SSRIs was withdrawn for cardiotoxicity [30]. Second, the sample number was calculated according to our primary outcome of PONV incidence. As a result, the sample may not have been adequately powered to detect inter-group differences in secondary outcomes, such as rate of severe PONV, and complication rates. Nevertheless, previous work from our group and others suggests that perioperative dexamethasone does not increase the incidence of postoperative infection in total hip and knee arthroplasty [11, 12, 31]. Third, all participants in our study were Chinese and most (67%) were women. Thus, our findings may not be widely generalizable, because female gender is a well-established risk factor for PONV [32]. Fourth, our postoperative analgesic regimen included extensive multimodal pain control drugs and modalities such as preemptive analgesic medication and periarticular injection, which may have introduced heterogeneity into our sample. However, the rest VAS pain score at postoperative 24 h and 48 h and requirement of rescue treatment for pain were comparable among the three groups (Table 5). Fifth, our study did not investigate whether the choice of PONV management regimen affected postoperative inflammatory marker levels and pain control. This should be explored in future work, since our previous study has shown that low-dose dexamethasone can relieve postoperative pain and postoperative nausea, as well as provide additional inflammatory control and improve clinical outcomes [28]. Lastly, our study excluded diabetic patients, so future work should examine whether our results can be generalized to this patient subpopulation.

Table 7 Adverse events and side effects

	Control (n = 80)	Dexa (n = 82)	Mosa + Dexa (n = 78)	p*
Long QT syndrome	0	0	0	NA
Diarrhea	0	1 (1.22%)	0	1.000
Abdominal pain	1 (1.25%)	0	1 (1.28%)	0.556
Dry mouth	2 (2.5%)	1 (1.22%)	2 (2.56%)	0.752
Insomnia	2 (2.5%)	3 (3.66%)	3 (3.85%)	0.908
Total	5 (6.25%)	5 (6.1%)	6 (7.69%)	0.906

Data presented as mean ± standard deviation. *Dexa* dexamethasone; *Mosa* mosapride
*p values were analyzed using Fisher's exact test

Conclusion

Prophylactic use of concurrent dexamethasone and oral mosapride can reduce overall incidence and severity of PONV, especially postoperative nausea, as well as increase complete response rates during the first 12 h after total hip and knee arthroplasty when compared with other patients. While it seemed that oral mosapride would not provide additional effect on reducing the rate of severe PONV when compared with dexamethasone alone. Preemptive oral mosapride can also improve postoperative appetite and bowel function.

Abbreviations

PONV: Postoperative nausea and vomiting; THA: Total hip arthroplasty; TKA: Total knee arthroplasty; ASA: American Society of Anesthesiologists; PACU: Post-anesthesia care unit; BMI: Body mass index

Acknowledgments
We thank Xiaowei Feng, M. D (Chengdu First People's Hospital, Chengdu, China) and A. Chapin Rodriguez, PhD for helpful suggestions on the manuscript. We also thank all the patients and staff who participated in this study.

Authors' contributions
Conceptualization, FXP; Methodology, JWX and YCC; Formal analysis, JM and QH; Investigation, YCC and JWX; Resources FXP; Data curation and Writing, YCC and JWX; Project administration and Funding Acquisition, FXP and JWX. All authors have read and approved the manuscript.

Author details
[1]Department of Orthopaedic Surgery, National Clinical Research Center for Geriatrics, West China Hospital, Sichuan University, No. 37 Guoxue Road, Chengdu, Sichuan Province 610041, People's Republic of China. [2]Department of Orthopaedic Surgery, The First Affiliated Hospital of Zhengzhou University, No. 1 East Jianshe Road, Zhengzhou 450052, People's Republic of China.

References
1. Kurtz S, Ong K, Lau E, Mowat F, Halpern M. Projections of primary and revision hip and knee arthroplasty in the United States from 2005 to 2030. J Bone Joint Surg Am. 2007;89(4):780–5. https://doi.org/10.2106/JBJS.F.00222.
2. Patel A, Pavlou G, Mujica-Mota RE, Toms AD. The epidemiology of revision total knee and hip arthroplasty in England and Wales: a comparative analysis with projections for the United States. A study using the National Joint Registry dataset. Bone Joint J. 2015;97-B(8):1076–81. https://doi.org/10.1302/0301-620X.97B8.35170.
3. Lin CJ, Williams BA. Postoperative nausea and vomiting in ambulatory regional anesthesia. Int Anesthesiol Clin. 2011;49(4):134–43. https://doi.org/10.1097/AIA.0b013e318216bf9c.
4. Sansonnens J, Taffe P, Burnand B, group ADSs. Higher occurrence of nausea and vomiting after total hip arthroplasty using general versus spinal anesthesia: an observational study. BMC Anesthesiol. 2016;16(1):44. https://doi.org/10.1186/s12871-016-0207-0.
5. Sculco PK, Pagnano MW. Perioperative solutions for rapid recovery joint arthroplasty: get ahead and stay ahead. J Arthroplast. 2015;30(4):518–20. https://doi.org/10.1016/j.arth.2015.01.036.
6. Kehlet H. Fast-track hip and knee arthroplasty. Lancet. 2013;381(9878):1600–2. https://doi.org/10.1016/S0140-6736(13)61003-X.
7. Gan TJ, Diemunsch P, Habib AS, Kovac A, Kranke P, Meyer TA, Watcha M, Chung F, Angus S, Apfel CC, Bergese SD, Candiotti KA, Chan MT, Davis PJ, Hooper VD, Lagoo-Deenadayalan S, Myles P, Nezat G, Philip BK, Tramer MR, Society for Ambulatory A. Consensus guidelines for the management of postoperative nausea and vomiting. Anesth Analg. 2014;118(1):85–113. https://doi.org/10.1213/ANE.0000000000000002.
8. Kranke P, Diemunsch P. The 2014 consensus guidelines for the management of postoperative nausea and vomiting: a leapfrog towards a postoperative nausea and vomiting-free hospital. Eur J Anaesthesiol. 2014; 31(12):651–3. https://doi.org/10.1097/EJA.0000000000000080.
9. Eberhart LH, Kranke P. Postoperative nausea and vomiting: is everything now solved or still more questions than answers? Eur J Anaesthesiol. 2016; 33(12):878–80. https://doi.org/10.1097/EJA.0000000000000527.
10. Ross-Adjie GM, Monterosso L, Bulsara M. Bowel management post major joint arthroplasty: results from a randomised controlled trial. Int J Orthop Trauma Nurs. 2015;19(2):92–101. https://doi.org/10.1016/j.ijotn.2014.04.002.
11. Xu B, Ma J, Huang Q, Huang ZY, Zhang SY, Pei FX. Two doses of low-dose perioperative dexamethasone improve the clinical outcome after total knee arthroplasty: a randomized controlled study. Knee Surg Sports Traumatol Arthrosc. 2018;26(5):1549–56. https://doi.org/10.1007/s00167-017-4506-x.
12. Lei YT, Xu B, Xie XW, Xie JW, Huang Q, Pei FX. The efficacy and safety of two low-dose peri-operative dexamethasone on pain and recovery following total hip arthroplasty: a randomized controlled trial. Int Orthop. 2018;42(3):499–505. https://doi.org/10.1007/s00264-017-3537-8.
13. Dorn S, Lembo A, Cremonini F. Opioid-induced bowel dysfunction: epidemiology, pathophysiology, diagnosis, and initial therapeutic approach. Am J Gastroenterol Suppl. 2014;2(1):31–7. https://doi.org/10.1038/ajgsup.2014.7.
14. Mine Y, Oku S, Yoshida N. Anti-emetic effect of mosapride citrate hydrate, a 5-HT4 receptor agonist, on selective serotonin reuptake inhibitors (SSRIs)-induced emesis in experimental animals. J Pharmacol Sci. 2013;121(1):58–66. https://doi.org/10.1254/jphs.12175fp.
15. Ganesan P, Sharma A, Mohanti BK, Gogia A. Protracted cisplatin-induced vomiting responding to mosapride. Indian J Cancer. 2010;47(1):73–4. https://doi.org/10.4103/0019-509X.58866.
16. Watcha MF, White PF. Postoperative nausea and vomiting. Its etiology, treatment, and prevention. Anesthesiology. 1992;77(1):162–84. https://doi.org/10.1097/00000542-199207000-00023.
17. Xiang Y, Ye W, Sun N, Jin X. Analgesic and sedative effects of Dezocine and midazolam during Vitrectomy. Curr Eye Res. 2016;41(11):1460–4. https://doi.org/10.3109/02713683.2015.1128551.
18. Reibaldi M, Fallico M, Longo A, Avitabile T, Astuto M, Murabito P, Minardi C, Bonfiglio V, Boscia F, Furino C, Rejdak R, Nowomiejska K, Toro M, Cennamo G, Cillino S, Rinaldi M, Fiore T, Cagini C, Russo A. Efficacy of three different prophylactic treatments for postoperative nausea and vomiting after Vitrectomy: a randomized clinical trial. J Clin Med. 2019;8(3). https://doi.org/10.3390/jcm8030391.
19. Gan TJ, Meyer T, Apfel CC, Chung F, Davis PJ, Eubanks S, Kovac A, Philip BK, Sessler DI, Temo J, Tramer MR, Watcha M, Department of Anesthesiology DUMC. Consensus guidelines for managing postoperative nausea and vomiting. Anesth Analg. 2003;97(1):62–71, table of contents. https://doi.org/10.1213/01.ane.0000068580.00245.95.
20. Habib AS, Gan TJ. Postoperative nausea and vomiting: then & now. Anesth Analg. 2012;115(3):493–5. https://doi.org/10.1213/ANE.0b013e318254285e.
21. Sinclair DR, Chung F, Mezei G. Can postoperative nausea and vomiting be predicted? Anesthesiology. 1999;91(1):109–18. https://doi.org/10.1097/00000542-199907000-00018.
22. Spies CM, Strehl C, van der Goes MC, Bijlsma JW, Buttgereit F. Glucocorticoids. Best Pract Res Clin Rheumatol. 2011;25(6):891–900. https://doi.org/10.1016/j.berh.2011.11.002.
23. Coutinho AE, Chapman KE. The anti-inflammatory and immunosuppressive effects of glucocorticoids, recent developments and mechanistic insights. Mol Cell Endocrinol. 2011;335(1):2–13. https://doi.org/10.1016/j.mce.2010.04.005.
24. D'Souza N, Swami M, Bhagwat S. Comparative study of dexamethasone and ondansetron for prophylaxis of postoperative nausea and vomiting in laparoscopic gynecologic surgery. Int J Gynaecol Obstet. 2011;113(2):124–7. https://doi.org/10.1016/j.ijgo.2010.11.022.
25. Lunn TH, Kehlet H. Perioperative glucocorticoids in hip and knee surgery - benefit vs. harm? A review of randomized clinical trials. Acta Anaesthesiol Scand. 2013;57(7):823–34. https://doi.org/10.1111/aas.12115.
26. Kardash KJ, Sarrazin F, Tessler MJ, Velly AM. Single-dose dexamethasone reduces dynamic pain after total hip arthroplasty. Anesth Analg. 2008;106(4):1253–7, table of contents. https://doi.org/10.1213/ANE.0b013e318164f319.
27. Koh IJ, Chang CB, Lee JH, Jeon YT, Kim TK. Preemptive low-dose dexamethasone reduces postoperative emesis and pain after TKA: a randomized controlled study. Clin Orthop Relat Res. 2013;471(9):3010–20. https://doi.org/10.1007/s11999-013-3032-5.
28. Lei Y, Huang Q, Xu B, Zhang S, Cao G, Pei F. Multiple low-dose dexamethasone further improves clinical outcomes following Total hip Arthroplasty. J Arthroplast. 2018;33(5):1426–31. https://doi.org/10.1016/j.arth.2017.11.057.
29. Ho J, Kuhn RJ, Smith KM. Update on treatment options for constipation. Orthopedics. 2008;31(6):570–4. https://doi.org/10.3928/01477447-20080601-12.
30. Bergeron R, Blier P. Cisapride for the treatment of nausea produced by selective serotonin reuptake inhibitors. Am J Psychiatry. 1994;151(7):1084–6. https://doi.org/10.1176/ajp.151.7.1084.
31. Richardson AB, Bala A, Wellman SS, Attarian DE, Bolognesi MP, Grant SA. Perioperative dexamethasone administration does not increase the incidence of postoperative infection in Total hip and knee Arthroplasty: a retrospective analysis. J Arthroplast. 2016;31(8):1784–7. https://doi.org/10.1016/j.arth.2016.01.028.
32. Gan TJ. Risk factors for postoperative nausea and vomiting. Anesth Analg. 2006;102(6):1884–98. https://doi.org/10.1213/01.ANE.0000219597.16143.4D.

Effect of sex differences in remifentanil requirements for inhibiting the response to a CO_2 pneumoperitoneum during propofol anesthesia

Chengwei Yang[1†], Yuanyuan Feng[2†], Sheng Wang[1], Mingming Han[1], Song Wang[1], Fang Kang[1], Xiang Huang[1] and Juan Li[1*]

Abstract

Background: A CO_2 pneumoperitoneum during a laparoscopic procedure causes violent hemodynamic changes. However, the remifentanil required to inhibit the cardiovascular response to a CO_2 pneumoperitoneum combined with propofol remains unknown. Moreover, the sex of the patient may influence the response to opioids, which can affect this requirement. The main objective of this study was to compare the required median effective concentration (EC_{50}) of remifentanil for inhibiting the cardiovascular response to a CO_2 pneumoperitoneum between female and male patients during propofol anesthesia.

Methods: The current study is an up-and-down sequential allocation trial. Forty-six patients with American Society of Anesthesiologists physical status I or II, a body mass index 18 to 30 kg/m^2, aged 20 to 60 years, and scheduled for laparoscopic surgery were enrolled. Induction of anesthesia was performed by target-controlled infusion. The effective effect-site concentration (Ce) of propofol was 4 μg/ml. The Ce of remifentanil was initially 4 ng/ml and then adjusted to a predetermined level after I-gel laryngeal mask airway insertion. The Ce of remifentanil for each patient was determined by the response of the previous patient using the modified Dixon "up-and-down" method. The first patient received remifentanil at 5.0 ng/ml Ce, and the step size between patients was 0.5 ng/ml.

Results: Patients characteristics including age, body mass index, American Society of Anesthesiologists physical status, type of surgery and surgery duration, were comparable between male and female patients. The EC_{50} of remifentanil required to inhibit the response to a CO_2 pneumoperitoneum based on the Dixon "up-and-down" method in women (4.17 ± 0.38 ng/ml) was significantly lower than that in men (5.00 ± 0.52 ng/ml) during propofol anesthesia ($P = 0.01$).

Conclusions: The EC_{50} of remifentanil required to inhibit the response to a CO_2 pneumoperitoneum was lower in women than in men during propofol anesthesia.

Keywords: Anesthesia, Pneumoperitoneum, Pharmacology, Remifentanil

* Correspondence: huamuzi1999@163.com
†Chengwei Yang and Yuanyuan Feng contributed equally to this work.
[1]Department of Anesthesiology, The First Affiliated Hospital of USTC, Division of Life Sciences and Medicine, University of Science and Technology of China, Hefei 230036, China

Background

Currently, laparoscopic surgery is widely used due to its minimal invasiveness, low postoperative pain, short length of hospitalization and rapid postoperative recovery [1, 2]. However, a CO_2 pneumoperitoneum during a laparoscopic procedure causes violent hemodynamic changes [3, 4]. Zou et al. [5] demonstrated that the response to a CO_2 pneumoperitoneum was even stronger than that to the surgical incision.

A combination of remifentanil and propofol is commonly used for total intravenous anesthesia. Remifentanil has a very short infusion time-related half-life and is suitable for continuous infusion [6]. Moreover, it can inhibit the stress reaction effectively. The onset and recovery time of propofol are rapid, making sedation easy to control [7, 8]. Although there have been several studies investigating the median effective concentration (EC_{50}) of remifentanil during propofol anesthesia in different situations [9–11], the remifentanil required to inhibit the cardiovascular response to a CO_2 pneumoperitoneum combined with propofol remains unknown.

Moreover, the sex of the patient may influence the response to analgesic treatment with opioids, which can affect these requirements [12–14]. Men seem to need more opioids to achieve the same effect than women [15]. A recent study showed that the remifentanil requirements for the insertion of a laryngeal mask airway were higher in men than in women [16]. Accordingly, we hypothesized that the sex of the patient may affect the remifentanil required to inhibit the cardiovascular response to a CO_2 pneumoperitoneum.

The main objective of this study was to compare the EC_{50} of remifentanil required to inhibit the cardiovascular response to a CO_2 pneumoperitoneum between female and male patients during propofol anesthesia.

Methods

The current study is an up-and-down sequential allocation trial. This study was approved by the Clinical Research Ethics Committee of Anhui Provincial Hospital (2016–110) and registered at http://www.chictr.org.cn (ChiCTR-IOR-17011906). Written informed consent was obtained from 46 patients undergoing elective laparoscopic surgery. The inclusion criteria were an age between 20 and 60 years old, an American Society of Anesthesiologists (ASA) physical status I or II and a body mass index (BMI) 18 to 30 kg/m^2. The exclusion criteria included a history of cardiac, pulmonary, renal or liver diseases, alcohol or drug abuse, current use of vasoactive drugs, and recent use of any drugs known to affect the sympathetic adrenergic response.

All patients fasted routinely before surgery and received no premedication. Electrocardiograms, pulse oxygen saturation, end-tidal CO_2 concentrations ($EtCO_2$), and invasive radial arterial pressures were monitored. A bispectral index (BIS) monitor (BIS VISTATM monitor, Aspect Medical Systems, Norwood, MA) was used to monitor the depth of anesthesia.

Before anesthesia, 15 kg/ml lactated Ringer's solution was administered and then maintained at a rate of 10 ml/kg/h. Patients were preoxygenated with 100% oxygen for 3 min. Induction of anesthesia was performed by a target-controlled infusion (TCI) pump (CP-730TCI; Inc., Beijing SLGO, China). The effective effect-site concentrations (Ce) of propofol (Marsh pharmacokinetic model) and remifentanil (Minto pharmacokinetic model) were 4 μg/ml and 4 ng/ml respectively. After loss of consciousness, 0.6 mg/kg rocuronium was injected intravenously, and then an I-gel laryngeal mask airway (LMA, size 3 for women, size 4 for men) was inserted. Mechanical ventilation was controlled with a tidal volume of 6–8 ml/kg and respiratory rate of 12–14 breaths per minute, maintaining the $P_{ET}CO_2$ within 35–45 mmHg. Three minutes after LMA insertion, the Ce of remifentanil was adjusted to a predetermined level. After maintaining the predetermined target Ce of remifentanil for at least 10 min, a CO_2 pneumoperitoneum was established with a Veress insufflation needle. The pneumoperitoneum pressure of the machine (Inc., Stryker, America) was maintained at 14 mmHg, and the CO_2 flow rate was 20 l per minute.

The Ce of remifentanil for each patient was determined by the response of the previous patient using the modified Dixon "up-and-down" method [17]. The first patient in each group received remifentanil at 5.0 ng/ml Ce, and the step size was 0.5 ng/ml. The response of patients to the CO_2 pneumoperitoneum was determined by another anesthesiologist blinded to the remifentanil concentrations as either positive or negative. If the increase in the mean arterial pressure (MAP) or heart rate (HR) was more than 20% of its baseline, the response was defined as positive. In contrast, a negative response was defined as an increase in the MAP or HR of less than 20% of its baseline [5]. Patients' MAP, HR and BIS values were recorded before induction, at baseline (defined as the average of 3 and 1 min measured values before the CO_2 pneumoperitoneum) and 1 and 3 min after a stable pneumoperitoneum pressure was maintained. The increase in the MAP or HR was the difference between the average of the 1 and 3 min measured values after CO_2 pneumoperitoneum and its baseline value. During this study, when the patient's HR was less than 50 beats per minute, 0.5 mg atropine was injected intravenously. A bolus of 6–10 mg ephedrine was administered intravenously if the MAP was less than 50 mmHg. These patients were excluded from our study. The study was continued until 6 negative/positive crossover pairs had occurred. After finishing this study, intravenous administration of propofol and remifentanil was used to maintain the BIS between 40 and 60, and to ensure that the change in the MAP and HR did not exceed 20% of their baseline values. A TOF monitor (Veryark-TOF, Guangxi, China) was used to determine neuromuscular blockade. Rocuronium (0.15 mg/kg) was intravenously injected to maintain muscle relaxation when T_1 twitch height reached 25% of the control.

Statistical analysis was performed using SPSS version 13.0 software (SPSS Inc., Chicago, IL). Data are expressed as the means ± standard deviations for continuous variables or the number (percentage) of patients. The EC_{50} of the remifentanil required to inhibit the cardiovascular response to a CO_2 pneumoperitoneum in each group was determined by calculating the average of the midpoint dose of each pair of patients after 6 negative/positive crossover points were obtained. The "up-and-down" data were also analyzed by probit analysis [18, 19], deriving the EC_{50} and the 95% effective effect-site concentration (EC_{95}) with their 95% confidence intervals (CIs). A t test was used to compare the EC_{50} values. Repeated measures analysis of variance was used to compare MAP, HR and BIS changes. All P values < 0.05 indicated significant differences.

Results

Twenty-three male and 23 female patients were enrolled in this study. One female patient was excluded due to a MAP < 50 mmHg. One male patient was excluded due to an HR < 50 beats/min. Finally, 44 patients (22 male, 22 female) completed the study. The patients characteristics are shown in Table 1. Age, BMI, ASA physical status, type of surgery and surgery duration were comparable between the males and females. However, height and weight were significantly lower in the females.

The sequences for negative and positive responses to the CO_2 pneumoperitoneum in the 2 groups are shown in Fig. 1. The EC_{50} of remifentanil required to inhibit a CO_2 pneumoperitoneum based on the Dixon "up-and-down" method in women (4.17 ± 0.38 ng/ml) was significantly lower than that in men (5.00 ± 0.52 ng/ml) during propofol anesthesia ($P = 0.01$).

Table 1 Patient Characteristics

	Male ($n = 22$)	Female ($n = 22$)	P
Age, years	38 ± 11	40 ± 10	0.56
Height, cm	172 ± 4	160 ± 5	<0.001
Weight, kg	69 ± 7	60 ± 10	0.001
BMI, kg/m^2	23.4 ± 2.6	23.5 ± 3.7	0.94
ASA physical status (I/II)	18/4	20/2	0.39
Type of surgery (LA/LC)	15/7	14/8	0.75
Surgery duration	58.4 ± 13.4	57.3 ± 18.5	0.82

Values are presented as the means±standard or numbers. *BMI* Body mass index, *ASA* American society of anesthesiologists, *LA* Laparoscopic appendectomy, *LC* Laparoscopic cholecystectomy

From the probit analysis, the EC_{50} and EC_{95} of remifentanil (95% confidence interval [CI]) were 4.30 (3.49–4.82) ng/ml and 5.27 (4.78–10.22) ng/ml in women and 5.16 (4.64–5.58) ng/ml and 6.19 (5.70–8.99) ng/ml in men, respectively (Fig. 2).

The MAP, HR and BIS values over time are shown in Table 2. The hemodynamic and BIS data were not significantly different between the sexes.

Discussion

The present study demonstrated that the EC_{50} of remifentanil required to inhibit the cardiovascular response to a CO_2 pneumoperitoneum in women (4.17 ± 0.38 ng/ml) was lower than that in men (5.00 ± 0.52 ng/ml) during propofol anesthesia.

The hemodynamic change induced by a CO_2 pneumoperitoneum during laparoscopic surgery is a challenge to anesthesiologists [3, 20]. Remifentanil intravenously combined with general anesthesia provides stable hemodynamics during laparoscopic surgery [21]. Moreover, remifentanil effectively decreases the sevoflurane concentration to block the sympathetic adrenergic response to the CO_2 pneumoperitoneum [5]. In this study, we were interested in exploring the EC50 of remifentanil required to inhibit the cardiovascular response to a CO_2 pneumoperitoneum stimulus in both sexes during propofol anesthesia.

To the best of our knowledge, this is the first study investigating the EC_{50} of remifentanil required to inhibit the cardiovascular response to a CO_2 pneumoperitoneum during propofol anesthesia. The EC_{50} of remifentanil required was higher than that measured by Albertin et al. (2.1 ng/ml) [9] or Wang et al. (3.09 ng/ml) [22]. The reason may be that a skin incision, which induces pain to the body surface and disappears fast, was used in their studies. This is consistent with Zou's experiment [5]. The influence of CO_2 pneumoperitoneum on the circulatory system is more complicated than that caused by a surgical incision. The increase in intra-abdominal pressure causes blood vessels to compress and reduces venous return, leading to a decrease in cardiac output. However, the increase in the partial pressure of CO_2 in arterial blood, which may cause hypercapnia, can induce a sympathetic adrenergic response. As a result, the CO_2 pneumoperitoneum causes an increase in blood pressure and heart rate [23, 24]. Furthermore, a continuous CO_2 pneumoperitoneum distends the peritoneum and elicits a much stronger response than a skin incision. Accordingly, the required EC_{50} of remifentanil would be increased.

Increasing numbers of studies have focused on the sex differences in the response to anesthetics, especially

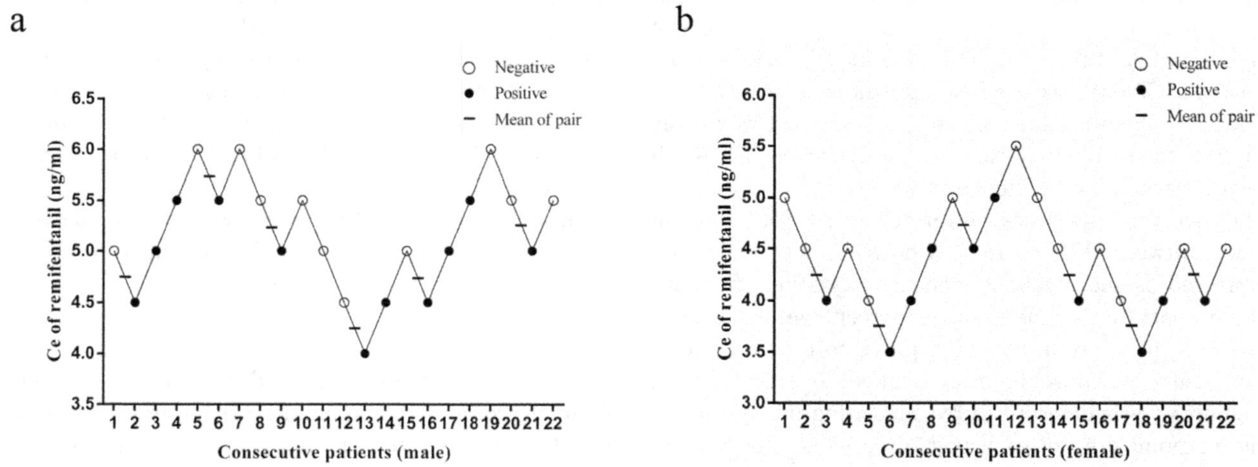

Fig. 1 Assessment of negative or positive responses to inhibit a CO_2 pneumoperitoneum under a predetermined Ce of remifentanil using the Dixon "up-and-down" method in 22 consecutive male patients (**a**) and 22 consecutive female patients (**b**). Horizontal bars represent crossover midpoints (negative to positive). The EC_{50} values of remifentanil required to inhibit the CO_2 pneumoperitoneum in the male group and the female group were 5.00 ± 0.52 ng/ml and 4.17 ± 0.38 ng/ml, respectively. EC_{50}, median effective concentration

opioids [12, 15, 16, 25]. In our study, the EC_{50} of remifentanil required to inhibit the cardiovascular response to a CO_2 pneumoperitoneum was lower in women than in men during propofol anesthesia. There are some possible explanations for this result. First, Zubieta et al. demonstrated that premenopausal females have significantly higher mu-receptor binding potential than males in the cortical and subcortical areas [26]. Females may have a significantly greater response to mu opioid-receptor agonists than males [15, 27]. However, some studies have reported no sex differences in the analgesic responses to mu opioid- receptor agonists [28, 29]. Differences in the opioids, drug doses or pain models used may contribute to the different results. Second, previous studies have demonstrated that men have higher cortisol responses than women after exposure to acute real-life psychological stress or controlled laboratory stress tasks [30, 31]. However, sex differences in the hypothalamus–

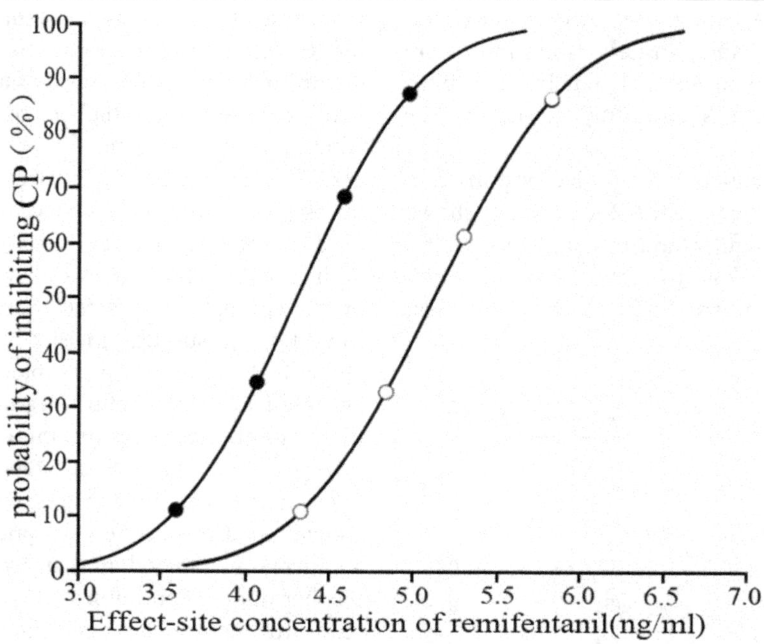

Fig. 2 Effect-site concentration and response curves from the probit analysis in male (o) and female (•) patients. The EC_{50} and EC_{95} of remifentanil (95% confidence interval) required to inhibit the CO_2 pneumoperitoneum were 4.30 (3.49–4.82) ng/ml and 5.27 (4.78–10.22) ng/ml in women and 5.16 (4.64–5.58) ng/ml and 6.19 (5.70–8.99) ng/ml in men, respectively. CP, CO_2 pneumoperitoneum; EC_{50}, median effective concentration; EC_{95}, 95% effective effect-site concentration

Table 2 Hemodynamic profiles and BISs during the CO_2 pneumoperitoneum

	Sex	Before induction	3 min before CP	1 min before CP	1 min after CP	3 min after CP
MAP, mmHg	Male	94 ± 11	73 ± 9	70 ± 8	87 ± 11	85 ± 11
	Female	92 ± 10	76 ± 11	70 ± 10	92 ± 13	88 ± 13
P		0.43	0.41	0.91	0.28	0.40
HR, beats/minute	Male	73 ± 8	61 ± 6	60 ± 6	68 ± 8	68 ± 8
	Female	76 ± 9	63 ± 7	60 ± 8	67 ± 11	66 ± 10
P		0.17	0.37	0.90	0.79	0.68
BIS	Male	96.3 ± 1.7	51.7 ± 6.4	49.7 ± 6.8	52.1 ± 6.5	51.8 ± 6.9
	Female	96.0 ± 1.4	52.1 ± 7.4	50.1 ± 7.7	53.0 ± 7.7	52.3 ± 8.1
P		0.51	0.83	0.85	0.69	0.83

Values are showed as the means±standard deviation. *MAP*, Mean arterial pressure; *HR* Heart rate, *BIS* Bispectral index, *CP* CO_2 pneumoperitoneum

pituitary–adrenal axis responses to stress remain controversial [32, 33]. Moreover, whether sex differences exist in response to a CO_2 pneumoperitoneum is unknown. Third, there is a sex difference in the activity of nonspecific esterase [34], which is responsible for metabolizing remifentanil. However, the specific esterase action on remifentanil remains unknown, and more research is needed.

According to a previous study, the EC_{95} (95%CI) of remifentanil required for successful LMA insertion in women and men was 3.38 (3.0–3.48) ng/ml and 3.94 (3.80–3.98) ng/ml, respectively, during propofol (Ce 3.5 μg/ml) anesthesia [16]. Therefore, the Ce of remifentanil was set at 4.0 ng/ml for LMA insertion. Furthermore, in our study, the heights and weights of the men were greater than those of the women. However, the influence of the differences in demographic data on our results may be small, as the Ce of remifentanil was calculated and adjusted by these covariates in the Minto model.

There are some limitations in our study. First, we did not take patients' blood samples to measure the actual Ce of remifentanil. Instead, we calculated the remifentanil Ce using the Minto pharmacokinetic model, which has been widely used with acceptable levels of inaccuracy and bias in clinical settings [35]. Second, we did not perform arterial blood gas analysis to determine whether hypercarbia existed during the period of the CO_2 pneumoperitoneum, which may have led to a sympathetic adrenergic response if the increased ventilation failed to compensate for the absorbed CO_2. However, a previous study demonstrated that for changes in the $P_{ET}CO_2$ above 43 and below 26 mmHg, the mean arterial pressure increased and decreased, respectively [36]. In our study, we maintained the $P_{ET}CO_2$ within 35–45 mmHg to minimize the impact on blood pressure. Third, for safety considerations, we excluded patients with low MAPs and HRs, which may have resulted in an overestimation of the EC_{50} of remifentanil because these patients were possibly more sensitive to the drugs given. Lastly, the EC_{95} of remifentanil calculated by the "up-and-down" method may not be a reliable value [37], and further research may be needed for clinical practice.

Conclusions

The EC_{50} of remifentanil required to inhibit the cardiovascular response to a CO_2 pneumoperitoneum was lower in women than in men during propofol anesthesia using the modified Dixon "up-and-down" method. Patient sex should be taken into consideration for appropriate dosing when using remifentanil for laparoscopic surgery.

Abbreviations

ASA: American society of anesthesiologists; BIS: Bispectral index; BMI: Body mass index; Ce: Effect-site concentration; CP: CO_2 pneumoperitoneum; EC_{50}: Median effective concentration; EC_{95}: 95% effective effect-site concentration; HR: Heart rate; LA: Laparoscopic appendectomy; LC: Laparoscopic cholecystectomy; LMA: Laryngeal mask airway; MAP: Mean arterial pressure

Acknowledgements

Not applicable.

Authors' contributions

CY and JL designed the study. SW1 (Sheng Wang), MH and FK recruited patients. SW2 (Song Wang) performed statistical processing. YF wrote the manuscript. XH and JL revised the manuscript. All authors read and approved the manuscript in its final version.

Author details

[1]Department of Anesthesiology, The First Affiliated Hospital of USTC, Division of Life Sciences and Medicine, University of Science and Technology of China, Hefei 230036, China. [2]Department of Hematology, The First Affiliated Hospital of USTC, Division of Life Sciences and Medicine, University of Science and Technology of China, Hefei 230031, China.

References

1. Khorgami Z, Shoar S, Anbara T, Soroush A, Nasiri S, Movafegh A, Aminian A. A randomized clinical trial comparing 4-port, 3-port, and single-incision laparoscopic cholecystectomy. J Invest Surg : Official J Acad Surg Res. 2014; 27(3):147–54.
2. Grace PA, Quereshi A, Coleman J, Keane R, McEntee G, Broe P, Osborne H, Bouchier-Hayes D. Reduced postoperative hospitalization after laparoscopic cholecystectomy. Br J Surg. 1991;78(2):160–2.

3. Mann C, Boccara G, Pouzeratte Y, Eliet J, Serradel-Le Gal C, Vergnes C, Bichet DG, Guillon G, Fabre JM, Colson P. The relationship among carbon dioxide pneumoperitoneum, vasopressin release, and hemodynamic changes. Anesth Analg. 1999;89(2):278–83.
4. Akca O. Optimizing the intraoperative management of carbon dioxide concentration. Curr Opin Anaesthesiol. 2006;19(1):19–25.
5. Zou ZY, Zhao YL, Yang XL, Zhang GY, Zhou HG. Effects of different remifentanil target concentrations on MAC BAR of sevoflurane in gynaecological patients with CO2 pneumoperitoneum stimulus. Br J Anaesth, 4. 2014;114:634–9.
6. Glass PS, Gan TJ, Howell S. A review of the pharmacokinetics and pharmacodynamics of remifentanil. Anesth Analg. 1999;89(4 Suppl):S7–14.
7. Sieg A, Beck S, Scholl SG, Heil FJ, Gotthardt DN, Stremmel W, Rex DK, Friedrich K. Safety analysis of endoscopist-directed propofol sedation: a prospective, national multicenter study of 24 441 patients in German outpatient practices. J Gastroenterol Hepatol. 2014;29(3):517–23.
8. Khan HA, Umar M, Tul-Bushra H, Nisar G, Bilal M, Umar S. Safety of non-anaesthesiologist-administered propofol sedation in ERCP. Arab J Gastroenterol : Official Publication Pan-Arab Assoc Gastroenterol. 2014;15(1):32–5.
9. Albertin A, Casati A, Federica L, Roberto V, Travaglini V, Bergonzi P, Torri G. The effect-site concentration of remifentanil blunting cardiovascular responses to tracheal intubation and skin incision during bispectral index-guided propofol anesthesia. Anesth Analg. 2005;101(1):125–30 table of contents.
10. Liu Z, Wang F, Wang W, Luo Y. Median effective concentration of remifentanil for the inhibition of laryngoscope-induced cardiovascular responses. Exp Ther Med. 2016;12(1):457–62.
11. Yoo JY, Kwak HJ, Lee KC, Kim GW, Kim JY. Predicted EC (5)(0) and EC (9)(5) of Remifentanil for smooth removal of a laryngeal mask airway under Propofol anesthesia. Yonsei Med J. 2015;56(4):1128–33.
12. Fillingim RB, Gear RW. Sex differences in opioid analgesia: clinical and experimental findings. Eur J Pain. 2004;8(5):413–25.
13. Craft RM. Sex differences in opioid analgesia: "from mouse to man". Clin J Pain. 2003;19(3):175–86.
14. Dahan A, Kest B, Waxman AR, Sarton E. Sex-specific responses to opiates: animal and human studies. Anesth Analg. 2008;107(1):83–95.
15. Sarton E, Olofsen E, Romberg R, den Hartigh J, Kest B, Nieuwenhuijs D, Burm A, Teppema L, Dahan A. Sex differences in morphine analgesia: an experimental study in healthy volunteers. Anesthesiol. 2000;93(5):1245–54 discussion 1246A.
16. Joe HB, Kim JY, Kwak HJ, Oh SE, Lee SY, Park SY. Effect of sex differences in remifentanil requirements for the insertion of a laryngeal mask airway during propofol anesthesia: a prospective randomized trial. Medicine. 2016; 95(39):e5032.
17. Dixon WJ. Staircase bioassay: the up-and-down method. Neurosci Biobehav Rev. 1991;15(1):47–50.
18. Han MM, Xue FS, Kang F, Huang X, Li J. Male requires a higher median target effect-site concentration of propofol for I-gel placement when combined with dexmedetomidine. Anaesth, Crit Care Pain Med. 2019;38(1):57–61.
19. Mustola S, Toivonen J. Effect-site concentration of remifentanil attenuating surgical stress index responses to intubation of the trachea. Anaesth. 2010; 65(6):581–5.
20. Joris JL, Noirot DP, Legrand MJ, Jacquet NJ, Lamy ML. Hemodynamic changes during laparoscopic cholecystectomy. Anesth Analg. 1993;76(5): 1067–71.
21. Watanabe K, Kashiwagi K, Kamiyama T, Yamamoto M, Fukunaga M, Inada E, Kamiyama Y. High-dose remifentanil suppresses stress response associated with pneumoperitoneum during laparoscopic colectomy. J Anesth. 2014; 28(3):334–40.
22. Wang JF, Xu XP, Yu XY, Li JB, Wu X, Chen JC, Hu XW, Deng XM. Remifentanil requirement for inhibiting responses to tracheal intubation and skin incision is reduced in patients with Parkinson's disease undergoing deep brain stimulator implantation. J Neurosurg Anesthesiol. 2016;28(4): 303–8.
23. Junghans T, Bohm B, Grundel K, Schwenk W. Effects of pneumoperitoneum with carbon dioxide, argon, or helium on hemodynamic and respiratory function. Arch Surg (Chicago, Ill : 1960). 1997;132(3):272–8.
24. Mas A, Saura P, Joseph D, Blanch L, Baigorri F, Artigas A, Fernandez R. Effect of acute moderate changes in PaCO2 on global hemodynamics and gastric perfusion. Crit Care Med. 2000;28(2):360–5.
25. Soh S, Park WK, Kang SW, Lee BR, Lee JR. Sex differences in remifentanil requirements for preventing cough during anesthetic emergence. Yonsei Med J. 2014;55(3):807–14.
26. Zubieta JK, Dannals RF, Frost JJ. Gender and age influences on human brain mu-opioid receptor binding measured by PET. Am J Psychiatry. 1999;156(6): 842–8.
27. Pud D, Yarnitsky D, Sprecher E, Rogowski Z, Adler R, Eisenberg E. Can personality traits and gender predict the response to morphine? An experimental cold pain study. Eur J Pain. 2006;10(2):103–12.
28. Romberg R, Olofsen E, Sarton E, den Hartigh J, Taschner PE, Dahan A. Pharmacokinetic-pharmacodynamic modeling of morphine-6-glucuronide-induced analgesia in healthy volunteers: absence of sex differences. Anesthesiol. 2004;100(1):120–33.
29. Olofsen E, Romberg R, Bijl H, Mooren R, Engbers F, Kest B, Dahan A. Alfentanil and placebo analgesia: no sex differences detected in models of experimental pain. Anesthesiol. 2005;103(1):130–9.
30. Kirschbaum C, Wust S, Hellhammer D. Consistent sex differences in cortisol responses to psychological stress. Psychosom Med. 1992;54(6):648–57.
31. Stroud LR, Salovey P, Epel ES. Sex differences in stress responses: social rejection versus achievement stress. Biol Psychiatry. 2002;52(4):318–27.
32. Kirschbaum C, Wust S, Faig HG, Hellhammer DH. Heritability of cortisol responses to human corticotropin-releasing hormone, ergometry, and psychological stress in humans. J Clin Endocrinol Metab. 1992;75(6):1526–30.
33. Back SE, Waldrop AE, Saladin ME, Yeatts SD, Simpson A, McRae AL, Upadhyaya HP, Contini Sisson R, Spratt EG, Allen J, et al. Effects of gender and cigarette smoking on reactivity to psychological and pharmacological stress provocation. Psychoneuroendocrinology. 2008;33(5):560–8.
34. Ciccone GK, Holdcroft A. Drugs and sex differences: a review of drugs relating to anaesthesia. Br J Anaesth. 1999;82(2):255–65.
35. Mertens MJ, Engbers FH, Burm AG, Vuyk J. Predictive performance of computer-controlled infusion of remifentanil during propofol/remifentanil anaesthesia. Br J Anaesth. 2003;90(2):132–41.
36. Kuznetsova DV, Kulikov VP. Cerebrovascular and systemic hemodynamic response to carbon dioxide in humans. Blood Press Monit. 2014;19(2):81–9.
37. Pace NL, Stylianou MP. Advances in and limitations of up-and-down methodology: a precis of clinical use, study design, and dose estimation in anesthesia research. Anesthesiol. 2007;107(1):144–52.

14

Outcomes of general anesthesia versus conscious sedation for stroke undergoing endovascular treatment

Teng-Fei Wan[1†], Rui Xu[2†], Zi-Ai Zhao[3], Yan Lv[3], Hui-Sheng Chen[3*] and Liang Liu[3*]

Abstract

Background: The impact of anesthesia strategy on the outcomes of acute ischemic stroke (AIS) patients undergoing endovascular treatment is currently controversy. Thus, we performed this meta-analysis to compare the differences of clinical and angiographic outcomes between general anesthesia (GA) and conscious sedation (CS).

Methods: A literature search in PubMed, Embase, and Web of Knowledge databases through February 2019 was conducted for related records on GA and CS of AIS undergoing endovascular treatment. The results of the studies were pooled and meta-analyzed with fixed- or random-effect model based on heterogeneity test in total and subgroup analyses.

Results: Twenty-three studies including 6703 patients were analyzed in this meta-analysis. We found that patients in the GA group have lower odds of favorable functional outcome (mRS scores ≤2) compared with the CS group (odds ratio [OR] = 0.62, 95% confidence interval [CI]: 0.49–0.77), and higher risk of mortality (OR = 1.68, 95% CI: 1.49–1.90), pneumonia (OR = 1.78, 95% CI: 1.40–2.26), symptomatic intracranial hemorrhage (OR = 1.64, 95% CI: 1.13–2.37). However, no significant differences were seen between the groups in the rate of recanalization (OR = 1.07, 95% CI: 0.89–1.28), vessel dissection or perforation (OR = 1.00, 95% CI: 0.98–1.03) and asymptomatic intracranial hemorrhage (OR = 1.19, 95% CI: 0.96–1.47). While in the RCT subgroup analysis, we found patients in the GA group does not show lower rate of favorable functional outcome compared with the CS group (OR = 1.84, 95% CI: 1.17–2.89). And there was no significant difference in the rate of mortality between GA and CS groups during RCT subgroup analysis (OR = 0.74, 95% CI: 0.43–1.27).

Conclusions: AIS patients performed endovascular treatment under GA compared with CS was associated with worse functional outcome and increased rate of mortality, but differences in worsened outcomes do not exist when one looks into the GA vs. CS RCTs. Moreover, these findings are mainly based on the retrospective studies and additional multi-center randomized controlled trials to definitively address these issues is warranted.

Keywords: Ischemic stroke, Anesthesia, Endovascular treatment, Meta-analysis

Background

Acute ischemic stroke (AIS) is one of the leading causes of death and long-term disability. The common therapy for AIS patients with large-vessel occlusion is endovascular treatment [1]. During the endovascular treatment, there are two types of anesthesia /sedation which are commonly used to make the AIS patients immobile, including general anesthesia (GA) and conscious sedation (CS). However, the understanding of the impact of GA or CS on the outcomes of endovascular treatment remains controversial. Previous observational studies report worse outcomes from GA than that from CS during endovascular treatment [2]. By contrast, there were some new randomized trials found that functional independence or worse tissue is either no different in the patients who had GA [3–5]. While the available previous meta-analysis studies revealed superior neurological outcome with CS compared with GA [2, 6, 7]. But those meta-analysis studies were limited by the small sample size and the

* Correspondence: chszh@aliyun.com; 18580763671@163.com
[†]Teng-Fei Wan and Rui Xu contributed equally to this work.
[3]Department of Neurology, the General Hospital of Northern Theater Command , No. 83 Wenhua Street, Shenyang 110016, Liaoning, China

included studies were not comprehensive. Besides, there are updated and larger randomized clinical trials have conducted. In light of the continuing debate and limitations among these studies, a new and comprehensive meta-analysis study is warranted. We aim to compare the outcomes of AIS patients with GA and CS during the procedures.

Methods

Search strategy

This systematic review and meta-analysis was conducted in accordance with the PRISMA (Preferred Reporting Items for Systematic Reviews and Meta-Analyses) statement. All published articles were searched without language restricted in the PubMed, Embase, and Web of Knowledge databases through February 2019. Key words were identified and in various relevant combinations as follows: endovascular OR 'fibrinolytic agents' OR thromboembolism OR catheter OR transcatheter OR thrombolysis OR fibrinolysis OR recanalization OR embolectomy OR thrombectomy AND "intracranial embolism" OR thrombosis OR stroke AND "conscious sedation" OR "general anesthesia". The updated literature search was conducted independently by two authors (L.L., T.-F. W.). All articles were retrieved and their references were manually screened to avoid missing out other relevant articles. If data could not be extracted in the original articles, we contacted the authors to obtain them.

Study selection

The eligible studies were evaluated by two authors (T.-F.W., L.L.) independently. Disagreement was resolved by discussion, and if necessary, by a third reviewer (H.-S. C).The inclusion criteria were as follows: (1) studies evaluating the outcomes of general anesthesia versus conscious sedation during endovascular therapy among acute ischemic stroke patients; (2) studies reporting mortality or functional outcome using the modified Rankin scale (mRS) for the general anesthesia and conscious sedation groups; and (3) the effect estimates of studies could be extracted or calculated from the available data. We excluded those studies with unavailable data to calculate or extract effect estimates. The abstracts from meeting proceedings, duplicate reports, case reports, reviews, comments, or animal studies were also excluded.

Data extraction

Two independent investigators (L.L., T.-F. W.) extracted following variables from the trials' primary texts to ensure the reliability of the results, including the first author's name, publication year, study period, country, inclusion criteria, exclusion criteria, outcomes, type of endovascular treatment, sample size, good outcomes (mRS scores ≤2 at 90 days) and other outcomes (including mortality, pneumonia, successful recanalization, symptomatic intracranial hemorrhage [sICH], asymptomatic intracranial hemorrhage [aICH], and vessel dissection or perforation) during the random trial. Disagreement was resolved by discussion, and if necessary, by a third reviewer (Z.-A. Z.).

Quality assessment

Quality assessment of the studies was performed by two independent reviewers (L.L., T.-F. W.). We used the Newcastle-Ottawa Scale to assess the risk of selection, comparability and exposure or outcome for case-control and cohort studies, respectively. Eight items were included to assess the quality of studies with a 9-star system. The quality score ranges from 0 to 9 stars, we judged trials as a low-quality report study while the score is 0–3 stars, while a high quality study score is at least 7 stars. And the study with 4–6 stars was defined as a moderate quality study [8]. Moreover, we used Cochrane risk of bias tool to evaluate the quality of included RCTs [9].

Statistical analysis

The outcomes in each included study, including favorable functional outcome (mRS scores ≤2 at 90 days), mortality, pneumonia, successful recanalization, sICH, aICH, and vessel dissection or perforation were extracted from primary trial results, succeeding secondary publications and their supplementary materials. For each study, odds ratios (ORs) were expressed with their 95% confidence intervals (CIs) for each outcome of interest and were calculated from patient numbers with each outcome categorized by different anesthesia type treatment. The random-effects meta-analysis (DerSimonian-Laird method) or fixed-effects meta-analysis (Mantel-Haenszel method) was used for pooling across studies and the statistical significance of pooled ORs and 95% CIs were determined with a Z test [10]. Moreover, which effects model we used was according to our heterogeneity test. To determine the degree of heterogeneity among the studies included in our meta-analysis, the I-squared (I^2) statistic and the Cochran Q test were used [11], with I^2 values less than 25% representing low heterogeneity, 25~50% representing moderate heterogeneity, and more than 75% representing high heterogeneity, respectively. When I^2 values was less than 50%and the P value of the Q test was more than 0.1 among the studies included in the meta-analysis, the fixed-effects model was used for pooling across studies. While the I^2 values was more than 50% and the P value of the Q test was less than 0.1, the random-effects model was used. Moreover, we performed sensitivity analysis by sequentially excluding each study that we have included to assess the stability of the results. To quantitate the publication bias across included studies, the Egger regression and Begg's methods were used [12, 13]. All statistical tests were performed with STATA software version 12.0 (StataCorp, College Station, TX, USA). Statistical significance was based on a *P* value < 0.05 in all analyses.

Results

Characteristics of eligible studies

The PRISMA flow diagram is shown in Fig. 1. In detail, total 2575 records were identified from PubMed, Web of Science and Embase. Of these, 1540 duplicated records and 993 unrelated records were excluded after reading the abstracts alone. Of the remaining 42 records, 19 records were excluded after further screen through full-text reading (10 records did not provide outcome of interest or available data, 6 reviews, and 3 abstracts). Finally, 23 records were eligible in our meta-analysis [3–5, 14–33], including 5 randomized controlled trials (RCTs) and 18 non-RCTs.

The characteristics of the included studies are presented in Table 1. These studies were published during 2010–2018. Ten of the 23 included studies were performed in the United States of America. The patients both in GA and CS groups have received endovascular treatment, such as IA /IV tPA, mechanical thrombectomy, stent and thromboaspiration. The baseline NIHSS scores of all patients were listed in Additional file 3: Table S1. All of the included studies were involved in the analysis of mortality rate. Majority of included studies provided information regarding the effect of GA versus CS on the incidence of mRS scores ≤2 at 90 days except for two studies [25, 28]. The results of the Newcastle-Ottawa Scale showed that 16 studies had high quality and 4 studies with a moderate quality, and no study had less than five pluses

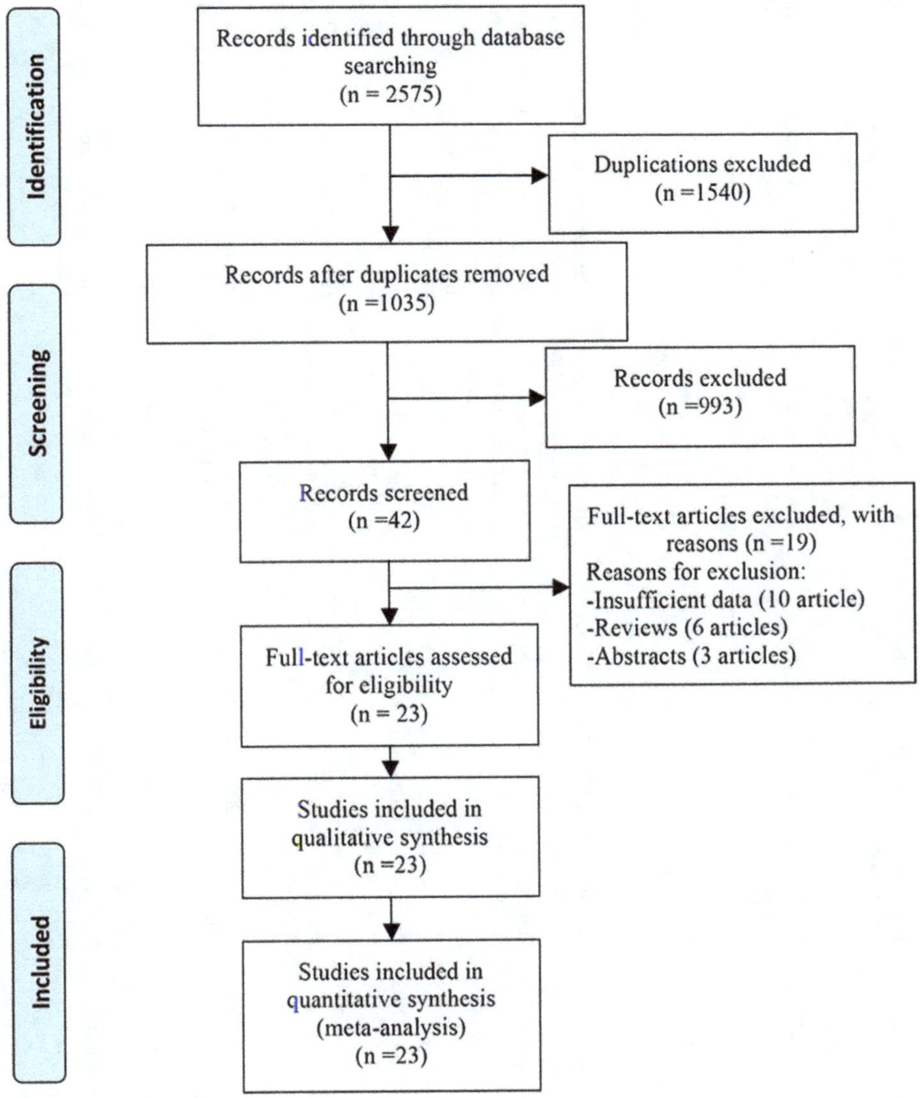

Fig. 1 Flow diagram of study identification

Table 1 Characteristics of the studies included in the meta-analysis

Author	Study design	Study Period	Country	Inclusion Criteria	Exclusion Criteria	Outcomes	Type of Endovascular Treatment	Sample Size (GA/CS)	Methodological quality[a]
Abou-Chebl et al. (2010)	Retrospective cohort study	2005–2009	USA	Anterior circulation AIS	Posterior circulation strokes; no intervention was performed	mRS and mortality on day 90	IA/IV tPA, mechanical thrombectomy, angioplasty	428/552	5
Jumaa et al. (2010)	Retrospective cohort study	2006–2009	USA	Middle cerebral artery–M1 segment occlusion treated with endovascular therapy	Vertebrobasilar occlusions; internal carotid artery terminus occlusion; M2 occlusion	mRS and mortality on day 90	IA/IV tPA and mechanical thrombectomy	53/73	7
Nichols et al. (2010)	Post hoc analysis of IMS II trial	NA	USA	Anterior circulation strokes and underwent angiography and/or intervention	Data were not available before or after angiography	Recanalization, mRS and mortality on day 90	IA/IV tPA, low-energy ultrasound	26/49	7
Sugg et al. (2010)	Retrospective cohort study	2007–2009	USA	AIS and underwent endovascular treatment within 8 h from symptom onset	NA	Recanalization, mRS and mortality on day 90	Mechanical thrombectomy	9/57	5
Davis et al. (2012)	Retrospective cohort study	2003–2009	Canada	AIS and received endovascular treatment	Management could not be determined	mRS and mortality on day 90	IA tPA and mechanical thrombectomy	48/48	7
Hassan et al. (2012)	Retrospective cohort study	2006–2010	USA	AIS and received endovascular treatment	The infarct burden was greater than or equal to one third of the middle cerebral artery territory	mRS and in-hospital mortality	IV tPA, endovascular technique not specified	53/83	5
Langner et al. (2013)	Retrospective cohort study	2005–2010	Germany	AIS and treated with endovascular therapy	NA	mRS and mortality	IA tPA and mechanical thrombectomy	19/105	8
Abou-Chebl et al. (2014)	Post hoc analysis of NASA registry	NA	North America	AIS and received endovascular treatment within 6 h from symptom onset	NA	mRS and mortality on day 90	IV tPA, mechanical thrombectomy	196/85	7
John, S et al. (2014)	Retrospective cohort study	2008–2012	USA	Anterior circulation AIS and treated with endovascular therapy	Posterior circulation AIS	In-hospital mortality and mRS on day 30	IV tPA, mechanical thrombectomy	91/99	9
Li et al. (2014)	Retrospective cohort study	2006–2012	USA	AIS and received endovascular treatment	NA	mRS and mortality	IA tPA, mechanical thrombectomy	35/74	8
Abou-Chebl et al. (2015)	Post hoc analysis of IMS III trial	2006–2011	USA	AIS, received IV tPA within 3 h and received endovascular treatment	Large regions of clear hypodensity on CT scan	mRS and in-hospital mortality	IV/IA tPA and mechanical thrombectomy	147/269	9
McDonald J.S et al. (2015)	Retrospective cohort study	2006–2013	USA	AIS and received mechanical thrombectomy	Patients who underwent another invasive surgery	In-hospital mortality and complications	IV tPA and mechanical thrombectomy	507/507	7
Van Den Berg L.A. et al. (2015)	Retrospective cohort study	2002–2013	Netherlands	Anterior circulation AIS	Patients lack of information	mRS and mortality	IA tPA and mechanical thrombectomy	70/278	7
Just, C. et al. (2016)	Retrospective cohort study	2000–2013	Canada	Underwent neuro-interventional stroke procedure	Aneurysm repair, carotid stenting, extracranial-intracranial bypass	mRS and mortality on day 90 and 180	IA tPA and mechanical thrombectomy, thromboaspiration	42/67	8

Table 1 Characteristics of the studies included in the meta-analysis *(Continued)*

Author	Study design	Study Period	Country	Inclusion Criteria	Exclusion Criteria	Outcomes	Type of Endovascular Treatment	Sample Size (GA/CS)	Methodological quality[a]
Berkhemer OA. et al. (2016)	Post hoc analysis of MR CLEAN	2010–2014	Netherlands	AIS patients who received mechanical thrombectomy or intra-arterial thrombolysis	Cerebral hemorrhage, coagulation abnormalities	mRS and mortality on day 90 and 180	IA tPA and mechanical thrombectomy, thromboaspiration	79/137	9
Schönenberger S et al. (2016)	RCT	2014–2016	Germany	Severe AIS, NIHSS> 10	diagnostic imaging results did not clearly depict site of vessel occlusion	NIHSS after 24 h, mRS and mortality on day 90	IA tPA and angioplasty, mechanical thrombectomy, thromboaspiration	73/77	NA
Bekelis, K. et al. (2017)	Retrospective cohort study	2009–2013	USA	AIS patients undergoing mechanical thrombectomy	NA	mortality in hospital	IV tPA, thromboaspiration	441/ 733	6
Lowhagen Henden, P. et al. (2017)	RCT	2013–2016	Sweden	Anterior circulation AIS, NIHSS> 10	Occlusion of posterior cerebral circulation	mRS and mortality on day 90 and 180	IV tPA, mechanical thrombectomy	45/45	NA
Slezak, A.et al. (2017)	Prospective study	2010–2015	Switzerland	Anterior circulation AIS	NA	mRS and mortality on day 90	IV tPA, mechanical thrombectomy	266/ 135	7
Simonsen, C. Z. et al. (2018)	RCT	2015–2017	Denmark	Anterior circulation AIS	Glasgow Coma Scale score < 9 or premorbid mRS score > 2	mRS and mortality on day 90 and 180	IA tPA, angioplasty, mechanical thrombectomy	65/63	NA
Peng et al. (2018)	Prospective study	2015.01–2015.08	China	Anterior circulation AIS	DWI lesion volume > 50 mL	Rates of successful recanalization and mRS on day 90	Interventional treatment with Solitaire	44/105	8
Omer F. Eker et al. (2018)	Post hoc analysis SWIFT PRIME trial	2013–2015	USA and Europe	Anterior circulation AIS	Subject who is contraindicated to IV t-PA	Rates of successful recanalization and mRS on day 90	Teated with Solitaire RevascularizationDevice and IV-tPA	32/65	8
Shanet et al. (2018)	Retrospective cohort study	2014–2016	China	Anterior circulation AIS	Received intra-arterial thrombolysis alone, with concomitant aneurysm or arteriovenous malformation	mRS and mortality on day 90	NA	114/ 114	8

[a]Newcastle Ottawa scale was designed to assess the quality of non-randomized studies. *GA* general anesthesia, *CS* conscious sedation, *AIS* acute ischemic stroke, *IA* intra-arterial, *IV* intra-venous, *tPA* tissue plasminogen activator, *mRS* modified Rankin Score, *NA* not available, *RCT* randomized controlled trial, *NIHSS* National Institute of Health Stroke Scale

on the Newcastle-Ottawa scale (Table 1). The results of quality assessment for RCTs were listed in Additional file 3: Table S2.

Outcomes

Six thousand seven hundred three patients were included in this meta-analysis in total, including 3820 patients in CS group and 2883 patients in GA group. The results of our meta-analysis suggested that GA patients have lower odds of favorable functional outcome (mRS scores ≤2) compared with CS patients (OR = 0.62, 95% CI: 0.49–0.77) (Fig. 2, Table 2). Moreover, GA was associated with a statistically significant higher risk of mortality (OR = 1.68, 95% CI: 1.49–1.90) (Fig. 3, Table 2), pneumonia (OR = 1.78, 95% CI: 1.40–2.26) (Table 2) and sICH (OR = 1.64, 95% CI: 1.13–2.37) (Table 2). However, there were no significant differences in the rate of recanalization (OR = 1.07, 95% CI: 0.89–1.28) (Table 2), vessel dissection or perforation (OR = 1.00, 95% CI: 0.98–1.03) (Table 2), aICH (OR = 1.19, 95% CI: 0.96–1.47) (Table 2) between the two groups.

While in the subgroup analysis, the rate of favorable functional outcome (mRS scores ≤2) in non-RCT subgroup also showed a statistically significant lower between CS and GA group (OR = 0.54, 95% CI: 0.44–0.66) but not in RCT subgroup (OR = 1.84, 95% CI: 1.17–2.89) (Fig. 2). Besides, GA was associated with significantly higher rate of mortality than CS in non-RCT subgroup (OR = 1.76, 95% CI: 1.55–1.99), but there was no significant difference in the rate of mortality between GA and CS groups during RCT subgroup analysis (OR = 0.74, 95% CI: 0.43–1.27) (Fig. 3).

Moreover, we have conducted an additional separate meta-analysis for high quality studies (quality scores

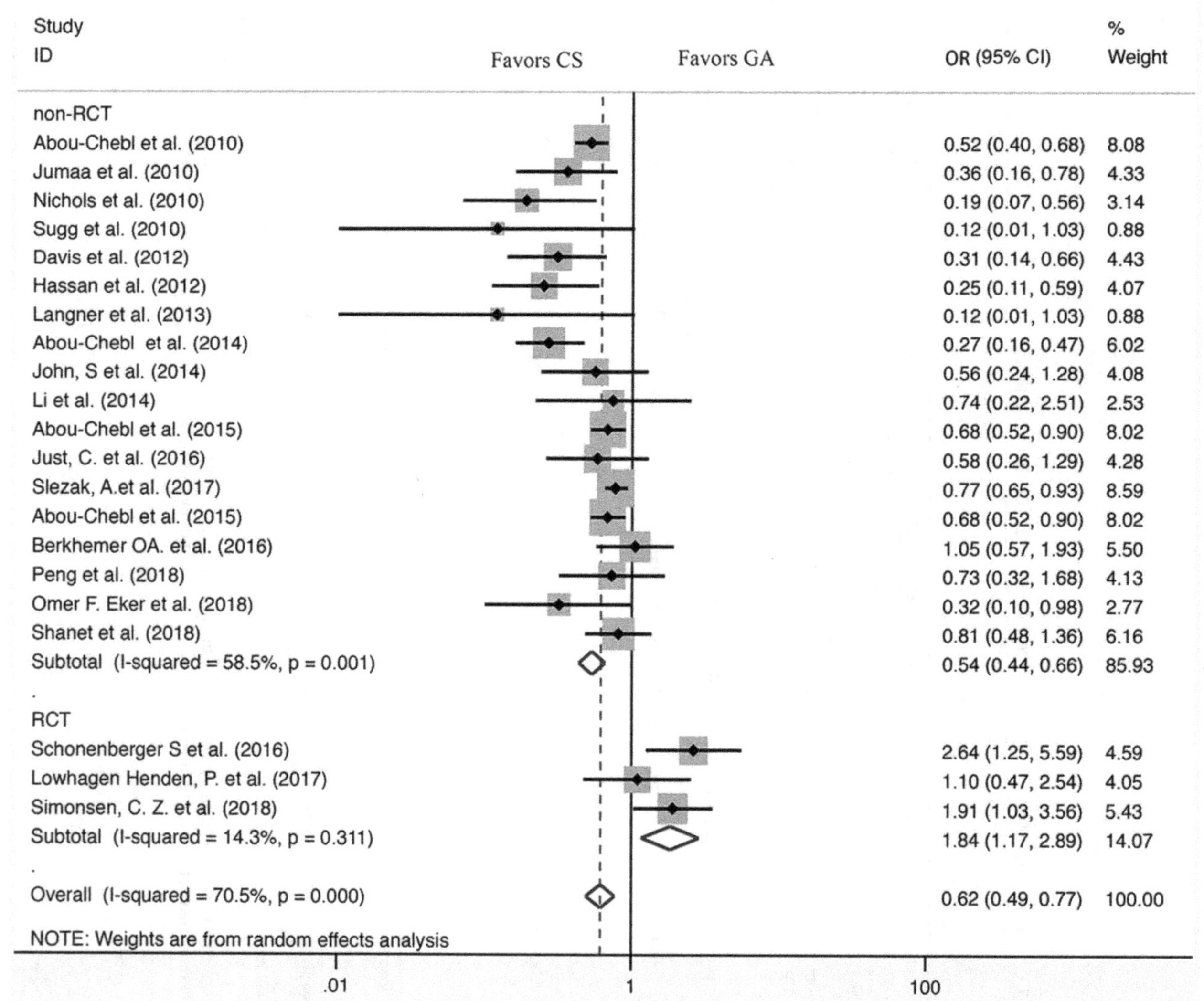

Fig. 2 Forest plot of meta-analysis results for good functional outcome (mRS ≤ 2). OR, odds ratio; CI, confidence interval

Table 2 Summary of meta-analysis results

Groups	Test of association				Heterogeneity		
	OR [95%CI]	*p* value	Model	Z	χ^2	*p* value	I^2 (%)
mRS score (0–2)	0.62 [0.49–0.77]	< 0.001	RE	4.16	67.83	< 0.001	70.5%
Mortality	1.68 [1.49–1.90]	< 0.001	FE	8.28	40.98	0.008	46.3%
Successful recanalization	1.07 [0.89–1.28]	0.943	FE	0.47	26.35	0.023	46.9%
Vessel dissection or perforation	1.00 [0.98–1.03]	0.010	FE	0.19	11.21	0.34	10.8%
sICH	1.64 [1.13–2.37]	0.010	RE	2.59	31.63	< 0.001	68.4%
aICH	1.19 [0.96–1.47]	0.116	FE	1.57	3.36	0.644	0.0%
Pneumonia	1.78 [1.40–2.26]	< 0.001	FE	4.67	7.95	0.539	0.0%

OR odds ratio, *CI* confidence interval, *mRS* modified Rankin Score, *RE* random effects, *FE* fixed effects, *sICH* symptomatic intracranial hemorrhage, *aICH* asymptomatic intracranial hemorrhage

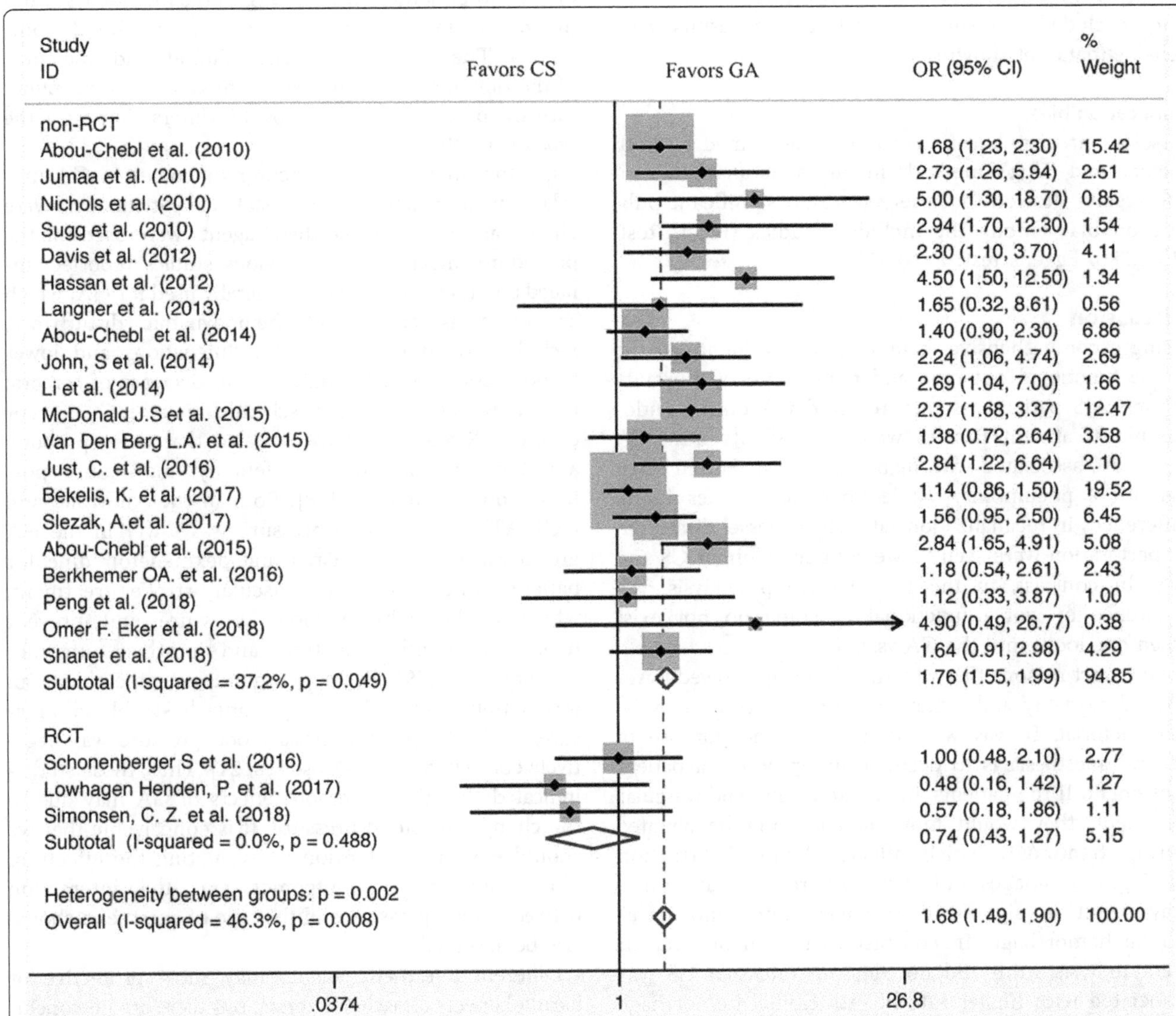

Fig. 3 Forest plot of meta-analysis results for the risk of mortality. OR, odds ratio; CI, confidence interval

≥7 and RCTs). We found the use of GA was also associated with poorer neurologic outcome at 90 days (OR = 0.64, 95% CI: 0.50–0.83) (Additional file 1: Figure S1) and higher mortality (OR = 1.83, 95% CI: 1.57–2.14) (Additional file 2: Figure S2) compared with CS.

Heterogeneity and sensitivity analysis

Obvious between-study heterogeneity (I^2 values more than 50%) was found for the following outcomes: good functional outcome (mRS scores ≤2) (I^2 = 70.5%) and sICH (I^2 = 68.4%). While no obvious heterogeneity (I^2 values less than 50%) was detected in death at 90 days (I^2 = 46.3%), successful recanalization (I^2 = 46.9%), pneumonia (I^2 = 0.0%), vessel dissection or perforation (I^2 = 0.0%) and aICH (I^2 = 0.0%).

Each study was removed sequentially to verify the effect of each individual study in our results. There are no other important changes in our pooled OR value after excluded any study. Therefore, our results were reliable (data not shown).

Publication bias

Assessment of publication bias was performed by both Egger's and Begg's methods in our meta-analysis. And the results showed that there were no significant publication bias among the included studies (Begg's test: $P = 0.780$, Egger's test: $P = 0.352$).

Discussion

Using a comprehensive meta-analysis, we identified the worse functional outcome and higher rate of mortality among AIS patients as they received GA during endovascular treatment. Besides, we found patients in the GA group are associated with higher rate of sICH and often had more pneumonia. While no clinically meaningful differences in recanalization rate, aICH, vessel dissection or perforation were seen between patients under CS and GA. In contrast, in the RCT subgroup analysis, the difference of worse functional outcome do not exist when one looks into the GA vs. CS.

The exact reasons that why the CS group showed lower rate of mortality and better functional outcome may be multifactorial. It was well known that the purpose of general anesthesia is to decrease intraprocedural patient movement. If the patients are awake during endovascular treatment, they would move casually and be agitated during treatment, which affects Digital Subtraction Angiography images and leads to wire perforation and may result in significant vascular injury and intracranial hemorrhage. In contrast to this theory, recent meta-analysis study did not demonstrate that CS was associated with higher rate of intracranial hemorrhage than GA [34]. Moreover, in our results, we found that patients in the GA group has a higher rate of sICH. Additionally, GA has been associated with significantly higher treatment costs ($46,444 VS $30,350) [24]. And GA may limit the ability of the interventionalist to assess neurological status during the procedure. Thus, these findings do not support GA as a safer and lower cost approach for endovascular thrombectomy treatment. Moreover, as one of main factors, delay of treatment was also commonly concerned. As the post hoc analysis of MR CLEAN showed, a longer delay for patients in the GA group was observed. Intra-arterial therapy was initiated sooner after symptom onset in patients treated with non-GA as compared with GA [28]. Recently, a meta-analysis from 5 randomized controlled trials also revealed that 1 hour of delay in door-to-puncture times could reduce 19% likelihood of regaining functional independence [35]. Thus, it is reasonable to assume that treatment delays during GA may result in a disadvantage. However, the detail of door-to-puncture times among all the included studies in this meta-analysis could not be obtained completely. Therefore, future trials should study the effect of the time delay from hospital admission to vessel puncture on outcomes and its possible interaction with the type of anesthesia.

On the other hand, the poorer outcomes in GA may related with the poorer clinical status in patients who were chosen and different anesthetic agents were used for the procedure under GA. As previous studies reported, inhaled anesthetic agents were generally used for GA, which are often associated with hemodynamic disturbance, including rapid blood pressure fluctuations and lower blood pressure, which would lead to decrease of cerebral bloodflow and exacerbate ischemic injury [36, 37]. For example, Reich et al. have revealed that using propofol and the induction dose of fentanyl may cause post induction hypotension [38]. Both in the AnStroke and GOLIATH trials, blood pressure was lower in the GA group [3, 4]. In contrast, using dexmedetomidine for patients undergoing endovascular stroke treatment, which could stabilize blood pressure and prevent hypotension with induction, and improve outcomes consequently [39]. Besides, a good outcome shows an association with a higher pre-anesthesia blood pressure, while the pre-anesthesia blood pressure was negatively correlated with GA use [18, 21]. Thus, those studies indicated that the deleterious effects of GA may due to the changes of blood pressure. It is conceivable that we should pay more attention to evaluating the effects of blood pressure on outcomes and the interaction between blood pressure and the type of anesthesia should also be observed.

Different anesthetic agents may show protective or harmful effects on ischemic brain, but there are no conclusive data about the neuroprotective properties of anesthetic agents to help recommending an anesthetic agent [40].

Numerous preclinical studies indicate that isoflurane shows neuroprotective effects in ischemic preconditioning and postconditioning by alleviating glutamate excitotoxicity and opening of potassium channels [41, 42]. Besides, intravenous propofol has also been suggested as a neuroprotective agent on ischemic stroke by many molecular pathways [43]. However, these findings were just demonstrated in nonhuman primate studies. A retrospective study for endovascular management of AIS suggested that volatile anesthetics are superior to intravenous agents, but this finding should be validated by a larger randomized controlled trial [44]. Thus, to minimize the confounding effects of different drugs during endovascular treatment, the same anesthetic agent should be used as both a general anesthetic and a sedative. Among the included studies in this meta-analysis, the specific data on the type of anesthetic agent used in the GA or CS patients are unavailable in most included studies, but the GOLIATH trial has used the propofol as both a general anesthetic and a sedative in the CS group [3].

Actually, the choice of GA or CS for a given AIS patient in clinical practice, which were mainly decided by the patient's physical status. For instance, the AIS patients with underlying medical comorbidities or stroke severity may be performed with GA as "medically indicated" [18]. Moreover, as Abou-Chebl et al. have stated that a major weakness of the retrospective study was that the association between GA and poor outcomes may be due to the AIS patients with aphasia or who were unable to follow commands and necessitated GA [24]. In non-randomized studies, the choice of GA or CS for a given AIS patient was most likely due to either technical concerns (difficulty of interventional procedure) or safety concerns (airway patency). Consequently, in the subgroup analysis of this study, we have revealed inconsistent findings between the randomized and non-randomized studies. These findings were also consistent with the previous meta-analyses by Jing R. and his colleagues, but our study have included more studies [7]. Taken together, the "medically indicated" highlights the problem of bias and may explain the reason that why the randomized and nonrandomized studies show marked discrepancy in results.

We must acknowledge that this study has several limitations. The design of included studies were various and the choice of CS or GA for a given AIS patient was not randomized for most of included studies. Thus, we conducted the subgroup analysis according to the design type of the included trials and the subgroup analysis showed inconsistent results, but we could not find the exact reasons for this discrepancy due to the lack of some of essential reported data (eg, the type and dose of anesthetic agents used, stroke location, time to treatment, baseline NIHSS scores). Although, parts of included studies have presented the baseline NIHSS scores for patients in GA and CS groups, we could not pool all the baseline NIHSS scores of patients for all included trials, because these studies presented data in different forms [mean (SD) or mean (IQR)] and the individual data were unobtainable. Moreover, in clinical practice, there was a lower rate of anterior circulation occlusions in the GA group than in the CS group. As a meta-analysis of individual patients with anterior circulation showed, outcomes were significantly better for patients who did not receive GA versus those who received GA [34]. However, we could not conduct the subgroup analyses according to those factors in the present study for relatively small or incomparable number of available studies.

Conclusions

In summary, the pooled data from this meta-analysis indicated that performing endovascular treatment under GA compared with CS was associated with worse functional outcome and increased rate of mortality. However, in the RCT subgroup analysis, differences in worsened outcomes do not exist between GA and CS group. Moreover, these findings are mainly based on the retrospective studies that did not randomize patients by anesthesia type. Thus, additional multi-center RCTs to definitively address these issues is warranted. In addition, to understand the exact reasons which cause the differences between the GA and CS when AIS patients are performed endovascular treatment, future studies should consider the underlying confounding factors (eg, door-to-puncture times, baseline NIHSS scores, blood pressure level).

Additional files

Additional file 1: Figure S1. Forest plot of meta-analysis results for good functional outcome (mRS ≤ 2) among the high quality studies. OR, odds ratio; CI, confidence interval.

Additional file 2: Figure S2. Forest plot of meta-analysis results for the risk of mortality among the high quality studies. OR, odds ratio; CI, confidence interval.

Additional file 3: Table S1. The baseline NIHSS scores of patients in each included trials. **Table S2.** Assessment of the methodological quality of included randomized trials using the Cochrane Collaboration's Tool.

Abbreviations

aICH: Asymptomatic intracranial hemorrhage; AIS: Acute ischemic stroke; CI: Confidence interval; CS: Conscious sedation; FE: Fixed effects; GA: General anesthesia; IA: Intra-arterial; IV: Intra-venous; mRS: Modified Rankin scale; NIHSS: National Institute of Health Stroke Scale; OR: Odds ratio; PRISMA: Preferred Reporting Items for Systematic Reviews and Meta-Analyses; RCT: Randomized controlled trial; RE: Random effects; sICH: Symptomatic intracranial hemorrhage; tPA: Tissue plasminogen activator

Acknowledgements

We thank the Miao Pu project of the Army Medical University (no. 2017R016) and the science and technology planning project of the Shenyang (no. 1901220) for the support of this research project.

Authors' contributions

LL and HSC conceived the study. TFW and ZAZ collected the data and drafted the manuscript. YL and RX revised the manuscript and language. RX conducted the subgroup analysis. All authors have read and approved the manuscript.

Author details

[1]Department of First Cadre Ward, the General Hospital of Northern Theater Command, No. 83 Wenhua Street, Shenyang 110016, Liaoning, China. [2]Department of Neurology, Xinqiao Hospital, the Army Medical University, NO. 183 Xinqiao mian street, Chongqing 400037, China. [3]Department of Neurology, the General Hospital of Northern Theater Command , No. 83 Wenhua Street, Shenyang 110016, Liaoning, China.

References

1. Meyers PM, Schumacher HC, Connolly ES Jr, Heyer EJ, Gray WA, Higashida RT. Current status of endovascular stroke treatment. Circulation. 2011; 123(22):2591–601.
2. Brinjikji W, Pasternak J, Murad MH, Cloft HJ, Welch TL, Kallmes DF, Rabinstein AA. Anesthesia-related outcomes for endovascular Stroke revascularization: a systematic review and meta-analysis. Stroke. 2017;48(10):2784–91.
3. Simonsen CZ, Yoo AJ, Sorensen LH, Juul N, Johnsen SP, Andersen G, Rasmussen M. Effect of general anesthesia and conscious sedation during endovascular therapy on infarct growth and clinical outcomes in acute ischemic Stroke: a randomized clinical trial. JAMA Neurol. 2018;75(4):470–7.
4. Lowhagen Henden P, Rentzos A, Karlsson JE, Rosengren L, Leiram B, Sundeman H, Dunker D, Schnabel K, Wikholm G, Hellstrom M, et al. General anesthesia versus conscious sedation for endovascular treatment of acute ischemic Stroke: the AnStroke trial (anesthesia during Stroke). Stroke. 2017;48(6):1601–7.
5. Schonenberger S, Uhlmann L, Hacke W, Schieber S, Mundiyanapurath S, Purrucker JC, Nagel S, Klose C, Pfaff J, Bendszus M, et al. Effect of conscious sedation vs general anesthesia on early neurological improvement among patients with ischemic Stroke undergoing endovascular Thrombectomy a randomized clinical trial. JAMA. 2016;316(19):1986–96.
6. Brinjikji W, Murad MH, Rabinstein AA, Cloft HJ, Lanzino G, Kallmes DF. Conscious sedation versus general anesthesia during endovascular acute ischemic stroke treatment: a systematic review and meta-analysis. Am J Neuroradiol. 2015;36(3):525–9.
7. Jing R, Dai HJ, Lin F, Ge WY, Pan LH. Conscious sedation versus general anesthesia for patients with acute ischemic Stroke undergoing endovascular therapy: a systematic review and meta-analysis. Biomed Res Int. 2018;2018:2318489.
8. Liang Y, Yang Z, Zhong R. Primary biliary cirrhosis and cancer risk: a systematic review and meta-analysis. Hepatology. 2012;56(4):1409–17.
9. Higgins JP, Altman DG, Gotzsche PC, Juni P, Moher D, Oxman AD, Savovic J, Schulz KF, Weeks L, Sterne JA. The Cochrane Collaboration's tool for assessing risk of bias in randomised trials. BMJ. 2011;343:d5928.
10. Borenstein M, Higgins JP. Meta-analysis and subgroups. Prev Sci. 2013; 14(2):134–43.
11. Higgins JP, Thompson SG, Deeks JJ, Altman DG. Measuring inconsistency in meta-analyses. BMJ (Clinical research ed). 2003;327(7414):557–60.
12. Egger M, Davey Smith G, Schneider M, Minder C. Bias in meta-analysis detected by a simple, graphical test. Bmj. 1997;315(7109):629–34.
13. Begg CB, Mazumdar M. Operating characteristics of a rank correlation test for publication bias. Biometrics. 1994;50(4):1088–101.
14. Abou-Chebl A, Lin R, Shazam Hussain M, Jovin TG, Levy EI, Liebeskind DS, Yoo AJ, Hsu DP, Rymer MM, Tayal AH, et al. Conscious sedation versus general anesthesia during endovascular therapy for acute anterior circulation stroke: preliminary results from a retrospective, multicenter study. Stroke. 2010;41(6):1175–9.
15. Jumaa MA, Zhang F, Ruiz-Ares G, Gelzinis T, Malik AM, Aleu A, Oakley JI, Jankowitz B, Lin R, Reddy V, et al. Comparison of safety and clinical and radiographic outcomes in endovascular acute stroke therapy for proximal middle cerebral artery occlusion with intubation and general anesthesia versus the nonintubated state. Stroke. 2010;41(6):1180–4.
16. Nichols C, Carrozzella J, Yeatts S, Tomsick T, Broderick J, Khatri P. Is periprocedural sedation during acute stroke therapy associated with poorer functional outcomes? J Neurointerv Surg. 2010;2(1):67–70.
17. Sugg RM, Jackson AS, Holloway W, Martin CO, Akhtar N, Rymer M. Is mechanical embolectomy performed in nonanesthetized patients effective? Am J Neuroradiol. 2010;31(8):1533–5.
18. Davis MJ, Menon BK, Baghirzada LB, Campos-Herrera CR, Goyal M, Hill MD, Archer DP, Calgary Stroke P. Anesthetic management and outcome in patients during endovascular therapy for acute stroke. Anesthesiology. 2012;116(2):396–405.
19. Hassan AE, Chaudhry SA, Zacharatos H, Khatri R, Akbar U, Suri MF, Qureshi AI. Increased rate of aspiration pneumonia and poor discharge outcome among acute ischemic stroke patients following intubation for endovascular treatment. Neurocrit Care. 2012;16(2):246–50.
20. Langner S, Khaw AV, Fretwurst T, Angermaier A, Hosten N, Kirsch M. Endovascular treatment of acute ischemic stroke under conscious sedation compared to general anesthesia - safety, feasibility and clinical and radiological outcome. Rofo. 2013;185(4):320–7.
21. Abou-Chebl A, Zaidat OO, Castonguay AC, Gupta R, Sun CH, Martin CO, Holloway WE, Mueller-Kronast N, English JD, Linfante I, et al. North American SOLITAIRE stent-retriever acute Stroke registry: choice of anesthesia and outcomes. Stroke. 2014;45(5):1396–401.
22. John S, Thebo U, Gomes J, Saqqur M, Farag E, Xu J, Wisco D, Uchino K, Hussain MS. Intra-arterial therapy for acute ischemic stroke under general anesthesia versus monitored anesthesia care. Cerebrovasc Dis. 2014;38(4):262–7.
23. Li F, Deshaies EM, Singla A, Villwock MR, Melnyk V, Gorji R, Yang ZJ. Impact of anesthesia on mortality during endovascular clot removal for acute ischemic stroke. J Neurosurg Anesthesiol. 2014;26(4):286–90.
24. Abou-Chebl A, Yeatts SD, Yan B, Cockroft K, Goyal M, Jovin T, Khatri P, Meyers P, Spilker J, Sugg R, et al. Impact of general anesthesia on safety and outcomes in the endovascular arm of interventional Management of Stroke (IMS) III trial. Stroke. 2015;46(8):2142–8.
25. McDonald JS, Brinjikji W, Rabinstein AA, Cloft HJ, Lanzino G, Kallmes DF. Conscious sedation versus general anaesthesia during mechanical thrombectomy for stroke: a propensity score analysis. J NeuroInterv Surg. 2015;7(11):789–94.
26. Van Den Berg LA, Koelman DLH, Berkhemer OA, Rozeman AD, Fransen PSS, Beumer D, Dippel DW, Van Der Lugt A, Van Oostenbrugge RJ, Van Zwam WH, et al. Type of anesthesia and differences in clinical outcome after intra-arterial treatment for ischemic Stroke. Stroke. 2015;46(5):1257–62.
27. Just C, Rizek P, Tryphonopoulos P, Pelz D, Arango M. Outcomes of general anesthesia and conscious sedation in endovascular treatment for Stroke. Can J Neurol Sci. 2016;43(5):655–8.
28. Berkhemer OA, van den Berg LA, Fransen PS, Beumer D, Yoo AJ, Lingsma HF, Schonewille WJ, van den Berg R, Wermer MJ, Boiten J, et al. The effect of anesthetic management during intra-arterial therapy for acute stroke in MR CLEAN. Neurology. 2016;87(7):656–64.
29. Bekelis K, Missios S, Mackenzie TA, Tjoumakaris S, Jabbour P. Anesthesia technique and outcomes of mechanical Thrombectomy in patients with acute ischemic Stroke. Stroke. 2017;48(2):361–6.
30. Slezak A, Kurmann R, Oppliger L, Broeg-Morvay A, Gralla J, Schroth G, Mattle HP, Arnold M, Fischer U, Jung S, et al. Impact of anesthesia on the outcome of acute ischemic Stroke after endovascular treatment with the Solitaire stent retriever. AJNR Am J Neuroradiol. 2017;38(7):1362–7.
31. Peng Y, Wu Y, Huo X, Wu P, Zhou Y, Li J, Liang F, Liu X, Pan Y, Miao Z, et al. Outcomes of anesthesia selection in endovascular treatment of acute ischemic Stroke. J Neurosurg Anesthesiol. 2019;31(1):43–9.
32. Eker OF, Saver JL, Goyal M, Jahan R, Levy EI, Nogueira RG, Yavagal DR, Bonafe A, investigators SP. Impact of anesthetic management on safety and outcomes following mechanical Thrombectomy for ischemic Stroke in SWIFT PRIME cohort. Front Neurol. 2018;9:702.
33. Shan W, Yang D, Wang H, Xu L, Zhang M, Liu W, Zi W, Hao Y, Xiong Y, Xu G, et al. General anesthesia may have similar outcomes with conscious sedation in Thrombectomy patients with acute ischemic Stroke: a real-world registry in China. Eur Neurol. 2018;80(1-2):7–13.
34. Campbell BCV, van Zwam WH, Goyal M, Menon BK, Dippel DWJ, Demchuk AM, Bracard S, White P, Davalos A, Majoie C, et al. Effect of general anaesthesia on functional outcome in patients with anterior circulation ischaemic stroke having endovascular thrombectomy versus standard care: a meta-analysis of individual patient data. Lancet Neurol. 2018;17(1):47–53.
35. Saver JL, Goyal M, van der Lugt A, Menon BK, Majoie CB, Dippel DW, Campbell BC, Nogueira RG, Demchuk AM, Tomasello A, et al. Time to treatment with endovascular Thrombectomy and outcomes from ischemic Stroke: a meta-analysis. JAMA. 2016;316(12):1279–88.
36. Schifilliti D, Grasso G, Conti A, Fodale V. Anaesthetic-related neuroprotection: intravenous or inhalational agents? CNS drugs. 2010; 24(11):893–907.

37. Steen PA. Inhalational versus intravenous anesthesia: cerebral effects. Acta Anaesthesiol Scand Suppl. 1982;75:32–5.
38. Reich DL, Hossain S, Krol M, Baez B, Patel P, Bernstein A, Bodian CA. Predictors of hypotension after induction of general anesthesia. Anesth Analg. 2005;101(3):622–8 table of contents.
39. Whalin MK, Lopian S, Wyatt K, Sun CH, Nogueira RG, Glenn BA, Gershon RY, Gupta R. Dexmedetomidine: a safe alternative to general anesthesia for endovascular stroke treatment. J Neurointerv Surg. 2014;6(4):270–5.
40. Crosby G, Muir KW. Anesthesia and neurologic outcome of endovascular therapy in acute ischemic stroke: MR (not so) CLEAN. Neurology. 2016;87(7):648–9.
41. Sun M, Deng B, Zhao X, Gao C, Yang L, Zhao H, Yu D, Zhang F, Xu L, Chen L, et al. Isoflurane preconditioning provides neuroprotection against stroke by regulating the expression of the TLR4 signalling pathway to alleviate microglial activation. Sci Rep. 2015;5:11445.
42. Lee JJ, Li L, Jung HH, Zuo Z. Postconditioning with isoflurane reduced ischemia-induced brain injury in rats. Anesthesiology. 2008;108(6):1055–62.
43. Zwerus R, Absalom A. Update on anesthetic neuroprotection. Curr Opin Anaesthesiol. 2015;28(4):424–30.
44. Sivasankar C, Stiefel M, Miano TA, Kositratna G, Yandrawatthana S, Hurst R, Kofke WA. Anesthetic variation and potential impact of anesthetics used during endovascular management of acute ischemic stroke. J Neurointerv Surg. 2016;8(11):1101–6.

15

Effects of desflurane and sevoflurane anesthesia on regulatory T cells in patients undergoing living donor kidney transplantation

Arpa Chutipongtanate[1], Sasichol Prukviwat[1], Nutkridta Pongsakul[2], Supanart Srisala[3], Nakarin Kamanee[1], Nuttapon Arpornsujaritkun[4], Goragoch Gesprasert[4], Nopporn Apiwattanakul[5], Suradej Hongeng[6], Wichai Ittichaikulthol[1], Vasant Sumethkul[7] and Somchai Chutipongtanate[2,8*]

Abstract

Background: Volatile anesthetic agents used during surgery have immunomodulatory effects which could affect postoperative outcomes. Recognizing that regulatory T cells (Tregs) plays crucial roles in transplant tolerance and high peripheral blood Tregs associated with stable kidney graft function, knowing which volatile anesthetic agents can induce peripheral blood Tregs increment would have clinical implications. This study aimed to compare effects of desflurane and sevoflurane anesthesia on peripheral blood Tregs induction in patients undergoing living donor kidney transplantation.

Methods: A prospective, randomized, double-blind trial in living donor kidney transplant recipients was conducted at a single center, tertiary-care, academic university hospital in Thailand during August 2015 – June 2017. Sixty-six patients were assessed for eligibility and 40 patients who fulfilled the study requirement were equally randomized and allocated to desflurane versus sevoflurane anesthesia during transplant surgery. The primary outcome included absolute changes of peripheral blood $CD4^+CD25^+FoxP3^+$Tregs which measured by flow cytometry and expressed as the percentage of the total population of $CD4^+$ T lymphocytes at pre-exposure (0-h) and post-exposure (2-h and 24-h) to anesthetic gas. *P*-value < 0.05 denoted statistical significance.

(Continued on next page)

* Correspondence: schuti.rama@gmail.com; somchai.chu@mahidol.edu
[2]Pediatric Translational Research Unit, Department of Pediatrics, Faculty of Medicine Ramathibodi Hospital, Mahidol University, Bangkok 10400, Thailand
[8]Department of Clinical Epidemiology and Biostatistics, Faculty of Medicine Ramathibodi Hospital, Mahidol University, Bangkok 10400, Thailand

(Continued from previous page)

Results: Demographic data were comparable between groups. No statistical difference of peripheral blood Tregs between desflurane and sevoflurane groups observed at the baseline pre-exposure ($3.6 \pm 0.4\%$ vs. $3.1 \pm 0.4\%$; $p = 0.371$) and 2-h post-exposure ($3.0 \pm 0.3\%$ vs. $3.5 \pm 0.4\%$; $p = 0.319$). At 24-h post-exposure, peripheral blood Tregs was significantly higher in desflurane group ($5.8 \pm 0.5\%$ vs. $4.1 \pm 0.3\%$; $p = 0.008$). Within group analysis showed patients receiving desflurane, but not sevoflurane, had 2.7% increase in peripheral blood Treg over 24-h period ($p < 0.001$).

Conclusion: This study provides the clinical trial-based evidence that desflurane induced peripheral blood Tregs increment after 24-h exposure, which could be beneficial in the context of kidney transplantation. Mechanisms of action and clinical advantages of desflurane anesthesia based on Treg immunomodulation should be investigated in the future.

Keywords: Clinical trial, Inhalation agent, Kidney transplant, Tregs, Volatile anesthesia

Background

Kidney transplantation is the best option for renal replacement therapy in patients with end-stage renal disease (ESRD), often restoring quality of life in ESRD patients. Allograft rejection, an immune-mediated process, is a common cause of transplant failure [1–4]. Evidence indicates $CD4^{+}CD25^{+}FoxP3^{+}$ cells, commonly known as regulatory T cells (Tregs), play a critical role in preventing graft rejection by suppression of recipient alloimmune response [5–8]. In healthy subjects, Tregs represent up to 5% of peripheral $CD4^{+}$ T cells [9–11]. In kidney transplant patients, high peripheral blood Tregs were associated with stable graft function. Low peripheral blood Tregs was associated with allograft rejection [12–17].

Currently, adoptive transfer of ex vivo expanded Tregs is a promising strategy to induce transplant tolerance and control graft rejection in kidney transplant recipients [18, 19]. It has been investigated for safety and feasibility in phase I trials, i.e., the ONE (NCT02091232) and TRACT (NCT02145325). Identifying Treg-friendly agents from pharmacologic choices in multiple steps of kidney transplant management may also offer an attractive therapeutic strategy [19]. Characterization of Tregs under various treatment conditions may help refine current preventive measures or identify novel therapeutic targets.

Volatile anesthetic agents are widely used for general anesthesia during kidney transplantation. A growing body of evidence from ex vivo and clinical studies [20–26] suggest desflurane and sevoflurane (halogenated ether inhaled agents) exhibit immunomodulatory effects (e.g., cell proliferation, activation, migration, cytokine production) on neutrophils, macrophages, natural killer cells, B and T lymphocytes. These effects may be mediated via activation of volatile anesthetic receptors (i.e., γ-aminobutyric acid type A receptor, nicotinic acetylcholine receptor, serotonin receptor and non-canonical β2-integrins) or via binding to surface adhesion molecules such as integrin leukocyte function associated antigen-1, which express differentially on peripheral blood leukocytes [25, 26]. However, effects of desflurane and sevoflurane on Treg immunomodulation is surprisingly overlooked and has only rarely been investigated. A better understanding of these effects would have translational potential. For example, the early Treg immunomodulation by anesthetic agents may help mitigating the initiation of alloimmune responses during the 24-h perioperative period, and works in conjunction with the standard immunosuppressive regimen to seamlessly maintain the graft survival in LDKT patients.

This interventional trial aims to compare the immunomodulatory effects of desflurane and sevoflurane anesthesia on peripheral blood Treg induction in patients undergoing living donor kidney transplantation (LDKT). Several plasma cytokines were measured as the surrogate outcomes of the volatile anesthetic effects on anti- and pro-inflammatory responses. Evidence from this study would support future investigation of volatile anesthetic agents as part of perioperative management with an aim to improve transplant outcomes.

Methods

Trial design and patient enrollment

This prospective, double-blind, randomized intervention trial was approved by the Ethical Clearance Committee on Human Rights Related to Research Involving Human Subjects, Faculty of Medicine Ramathibodi Hospital, Mahidol University (protocol ID 045823) and the protocol was registered to ClinicalTrials.gov (identifier NCT02559297) on September 22, 2015. Patients aged ≥18 years old who received their first living donor kidney transplantation at Ramathibodi Hospital were included in the study. Patients were excluded for hyperacute graft rejection, currently on immunosuppressive drugs due to underlying diseases, receiving blood products during 24-h perioperative period, or patient refusal to participate in the study at any time point. Informed consent was obtained from all subjects. No interim analysis was performed during the trial. This study followed the CONSORT reporting guideline [27].

Randomization

Randomization was generated in a 1:1 allocation with a block size of 8 and the random number was put in a sealed envelope. Patients were randomly assigned to either desflurane or sevoflurane intervention by drawing a sealed envelope. Randomization took place on the day of surgery just prior to initiation of anesthesia.

Blinding

Subjects and outcome assessors (including laboratory technicians and all investigators except the designated research coordinator) were blinded to group allocation throughout surgery, laboratory investigation and data collection. Blinding was uncovered at the time of data analysis.

Interventions

Patients were randomly assigned to receive desflurane or sevoflurane for the maintenance phase of anesthesia. In addition to the randomized inhalation agents, patients received the same regimen of 1–2 mg of midazolam for premedication and intravenous anesthetic agents including 1–2 mcg kg^{-1} of fentanyl, 1–2 mg kg^{-1} of propofol and 0.5–0.6 mg kg^{-1} of atracurium for induction of anesthesia and intubation. A balance anesthesia technique was used for maintenance phase. The inhalation agent (sevoflurane or desflurane) was used in conjunction with 50% nitrous oxide in oxygen. Ventilation was adjusted to maintain normocarbia. End-tidal anesthetic gas monitoring was used to ensure 1.0–1.5 minimum alveolar concentration (MAC) of the inhalation agent during maintenance phase in both groups.

During anesthesia, blood pressure, heart rate, oxygen saturation, $ETCO_2$, and temperature were monitored and recorded. Blood pressure was maintained within 20% of baseline values. Hypotension was managed by intravenous fluid and ephedrine IV bolus as needed. Total doses of intravenous medications were recorded. All patients in both interventions were transferred to the kidney transplant unit for postoperative care.

Blood sample collection

Venipuncture was performed at three time-points; pre-exposure (0-h) and post-exposure (2-h, and 24-h) to inhalation agents. Two tubes of 0.5-ml EDTA blood were collected at each time point, one for Treg enumeration and the other for cytokine measurement.

Outcome measures

The primary outcome was the absolute change in number of peripheral blood $CD4^+CD25^+FoxP3^+$Tregs, which was measured by flow cytometry and expressed as the percentage of the total population of $CD4^+$ T lymphocytes at pre-exposure (0-h) and post-exposure (2-h and 24-h) to anesthetic gas. A secondary outcome was the plasma level of anti-inflammatory cytokine IL-10 (the major cytokine produced by Tregs), TGF-β1 (anti-inflammatory cytokines produced by many types of cells and required for Tregs differentiation), and pro-inflammatory cytokines produced by T helper (Th) 1/Th2, i.e., GM-CSF, IFN-ɣ, IL-2, IL-4, IL-5, IL-12, IL-13 and TNF-α, which measured by multiplex immunoassay. All measurements were performed in triplicate.

Treg enumeration by flow cytometry

Peripheral blood mononuclear cells (PBMC) were isolated by density gradient centrifugation. Approximately 5×10^5 cells were suspended in 20 µL phosphate buffer saline (PBS) in the presence of cell surface marker antibodies (APC-CD4, PE-Cy7-CD25) (#MHCD0404, #25–0259-41; ThermoFisher, Florence, KY), mixed well and incubated at room temperature for 15 min. Thereafter, cells were permeabilized and intracellularly stained using FoxP3-FITC antibody (#11–4776-42; ThermoFisher). Flow cytometry (BD FACSVerse with BD FACSuite software; BD Bioscience, San Jose, CA) was used to measure the number of Tregs, expressed as a percentage of $CD4^+CD25^+FoxP3^+$ T cells among the $CD4^+$ cell population. The estimated number of CD4 + cells and Treg were calculated by determining the ratio of CD4 + cell count and CD4 + CD25 + FoxP3 + cell count, respectively, to the total count in the flow cytometry, and then multiplied by the number of white blood cells measured from the complete blood count (CBC) which ordered at the pre-operative and post-operative evaluations.

Cytokine measurement by multiplex immunoassay

Multiplex cytokine immunoassay was performed by BioPlex-200 system (Bio-Rad, Hercules, CA). GM-CSF, IFN-ɣ, IL-2, IL-4, IL-5, IL-10, IL-12, IL13, and TNF-α were detected by BioPlex Pro human cytokine Th1/Th2 assay (Bio-Rad), and TGF-β1 was measured by single-plex custom assay (Bio-Rad) as the manufacturer's instruction.

Sample size estimation and statistical analysis

There was no data related to sevoflurane and desflurane anesthesia on Treg immunomodulation available at the initiation of the study. Nevertheless, Pirbudak Cocelli L et al. [21], showed that sevoflurane and desflurane anesthesia caused a significant difference in total lymphocyte count at 2-h post-induction in patients undergoing abdominal surgery. Since Treg is a subset of lymphocytes, our study then adopted mean difference and standard deviation to calculate the effect size. The nQuery Advisor program was applied for sample size calculation. Accordingly, at least 40 patients (20 patients per group) were required to determine statistically significant mean difference between groups (the effect size of 0.915, alpha = 0.05 and power = 80%).

Statistical analysis was performed by Excel and R packages. Data were reported in number, percentage, mean ± SD (or SEM) or median [IQR] as appropriate. Parametric and non-parametric tests were used, as appropriate, to determine difference between groups. ANOVA with Tukey *post-hoc* test was performed for multiple comparison. *P*-value < 0.05 was considered to be statistically significant.

Results

Baseline characteristics

Figure 1 shows the flow of the participants in this study. A total of 66 patients were assessed for eligibility and 46 patients who met inclusion criteria were recruited during August 10, 2015 to June 3, 2017 for randomization and allocation to the intervention. Six patients who met exclusion criteria after allocation due to receiving perioperative blood products were excluded. Table 1 shows demographic and clinical data for the 40 patients enrolled in this study. Most variables, including recipient factors, donor factors, protocol immunosuppressive regimens, intraoperative parameters, the dosage of intravenous anesthesia were not significantly different between the intervention groups. Donor age and the estimated blood loss were slightly lower in patients receiving desflurane anesthesia. Factors contributing to ischemic-reperfusion injury, i.e., cold and warm ischemic time, were comparable between groups. Also, anesthesia time was not different between groups (279 ± 42 min vs. 303 ± 45 min, $p = 0.098$). Given that the depth of sevoflurane and desflurane anesthesia was maintained at 1.0–1.5 MAC for each arm, this finding supported that patients were exposed to inhalation agents equally (Table 1).

Effects of Desflurane and Sevoflurane anesthesia on Tregs in LDKT recipients

Figure 2a demonstrates the gating strategy of flow cytometry and Fig. 2b shows the effects of sevoflurane and desflurane anesthesia on $CD4^{+}CD25^{+}FoxP3^{+}$ Tregs in peripheral blood of LDKT recipients ($n = 20$ per group). No significant difference of peripheral blood Tregs (mean ± SEM) was observed at pre-exposure (3.6 ± 0.4% vs. 3.1 ± 0.4%; $p = 0.371$) and 2-h post-exposure (3.0 ± 0.3% vs 3.5 ± 0.4%; $p = 0.319$) between desflurane and sevoflurane, respectively. However, at 24-h post-exposure, desflurane group had significantly higher peripheral blood Tregs as compared to sevoflurane group (5.8 ± 0.5% vs. 4.1 ± 0.3%; $p = 0.008$) (Fig. 2b). Within-group analysis showed that the patients receiving desflurane had 2.7% increase in Tregs over 24-h period ($p <$

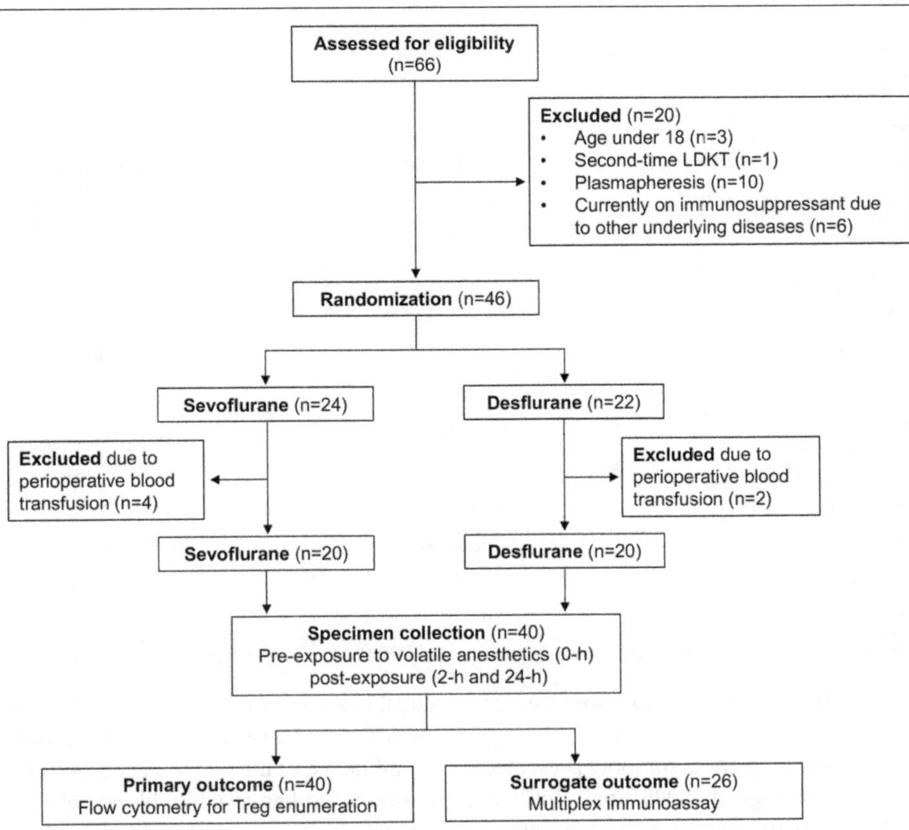

Fig. 1 Flow diagram of study participants

Table 1 Demographic data of LDKT recipients enrolled into the study. If not indicated otherwise: n (%)

Characteristics	Sevoflurane (**n** = 20)	Desflurane (**n** = 20)	**P**-value
Recipient			
Age (year), mean ± SD	37.6 ± 10.5	42.3 ± 10.6	0.163
Gender, male	13 (65)	15 (75)	0.490
BMI (kg/m^2), median [IQR]	21.8 [19.2, 24.4]	22.3 [21.5, 25.1]	0.301
Hypertension	18 (90)	19 (95)	0.999
Diabetes mellitus	4 (20)	0 (0)	0.106
ADPKD	1 (5)	0 (0)	0.999
Hemodialysis	18 (90)	15 (75)	0.407
Peritoneal dialysis	2 (10)	5 (25)	0.407
Baseline creatinine (mg/dL), median [IQR]	7.7 [5.4, 11.8]	7.2 [5.2, 12.9]	0.797
Pretransplant PRA (%), median [IQR]	0 [0, 0]	0 [0, 0]	0.999
HLA-A + B + DR mismatch, median [IQR]	1 [1, 1.5]	3 [1, 3]	0.371
White blood cell count (cells/mL), mean ± SD	6130 ± 2157	5838 ± 2072	0.665
Lymphocyte (%), mean ± SD	21.4 ± 6.7	22.8 ± 9.2	0.586
Donor			
Age (year), mean ± SD	44.8 ± 12.8	36.1 ± 11.3	0.029
Gender, male	7 (35)	6 (30)	0.736
Donor warm ischemic time (min), median [IQR]	3.0 [2.0, 4.0]	3.0 [2.0, 5.3]	0.519
Cold ischemic time (min), median [IQR]	26.5 [18.0, 31.5]	26.5 [19.5, 40.8]	0.432
Protocol immunosuppressive drug			
Tacrolimus	8 (40)	11 (55)	0.342
Cyclosporin A	3 (15)	2 (10)	0.999
Tacrolimus *plus* basiliximab	7 (35)	5 (25)	0.490
Cyclosporin A *plus* basiliximab	2 (10)	2 (10)	0.999
Intraoperative variable			
Recipient warm ischemic time (min), median [IQR]	37.5 [31.5, 44.5]	35.5 [30.0, 41.3]	0.647
Estimated blood loss (mL), mean ± SD	348 ± 124	250 ± 129	0.020
Intravenous fluid (mL), mean ± SD	3716 ± 869	3968 ± 979	0.396
Intravenous ephedrine (mg), median [IQR]	0.0 [0.0, 7.5]	0.0 [0.0, 12.8]	0.701
Intravenous anesthesia			
Propofol (mg), median	175.0 [127.5,	200.0 [170.0,	0.26
[IQR]	200.0]	200.0]	2
Fentanyl (mcg), median	100.0 [100.0,	100.0 [100.0,	0.76
[IQR]	150.0]	156.3]	7
Morphine (mg), median [IQR]	5.5 [3.0, 7.3]	6.0 [3.0, 10.0]	0.678
Midazolam (mg), median [IQR]	2.0 [0.0, 2.1]	2.0 [0.0, 2.5]	0.650
Atracurium (mg), median [IQR]	90.0 [80.0, 110.0]	92.5 [85.0, 101.3]	0.643
Anesthesia time (min)	279 ± 42	303 ± 45	0.098

Abbreviations: *ADPKD* Autosomal dominant polycystic kidney disease, *BMI* Body mass index, *HLA* Human leukocyte antigen, *PRA* Panel reactive antibodies

0.001) (Fig. 2b), while this effect was not observed in sevoflurane group.

Although peripheral blood Treg are commonly presented in the literatures as the percentage of CD25$^+$FoxP3$^+$cells in the CD4$^+$cell population, one argument was that the increment in Treg percentage might be corresponding to the global changes of leukocytes or CD4$^+$ T cells in response of surgical procedure and postoperative inflammation but not the influence of inhalation agents. To address this issue, the absolute number of white blood cells (as measured by the complete blood count), and the calculated numbers of CD4+ T cells and CD4$^+$CD25$^+$FoxP3$^+$ Tregs (details in the

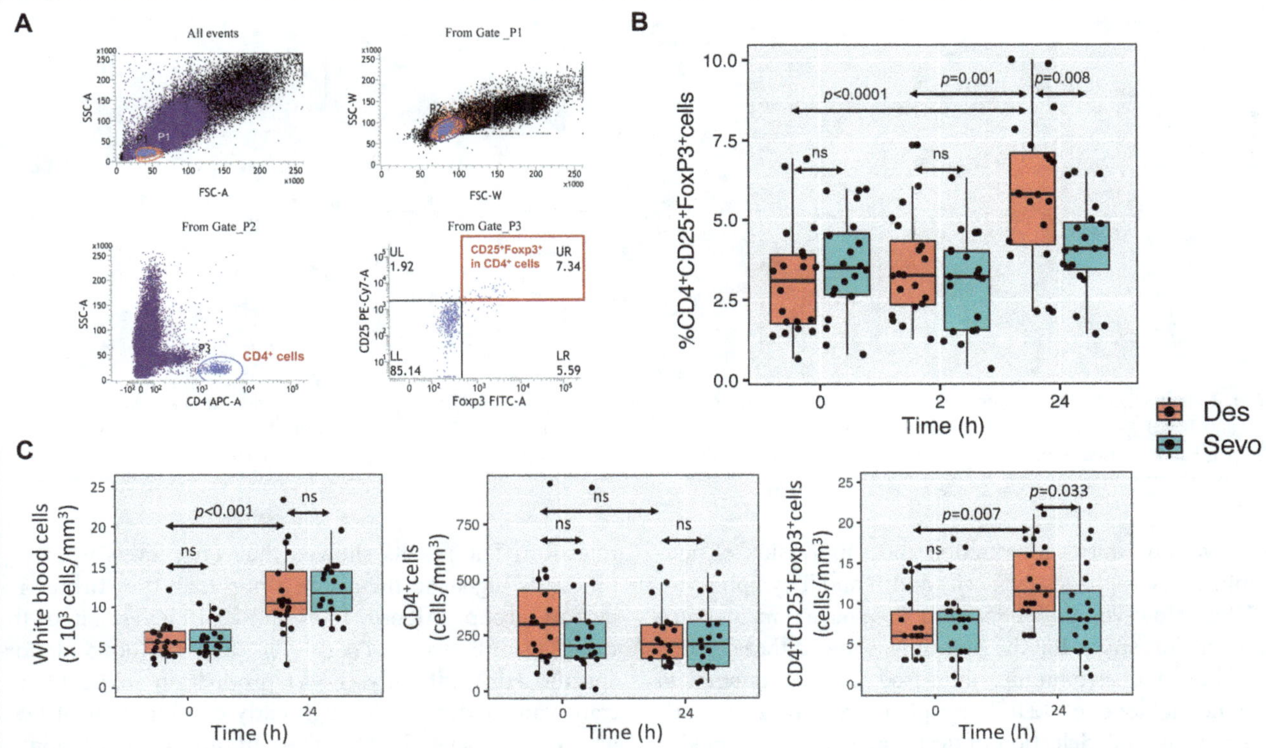

Fig. 2 Effects of desflurane and sevoflurane anesthesia on the CD4 + CD25 + FoxP3+ Tregs ($n = 20$ per group). **a** Representative gating strategy of Treg enumeration. **b** The percentage of Treg in the CD4 + cell population. **c** The absolute number of white blood cells (left), and the calculated numbers of CD4 + cells (center) and Treg (right), in peripheral blood (details in the Method section). The result showed that the LDKT patients who received desflurane anesthesia, but not sevoflurane, had significantly increased Tregs in the peripheral blood at 24-h post-exposure. All experiments were performed in triplicate. Des, desflurane; NS, not significant; Sevo, sevoflurane

Method section), were shown in Fig. 2c. Postoperative leukocytosis was observed in both groups as expected (Fig. 2c, the left panel), while the number of CD4+ T cells were not significantly changed during 24-h perioperative period (Fig. 2c, the center panel). Consistently, the number of Tregs (median [IQR]) were comparable between groups at the baseline (7 [6, 11] vs. 8 [4, 9] cells/mm^3; $p = 0.780$) and were significantly higher in desflurane group (12 [9, 16] vs. 8 [4, 12] cells/mm^3; $p = 0.033$) at 24-h post-exposure (Fig. 2c, the right panel). This finding suggested the effect of desflurane anesthesia on the peripheral blood Treg induction during 24-h postoperative period.

Plasma cytokine levels were measured by multiplex immunoassay as a surrogate outcome of immunomodulation possibly influenced by inhalation agents ($n = 26$, 12 sevoflurane and 14 desflurane). Although there was no statistically significant difference between groups in any cytokine, a trend of increased IL-10 was observed in desflurane group as compared to sevoflurane group at 24-h post-exposure (27.5 [17.6, 34.4] vs. 17.8 [11.4, 22.3] pg/mL; $p = 0.12$) (Fig. 3 and Supplementary Table 1). IL-10, the signature anti-inflammatory cytokine produced by Tregs, had an upward trend (1.67-time increased at 24-h as compared to the baseline pre-exposure) in the patients receiving desflurane, whereas other cytokines seemed to be unchanged over the 24-h period (Fig. 3 and Supplementary Table 1). The transient drop of measured cytokines at 2-h was potentially associated with intraoperative factors, e.g., intravenous fluid administration, but not directly influenced by inhalation agents.

An increased trend of plasma IL-10 in the desflurane group was in line with previous results (Fig. 2) and suggested that desflurane anesthesia was associated with IL-10-producing Tregs induction in LDKT patients during the perioperative period. Matched-pair data of Tregs and plasma IL-10 levels in 26 patients (14 desflurane, 12 sevoflurane) were analyzed to observe this immunophenotypic response. Scatter plot showed a positive relationship between Tregs and IL-10 fold changes over 24-h period (Fig. 4a), in which the proportion of patients with increased Tregs and IL-10 immunophenotypic response was higher in the desflurane group (Fig. 4b). Taken together, our findings revealed that desflurane anesthesia induced IL-10-producing Tregs in LDKT recipients over 24-h postoperative period.

Discussion

Increasing evidence suggests that volatile anesthetic agents exhibit immunomodulatory effects linked to innate and

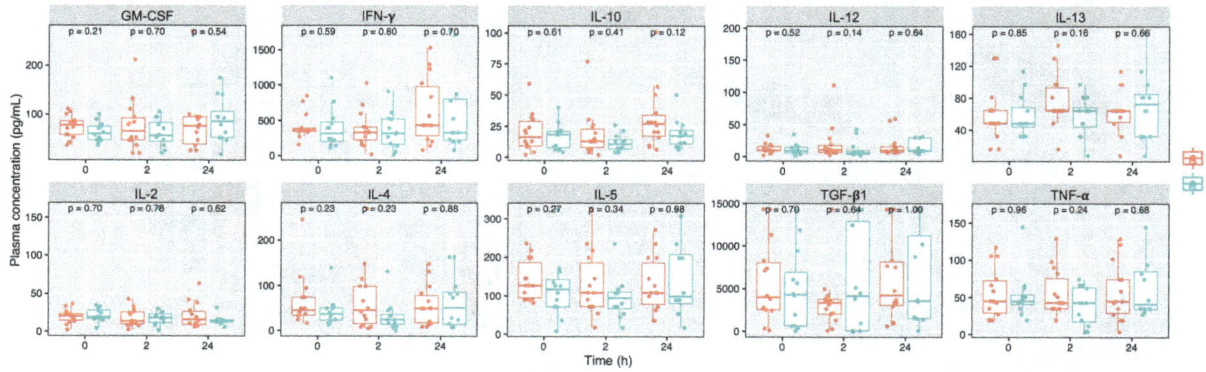

Fig. 3 Plasma cytokines were measured by multiplex cytokine immunoassay. Box plots exhibited plasma levels of anti-inflammatory cytokines IL-10 and TGF-β1, and pro-inflammatory cytokines GM-CSF, IFN-γ, IL-2, IL-4, IL-5, IL-12, IL-13 and TNF-α ($n = 26$; 14 desflurane, 12 sevoflurane). IL-10 showed an increased trend over 24-h period in patients receiving desflurane anesthesia. Des, desflurane; Sevo, sevoflurane

adaptive immunity via induction and suppression of neutrophils, macrophages, NK cells and B and T lymphocytes [25, 26]. However, their effects on Treg have remained unknown. This study, for the first time, showed that desflurane, but not sevoflurane, increased Treg frequency in peripheral blood of LDKT recipients during 24-h perioperative period. Selection of desflurane anesthesia in kidney transplantation may have additional benefits to kidney graft outcome, particularly preventing allograft rejection.

Studies showed that kidney transplant patients who maintained a high level of peripheral blood Tregs were associated with better outcomes [14, 15, 28]. San Segundo D, et al. [14], reported that among 90 kidney transplant recipients, patients who maintained high levels (above 70th percentile) of peripheral blood Tregs at both 6 and 12 months had a better prognosis in the aspect of long-term graft survival after 4 and 5 years follow-up. Liu L, et al. [15], compared peripheral blood Treg levels between 42 patients with stable kidney graft function and ten patients who suffered from chronic rejection. The results showed that Treg levels were significantly higher in the stable group than the chronic rejection group. Alberu J, et al. [28], investigated the association between Treg levels and de novo donor-specific HLA-antibody (DSA) production in 53 kidney transplant patients. Although early development of DSA was not associated with Treg numbers, at 12 months after kidney transplant DSA-negative patients had higher number of peripheral blood Treg.

The mechanisms for which higher peripheral blood Tregs help prevention of allograft rejection and maintenance of transplant tolerance meet the same concept of peripheral regulation in autoimmune reaction [18, 29–32]. On a cellular basis, Tregs utilize four modes of action in peripheral regulation including [29–32]; i) secretion or generation of inhibitory cytokines (e.g., IL-10, IL-35, TGF-β and adenosine); ii) direct killing of targets through Granzyme A/B and perforin-dependent cytolysis; iii) IL-2 consumption through high IL-2R expression which leads to cytokine-mediated deprivation and

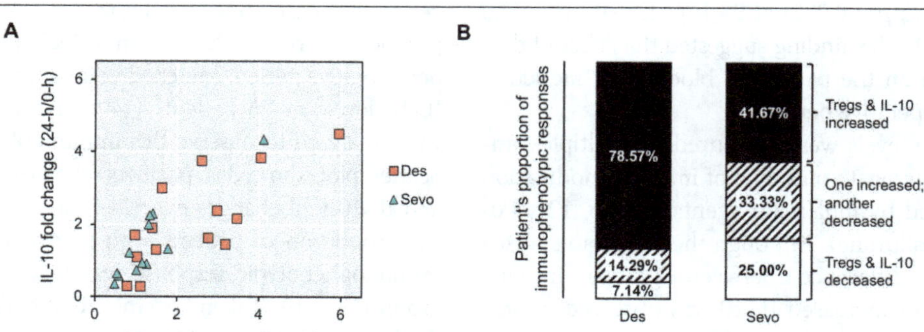

Fig. 4 Matched-pair data analysis of Tregs and IL-10 ($n = 26$; 14 desflurane, 12 sevoflurane). Fold change was calculated by Tregs (or IL-10) measured at 24-h divided by that of pre-exposure (0-h) in the same patient, in which fold change > 1 indicated upregulation and fold change < 1 was downregulation. **a** Scatter plot exhibited the positive relationship between Tregs and IL-10 fold changes. **b** Bar plots showed a higher proportion of co-increased Tregs and IL-10 immunophenotypic response in patients receiving desflurane anesthesia. Des, desflurane; Sevo, sevoflurane

apoptosis of effector cells; and iv) direct interaction with CTLA-4, LAG-3 and PD1 molecules. Although accumulating evidence would favor contact-dependent mechanisms over non-contact/secretory component alone, these different mechanisms should work in concert to control various immune effector cells and regulate different inflammatory settings [29–32]. Given that breadth of regulatory function on autoimmunity and self-tolerance, changes in peripheral blood Tregs in kidney transplant recipients may shift the balance between allograft rejection and transplant tolerance.

According to these lines of evidence, the increment of Tregs and IL-10 (Figs. 2, 3 and 4) after exposure to desflurane anesthesia should be beneficial to graft outcomes in LDKT recipients. In fact, several drugs routinely used in general anesthesia (besides volatile anesthetic agents) have immunomodulatory properties [25, 26]. It is possible that some of them have positive effects on Tregs. Synergistic effects of multiple Treg-modulated agents may provide a better transplant outcome. Understanding how anesthetic agents exhibit varied effects on the immune system, particularly on Tregs, is important for future development of perioperative medicine in kidney transplantation.

This study was associated with several limitations. First, clinical outcomes, such as short-term and long-term graft survival, that were associated with Treg immunomodulation of desflurane anesthesia were not investigated. Graft survival is influenced by various factors (such as adequacy and toxicity of immunosuppressive drugs, presence of donor-specific antigen, PRA levels, numbers of HLA mismatch). These factors, together with Treg immunomodulation of desflurane, should be taken into account in future studies. Secondly, plasma cytokine levels were measured in 26 out of 40 patients (2/3 of total population in this study) due to the limited budget. A non-significant difference of cytokines between intervention groups may be due to a lack of statistical power, but at least, the upward trend of plasma IL-10 was observed, given the supportive evidence that desflurane anesthesia induced peripheral blood Tregs with potential IL-10 production. Third, the mechanisms of action (MoA) that drive desflurane-Treg immunomodulation were not defined and not the focus of this study. Further studies to characterize receptors and downstream signaling pathways that are responsible for desflurane-Treg effects would give some insight into a new MoA class of volatile anesthetic agent or a new biological process that facilitates transplant tolerance in LDKT recipients.

Conclusion

In summary, desflurane had the advantage over sevoflurane as the inhalation anesthetic in LDKT patients regarding the increment of peripheral blood Tregs. Further research focused on clinical outcomes and pharmacological actions of desflurane on Treg immunomodulation has translational potential, which could eventually benefit LDKT recipients.

Abbreviations

ADPKD: Autosomal dominant polycystic kidney disease; BMI: Body mass index; ESRD: End-stage renal disease; HLA: Human leukocyte antigen; LDKT: Living donor kidney transplantation; MoA: Mechanisms of action; PRA: Panel reactive antibodies; Th1: T helper 1; Th2: T helper 2; Tregs: Regulatory T cells

Acknowledgments

We are grateful to all staff of the Ramathibodi Kidney Transplant Project. SC was financially supported by Faculty Staff Development Program of Faculty of Medicine Ramathibodi Hospital, Mahidol University, for his research activities.

Authors' contributions

AC and SC initiated the conception. AC, NOA, GG, WI, VS, SC developed the design. SP performed patient recruitment, randomization, and allocation. AC and WI performed anesthesia intervention. NUA, GG, VS provided medical care and surgical operation. NP, SS, NK, NOA, SH, SC performed Treg enumeration and cytokine measurement. AC, SP, SC analyzed data, prepared figures and tables. AC and SP wrote the manuscript. NP, SS, NK, NOA, GG, NUA, SH, WI, VS, SC revised the manuscript. All authors read and approved the final version to be published.

Author details

[1]Department of Anesthesiology, Faculty of Medicine Ramathibodi Hospital, Mahidol University, Bangkok 10400, Thailand. [2]Pediatric Translational Research Unit, Department of Pediatrics, Faculty of Medicine Ramathibodi Hospital, Mahidol University, Bangkok 10400, Thailand. [3]Research Center, Faculty of Medicine Ramathibodi Hospital, Mahidol University, Bangkok 10400, Thailand. [4]Vascular and Transplantation Unit, Department of Surgery, Faculty of Medicine Ramathibodi Hospital, Mahidol University, Bangkok 10400, Thailand. [5]Division of Infectious Disease, Department of Pediatrics, Faculty of Medicine Ramathibodi Hospital, Mahidol University, Bangkok 10400, Thailand. [6]Division of Hematology and Oncology, Department of Pediatrics, Faculty of Medicine Ramathibodi Hospital, Mahidol University, Bangkok 10400, Thailand. [7]Division of Nephrology, Department of Medicine, Faculty of Medicine Ramathibodi Hospital, Mahidol University, Bangkok 10400, Thailand. [8]Department of Clinical Epidemiology and Biostatistics, Faculty of Medicine Ramathibodi Hospital, Mahidol University, Bangkok 10400, Thailand.

References

1. Josephson MA. Monitoring and managing graft health in the kidney transplant recipient. Clin J Am Soc Nephrol. 2011;6:1774–80.
2. Goldberg RJ, Weng FL, Kandula P. Acute and chronic allograft dysfunction in kidney transplant recipients. Med Clin North Am. 2016;100:487–503.
3. Hara S. Banff 2013 update: pearls and pitfalls in transplant renal pathology. Nephrology. 2015;20(Suppl 2):2–8.
4. Halloran PF, Reeve JP, Pereira AB, Hidalgo LG, Famulski KS. Antibody-mediated rejection, T cell-mediated rejection, and the injury-repair response: new insights from the Genome Canada studies of kidney transplant biopsies. Kidney Int. 2014;85:258–64.
5. Graca L, Cobbold SP, Waldmann H. Identification of regulatory T cells in tolerated allografts. J Exp Med. 2002;195:1641–6.
6. Edozie FC, Nova-Lamperti EA, Povoleri GA, Scottà C, John S, Lombardi G, et al. Regulatory T-cell therapy in the induction of transplant tolerance: the issue of subpopulations. Transplantation. 2014;98:370–9.
7. Hu M, Wang YM, Wang Y, Zhang GY, Zheng G, Yi S, et al. Regulatory T cells in kidney disease and transplantation. Kidney Int. 2016;90:502–14.
8. Tang Q, Vincenti F. Transplant trials with Tregs: perils and promises. J Clin Invest. 2017;127:2505–12.
9. de St Groth BF. Regulatory T-cell abnormalities and the global epidemic of immuno-inflammatory disease. Immunol Cell Biol. 2012;90:256–9.

10. Stelmaszczyk-Emmel A, Zawadzka-Krajewska A, Szypowska A, Kulus M, Demkow U. Frequency and activation of CD4+CD25 FoxP3+ regulatory T cells in peripheral blood from children with atopic allergy. Int Arch Allergy Immunol. 2013;162:16–24.
11. Srisala S, Pongsakul N, Sahakijpicharn T, Hongeng S, Chutipongtanate S, Apiwattanakul N. Capillary blood as an alternative specimen for enumeration of percentages of lymphocyte subsets. BMC Res Notes. 2019; 12:633. https://doi.org/10.1186/s13104-019-4659-4.
12. Shan J, Guo Y, Luo L, Lu J, Li C, Zhang C, et al. Do CD4+ Foxp3+ Treg cells correlate with transplant outcomes: a systematic review on recipients of solid organ transplantation. Cell Immunol. 2011;270:5–12.
13. Karczewski M, Karczewski J, Kostrzewa A, Wiktorowicz K, Glyda M. The role of Foxp3+ regulatory T cells in kidney transplantation. Transplant Proc. 2009; 41:1527–9.
14. San Segundo D, Fernández-Fresnedo G, Rodrigo E, Ruiz JC, González M, Gómez-Alamillo C, et al. High regulatory T-cell levels at 1 year posttransplantation predict long-term graft survival among kidney transplant recipients. Transplant Proc. 2012;44:2538–41.
15. Liu L, Deng S, Teng L, Fu Q, Wang C, He X. Absolute of CD4(+)CD25(+)FOXP3(+) regulatory T-cell count rather than its ratio in peripheral blood is related to long-term survival of renal allografts. Transplant Proc. 2012;44: 284–6.
16. Ma L, Zhang H, Hu K, Lv G, Fu Y, Ayana DA, et al. The imbalance between Tregs, Th17 cells and inflammatory cytokines among renal transplant recipients. BMC Immunol. 2015;16:56. https://doi.org/10.1186/s12865-015-0118-8.
17. Carmona-Escamilla MA, Queipo G, García-Mosqueda LA, García-Covarrubias L, Fonseca-Sánchez MA, Villanueva-Ortega E, et al. Peripheral blood regulatory T cells are diminished in kidney transplant patients with chronic allograft nephropathy. Transplant Proc. 2018;50:444–8.
18. Hutchinson JA, Geissler EK. Now or never? The case for cell-based immunosuppression in kidney transplantation. Kidney Int. 2015;87:1116–24.
19. Zwang NA, Leventhal JR. Cell therapy in kidney transplantation: focus on regulatory T cells. J Am Soc Nephrol. 2017;28:1960–72.
20. Schneemilch CE, Hachenberg T, Ansorge S, Ittenson A, Bank U. Effects of different anaesthetic agents on immune cell function in vitro. Eur J Anaesthesiol. 2005;22:616–23.
21. Pirbudak Cocelli L, Ugur MG, Karadasli H. Comparison of effects of low-flow sevoflurane and desflurane anesthesia on neutrophil and T-cell populations. Curr Ther Res Clin Exp. 2012;73:41–51.
22. Koksoy S, Sahin Z, Karsli B. Comparison of the effects of desflurane and bupivacaine on Th1 and Th2 responses. Clin Lab. 2013;59:1215–20.
23. Zhang T, Fan Y, Liu K, Wang Y. Effects of different general anaesthetic techniques on immune responses in patients undergoing surgery for tongue cancer. Anaesth Intensive Care. 2014;42:220–7.
24. Liu S, Gu X, Zhu L, et al. Effects of propofol and sevoflurane on perioperative immune response in patients undergoing laparoscopic radical hysterectomy for cervical cancer. Medicine. 2016;95:e5479. https://doi.org/10.1097/MD.0000000000005479.
25. Stollings LM, Jia LJ, Tang P, Dou H, Lu B, Xu Y. Immune modulation by volatile anesthetics. Anesthesiology. 2016;125:399–411.
26. Yuki K, Eckenhoff RG. Mechanisms of the immunological effects of volatile anesthetics: a review. Anesth Analg. 2016;123:326–35.
27. Schulz KF, Altman DG, Moher D, for the CONSORT Group. CONSORT 2010 statement: updated guidelines for reporting parallel group randomised trials. Trials. 2010;11(1):32.
28. Alberu J, Vargas-Rojas MI, Morales-Buenrostro LE, Crispin JC, Rodríguez-Romo R, Uribe-Uribe NO, et al. De novo donor-specific HLA antibody development and peripheral CD4(+)CD25(high) cells in kidney transplant recipients: a place for interaction? J Transp Secur. 2012;2012:302539. https://doi.org/10.1155/2012/302539.
29. Vignali DA, Collison LW, Workman CJ. How regulatory T cells work. Nat Rev Immunol. 2008;8:523–32.
30. Li Z, Li D, Tsun A, Li B. FOXP3+ regulatory T cells and their functional regulation. Cell Mol Immunol. 2015;12:558–65.
31. Gianchecchi E, Fierabracci A. Inhibitory receptors and pathways of lymphocytes: the role of PD-1 in Treg development and their involvement in autoimmunity onset and cancer progression. Front Immunol. 2018;9:2374. https://doi.org/10.3389/fimmu.2018.02374.
32. Vanichapol T, Pongsakul N, Srisala S, Apiwattanakul N, Chutipongtanate S, Hongeng S. Suppressive characteristics of umbilical cord blood-derived regulatory T cells after ex vivo expansion on autologous and allogeneic T effectors and various lymphoblastic cells. J Immunother. 2019;42:110–8.

16

Intravesical dexmedetomidine instillation reduces postoperative catheter-related bladder discomfort in male patients under general anesthesia

Hong Chen[†], Bin Wang[†], Qin Li, Juan Zhou, Rui Li and Ye Zhang[*]

Abstract

Background: The catheter-related bladder discomfort (CRBD) of male patients is a common clinical problem, albeit lacking effective solutions. The present study aimed to investigate whether intravesical dexmedetomidine instillation alleviates the postoperative urinary discomfort in male patients with catheter under general anesthesia.

Methods: This single-blinded, prospective, randomized study included a total of 167 male patients American Society of Anesthesiologists (ASA) physical status I-II scheduled for surgery under general anesthesia were allocated to two groups: 84 in the dexmedetomidine group and 83 in the control group. Dexmedetomidine group patients received intravesical instillation of the drug 0.5 μg/kg and normal saline 20 mL, while the control group received intravesical instillation of 20 mL normal saline. The catheter was clamped for 30 min after intravesical instillation for all patients. CRBD scores and urethra pain numerical rating scale (NRS) scores were measured at admittance to post-anesthesia care unit (PACU) (T0), intravesical instillation (T1), 30 min (T2), 60 min (T3), 2 h (T4) after intravesical instillation, discharged from PACU (T5), and 6 h (T6) and 24 h (T7) after the operation. Patient satisfaction at discharge from PACU and 24 h post-operation were compared between the two groups.

Results: CRBD scores and urethra pain NRS scores after 30 min of intravesical dexmedetomidine instillation to 24 h post-operation were significantly lower than the control group ($p < 0.001$), and patient satisfaction was higher at discharge from PACU and 24 h post-operation ($p < 0.001$). No differences were detected in Steward score out of PACU ($p = 0.213$) and from the time of the end of operation to fully awake ($p = 0.417$).

Conclusion: Intravesical dexmedetomidine instillation reduces postoperative urinary discomfort and urethra pain and improves satisfaction in male patients under general anesthesia.

Keywords: Dexmedetomidine, Intravesical instillation, Catheter-related bladder discomfort, General anesthesia

* Correspondence: zhangye_hassan@sina.com
[†]Hong Chen and Bin Wang contributed equally to this work.
Department of Anesthesiology and Perioperative Medicine, The Second Affiliated Hospital of Anhui Medical University, 678# Furong Road, Hefei, Anhui Province, China

Background

Catheter-related bladder discomfort (CRBD) after the operation is a common adverse reaction; however, many surgery patients need an indwelling catheter during or after the operation. The incidence of CRBD is 47–90% [1, 2], and catheter maladjustment is common, especially in male patients [3, 4]. Reportedly, 27–55% of the patients experience moderate or severe catheter-related bladder discomfort symptoms in the post-anesthesia care unit (PACU) [3, 5]. CRBD leads to restlessness, delirium, decreased satisfaction, and a rise in postoperative complications, such as incision rupture, bleeding, hemodynamic instability, the severity of coronary heart disease [1]. Thus, how to relieve postoperative CRBD, reduce the incidence of related complications, improve patient satisfaction, and shorten the time of anesthesia recovery observation has become needs to be resolved urgently in clinical practice [6–9].

Dexmedetomidine is a type of high selective adrenergic α-2 receptor agonist, which has the effects of sedation, analgesia, and anti-anxiety. Several studies have confirmed that dexmedetomidine can reduce the incidence of postoperative agitation and delirium [10–14]. Moreover, dexmedetomidine might reduce bladder contractility via α-2 receptor agonism, M3 muscarinic receptor antagonism [15–17], and the incidence and severity of catheter-related bladder discomfort after general anesthesia [16, 18–21]. These studies were based on the intravenous administration of dexmedetomidine, which increases the risk of arrhythmia [22].

A large number of studies [23–25] showed that intravesical instillation is an effective way of drug administration, which exerts an obvious effect on the treatment of bladder-related diseases. Concurrently, the intravesical instillation of drugs can reduce the systemic response. However, whether dexmedetomidine can be used by intravesical instillation to reduce CRBD and improve the tolerance to indwelling catheter has not yet been reported. Thus, the present study aimed to investigate whether intravesical dexmedetomidine instillation can alleviate the postoperative urinary discomfort in male patients with general anesthesia.

Methods

Study design

This single-center, single-blinded, prospective, randomized study was approved by the Institutional Review Board and Hospital Research Ethics Committee of the Second Affiliated Hospital of Anhui Medical University [No. PJ-YX2018–004 (F2)]. The protocol of the study was registered in the Chinese Clinical Trial Registry (No. ChiCTR1800016429) and executed in accordance with the CONSORT checklist. Each patient provided written informed consent before participation in the study. Patients can withdraw from the study at any time according to their wishes. All patients were enrolled between June 2018 and April 2019. The inclusion criteria were as follows: male patients aged 18–70 years and American Society of Anesthesiologists (ASA) physical status I-II undergoing elective surgery, scheduled general anesthesia, and intraoperative catheter insertion. The exclusion criteria were as follows: urology patients, end-stage renal disease, pathological obesity, central nervous system dysfunction, chronic pain, cerebral infarction, mental disorder of consciousness, change in surgical and anesthesia plans, without CRBD when admitted to PACU. In this single-blinded study, patients were blinded to the group allocation. However, it was not blinded to anesthesiologists, PACU nurses, surgeons and ward nurses because this information is important for perioperative management of patients.

Sample size

PASS 11.0 software was used to compare the mean of two independent samples. According to the pre-experiment CRBD score, the mean value of the control group was 2.25, and the standard deviation was 0.66. The mean value of the dexmedetomidine group was 1.9 and the standard deviation was 0.67. Set α as 0.05, β as 0.9, using bilateral test, the sample size of each group is 75. Increase the sample size 20% to prevent the sample drop-out, so we chose 90 patients in each group.

Patient randomization

Male patients with CRBD into PACU were randomly divided into two groups with an allocation ratio of 1:1 according to the computerized randomization table in a blinded manner. Random numbers to each patient while the nurses collected postoperative data from the patients.

Anesthesia application

The surgery and anesthesia program of the patient was similar to that of the other patients. Electrocardiography (ECG), peripheral oxygen saturation (SpO_2), non-invasive blood pressure (NBP), and respiratory rate (RR) were monitored routinely after the patients were admitted to the operating room. The vein channel was established with a 22-gauge indwelling needle. Oxygen was inhaled by mask (oxygen flow rate was 4–5 L/min). Midazolam 0.025 mg/kg, sufentanil 2–4 μg/kg, etomidate 1–2 mg/kg, and rocuronium 0.9 mg/kg were injected intravenously for anesthesia induction. After intubation, a ureteral catheter was used for catheterization, followed by anesthesia maintenance propofol 2–4 mg/kg/h, remifentanil 10–20 μg/kg/h, and continued addition of cisatracurium to maintain muscle relaxation. At the end of the operation, the muscle relaxation and consciousness of the patient were restored, the tracheal tube was removed and sent to PACU for observation.

Catheterization

After induction of anesthesia, 16F latex ureteral catheter (Huaxing Medical Equipment Co., Ltd., China) was used for all participants. Catheterization was performed by surgeons with more than 5 years experience. The operation process must be as gentle as possible, and the whole process was sterile. Before catheterization, paraffin oil fully lubricated the catheter. After the successful placement of the catheter, 10 mL of normal saline was injected into the cuff balloon to prevent catheter slippage. After catheterization, the catheter was fixed on the inside of the thigh to prevent urinary tract injury caused by catheter pulling.

Interventions

As a safe and widely used drug, intravesical dexmedetomidine instillation method has been approved by the Institutional Review Board and Hospital Research Ethics Committee of the Second Affiliated Hospital of Anhui Medical University. In the dexmedetomidine group, 0.5 μg/kg dexmedetomidine was solubilized in 20 mL normal saline infused from the ureteral catheter to bladder for intravesical dexmedetomidine instillation. In the control group, 20 mL of normal saline was infused from the ureteral catheter to the bladder. After instillation, the ureteral catheter was clipped for 30 min and then unclipped.

Assessments

The primary outcome endpoint was CRBD score, and the second outcome endpoint was urethra pain NRS score and patient's satisfaction. The duration of anesthesia, the time length of operation, the time from the end of the operation to full consciousness, and patient characteristics were recorded. Mean arterial pressure (MAP), heart rate (HR), RR, SpO_2, CRBD score, and urethra pain NRS score were recorded when the patient was sent to PACU (T0), the time of intravesical instillation with dexmedetomidine or normal saline (T1), 30 min after intravesical instillation (T2), 1 h after intravesical instillation (T3), 2 h after intravesical instillation (T4), the time point of leaving PACU (T5), 6 h after operation (T6), and 24 h after opertaion (T7). The NRS score of urethra pain and the complications after intravesical instillation were also recorded. The patient satisfaction score were recorded when leaving PACU and 24 h after the operation. The NRS score was used for the assessment of urethra pain in both groups. CRBD score: 0 point, patients have no discomfort at all; 1 point, patients have slight discomfort, only when asked to show discomfort; 2 points, patients have moderate discomfort, frequency of urination, the urgency of urination, feeling of lower abdominal distension, which is not easy to bear; 3 points, the patient had severe discomfort, intolerable distension, urethral pain, frequent urination with strong restlessness, and needed to be removed. Ramsay score: 1 point, the patient is restless and fidgety; 2 points, the patient is quiet and cooperative; 3 points, the patient is sleepy and can follow the instructions; 4 points, the patient is in a sleep state and can wake up; 5 points, the respiratory response of the patient is slow; 6 points, the patient is deep asleep and has no response to stimulation. Patient satisfaction score is consisting of integers from 1 point to 5 points: 1 point means dissatisfied and 5 points mean very satisfied. The urethra pain NRS scores consists of integers from 0 to 10 points; 0 point means no urethra pain, and 10 points indicate intense urethra pain. Subsequently, the patients selected an integer to describe the intensity of their urethra pain while using a ureteral catheter.

Statistical analysis

SPSS software (version 22.0, Chicago, USA) was used for statistical analysis. The age, weight, blood, and other measurement data of patients were presented as mean ± standard deviation. The ASA classification data were expressed as counts. Student's *t*-test or the Mann-Whitney U test was used for continuous variables, such as age and weight. The χ^2 or Fisher's exact tests were assessed for categorical variables, such as ASA grade and patient satisfaction score. ANOVA was used for the comparison of MAP, HR, SpO_2, and other data at different time points. p-value < 0.05 was accepted as statistically significant.

Results

Study demographics

A total of 289 male patients were screened in this study, of which, 109 cases were excluded; among them, 96 did not present CRBD, 6 were not meeting the other incultion criteria, 5 refused to participate in the study, and 2 were excluded for other reasons. A total of 180 male patients with CRBD were randomly and equally divided into both groups when into PACU. Six cases in the dexmedetomidine group and 7 cases in the control group did not complete the experiment because transfer to intensive care unit (2 cases), delirium (10 cases), or catheter falls off (1 cases). None of the patients were lost follow-up. Finally, 84 patients in the dexmedetomidine group and 83 patients in the control group were included in the analysis (Fig. 1). The incidence of CRBD was 65.2%.

No significant difference was detected between the two groups in age, weight, ASA grade, duration of operation, duration of anesthesia, Steward's score when

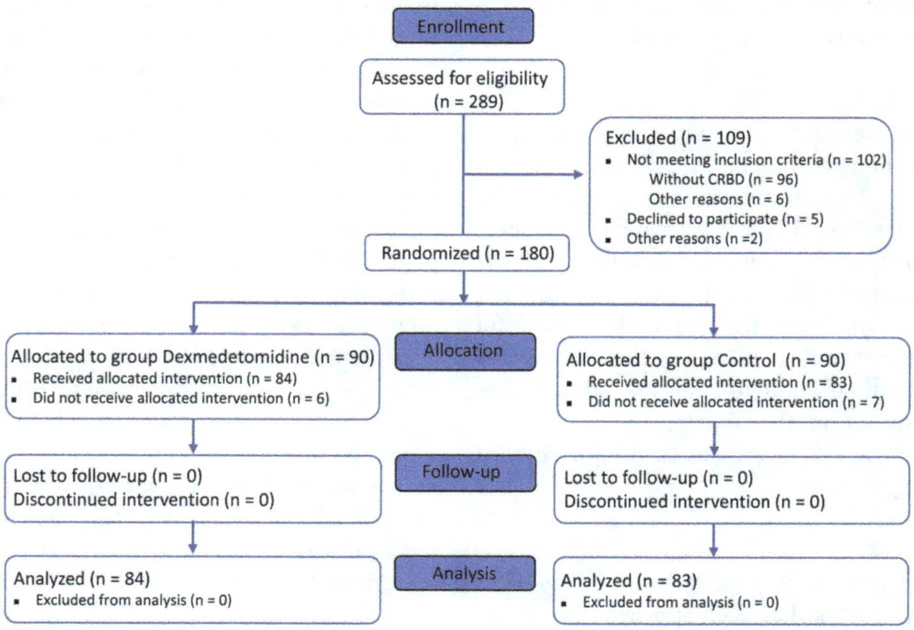

Fig. 1 Schematic of the study with a CONSORT diagram. CRBD, catheter-related bladder discomfort

leaving PACU, the time length of operation end to fully awake, catheter removal time (Table 1) and type of operation. There was no significant difference was observed in HR, RR, MAP, and SpO_2 in the two groups from T0 to T7 (Table 2), as well as no complications, occurred in either of the groups. Systematic pain NRS score decreased at T4.

CRBD and urethra pain NRS scores

Compared to the control group, the CRBD in the dexmedetomidine group was significantly improved at T3, T4, T5, T6, and T7 ($p < 0.001$) (Fig. 2a), while the urethra pain NRS scores of patients was significantly decreased ($p < 0.001$) (Fig. 2b).

Patient's satisfaction

Compared to the control group, the patient's satisfaction in the dexmedetomidine group in PACU (Fig. 3a) and 24 h post-operation (Fig. 3b) increased significantly ($p < 0.001$).

Discussion

In the present study, we observed that 0.5 μg/kg dexmedetomidine intravesical instillation can significantly

Table 1 Descriptive variables of the control group and dexmedetomidine group

	Control (*n* = 83)	Dexmedetomidine (*n* = 84)	*p*-value
Age (year)	51.2 ± 13.2	54.7 ± 12.5	0.076
Weight (kg)	68.1 ± 10.5	68.3 ± 11.1	0.919
ASA grade (I/II)	7/76	9/75	0.617
Time length of operation (min)	146.6 ± 70.8	160.2 ± 62.7	0.193
Time length of anesthesia (min)	175.2 ± 72.2	190.2 ± 67.6	0.122
Steward score out of PACU	5.98 ± 0.15	5.95 ± 0.21	0.213
Time length of operation end to fully awake (min)	13.6 ± 6.5	14.9 ± 7.3	0.417
Ureteral catheter removal time (6–12 h/12–24 h/more than 24 h after operation)	12/46/25	9/38/37	0.173
Operation type (general surgery/thoracic surgery/orthopedics/otolaryngology/stomatology/ plastic surgery)	33/14/31/5/0/0	31/20/23/7/1/2	0.343
The number of patients receiving postoperative analgesia treatment	22 (26.5%)	21 (25.0%)	0.482

Values are presented as mean (standard deviation) or counts
ASA American society of anesthesiologists

Table 2 Patients vital signs of group Dexmedetomidine ($n = 84$) and group Control ($n = 83$) at different time points

	Group	T0	T1	T2	T3	T4	T5	T6	T7
HR	Control	76.6 ± 15.4	75.9 ± 15.0	77.4 ± 14.7	79.0 ± 14.0$^{\#\#}$	80.1 ± 14.3$^{\#\#}$	80.9 ± 14.2$^{\#\#}$	80.2 ± 12.4$^{\#\#}$	79.7 ± 12.5$^{\#}$
	Dexmedetomidine	75.6 ± 15.2	75.4 ± 15.1	75.8 ± 14.5	77.8 ± 13.9$^{\#}$	79.1 ± 14.3$^{\#\#}$	79.1 ± 14.1$^{\#}$	78.7 ± 11.0$^{\#}$	79.7 ± 12.5
RR	Control	18.8 ± 1.1	18.8 ± 1.1	18.9 ± 1.3	19.2 ± 1.0$^{\#\#}$	19.1 ± 1.0	19.1 ± 0.9$^{\#}$	19.1 ± 0.9$^{\#}$	18.9 ± 0.9
	Dexmedetomidine	18.8 ± 1.5	18.7 ± 1.2	18.5 ± 1.2	18.5 ± 1.4	18.7 ± 1.1	19.0 ± 1.0	18.7 ± 0.8	18.8 ± 0.8
MAP	Control	98.9 ± 16.1	97.9 ± 14.4	97.8 ± 14.5	97.3 ± 14.4	95.6 ± 14.4$^{\#}$	94.3 ± 12.7$^{\#\#}$	91.4 ± 11.5$^{\#\#}$	89.6 ± 10.5$^{\#\#}$
	Dexmedetomidine	98.4 ± 15.2	97.7 ± 15.5	95.4 ± 14.3$^{\#\#}$	94.8 ± 14.2$^{\#\#}$	94.1 ± 12.8$^{\#\#}$	92.8 ± 12.3$^{\#\#}$	91.5 ± 10.6$^{\#\#}$	89.6 ± 8.6$^{\#\#}$
SPO_2	Control	98.7 ± 1.1	98.9 ± 1.2	98.6 ± 1.3	98.7 ± 1.2	98.7 ± 1.1	98.6 ± 1.2	98.3 ± 1.0$^{\#\#}$	98.3 ± 0.7$^{\#\#}$
	Dexmedetomidine	98.7 ± 1.8	98.9 ± 1.4	98.8 ± 1.4	98.8 ± 1.4	98.8 ± 1.1	98.8 ± 1.1	98.4 ± 0.9	98.3 ± 0.7
Systemic pain NRS score	Control	3.2 ± 1.2	3.1 ± 1.1	2.5 ± 0.7$^{\#\#}$	2.4 ± 0.7$^{\#\#}$	2.3 ± 0.7$^{\#\#}$	2.2 ± 0.7$^{\#\#}$	2.3 ± 1.0$^{\#\#}$	1.4 ± 0.9$^{\#\#}$
	Dexmedetomidine	3.0 ± 1.1	2.9 ± 1.0	2.5 ± 0.8$^{\#\#}$	2.2 ± 0.7$^{\#\#}$	2.1 ± 0.6$^{\#\#*}$	2.0 ± 0.6$^{\#\#}$	2.2 ± 1.4$^{\#\#}$	1.3 ± 0.8$^{\#\#}$

$^{*}p$-value < 0.05 compared to the same time of Group Control ($^{*}p$-value = 0.021)
$^{\#}p$-value < 0.05 compared to T0; $^{\#\#}p$-value < 0.01 compared to T0
Values are presented as mean ± standard deviation
MAP Mean arterial pressure, *HR* Heart rate, *RR* Respiratory rate, SpO_2 Pulse oximetry. Time course, the time point of the patient sent to PACU (T0), intravesical instillation (T1), 30 min after intravesical instillation (T2), 1 h after intravesical instillation (T3), 2 h after intravesical instillation (T4), leaving PACU (T5), 6 h after the operation (T6), 24 h after the operation (T7)

reduce the symptoms of postoperative catheter-related bladder discomfort and the urethral pain caused by catheter in male patients who received general anesthesia, and consequently, their satisfaction was improved. The improvement of these symptoms can sustain from 0.5–24 h after intravesical dexmedetomidine instillation.

CRBD is common in PACU, especially male patients [26]. Therefore, in this study, we included male patients as the study subject, and the incidence of CRBD was 65.2%, which was consistent with that reported previously [1, 2, 26]. The high incidence of CRBD in male patients might be related to the anatomical characteristics, such as the long urethra and large catheter [26]. Because several urological operations need to operate on the urethra, which markedly impacts this study, and the degree of impact is different, so this study was not included in the urological patients. In the clinical practice, to deal with bladder catheter pain, we often scribble lidocaine cream at the urethral orifice, meanwhile intravenous analgesic drugs, such as fentanyl, flurbiprofen axetil could also be used, but the effect is not ideal.

In this study, we observed that intravesical dexmedetomidine instillation can significantly reduce the symptoms of postoperative CRBD according to the following underlying mechanism. Alpha 2-adrenoceptor, i.e., the α2A-subtype, is expressed in the bladder, urethra, and prostate. The intra-arterial administration of an α-2 agonist reduced the micturition pressure, bladder capacity, and micturition volume [27, 28]. dexmedetomidine is a high selective adrenergic α-2 receptor agonist which may reduce the micturition pressure, bladder capacity, and micturition volume. There are several muscarinic receptors in bladder epithelium and efferent nerves,

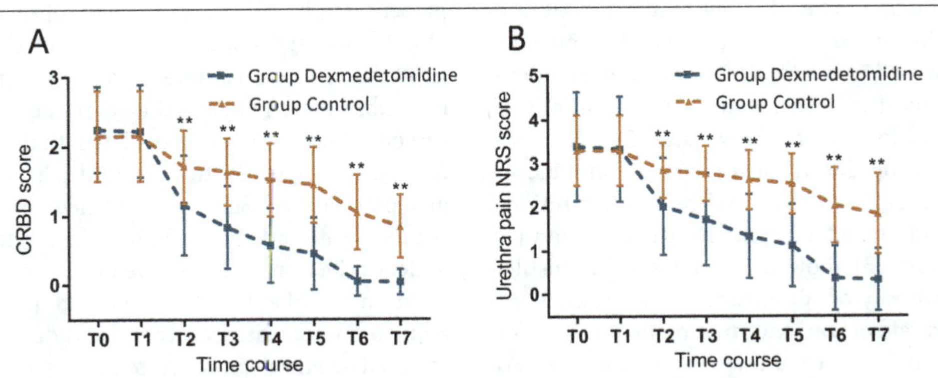

Fig. 2 Bladder stimulation scale (Fig. 2a) and urethra pain NRS score (Fig. 2b) in dexmedetomidine and control groups at various time points. CRBD, catheter-related bladder discomfort. Time course, the time point at which the patient sent to PACU (T0), intravesical instillation (T1), 30 min after intravesical instillation (T2); 1 h after intravesical instillation (T3), 2 h after intravesical instillation (T4), leaving PACU (T5), 6 h after operation (T6), 24 h after operation (T7); **p < 0.001

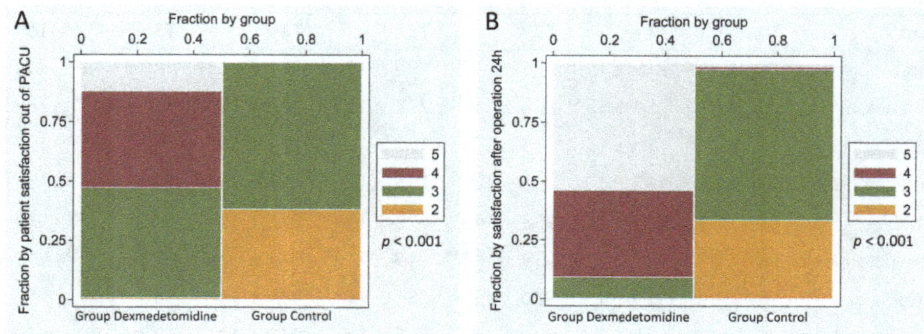

Fig. 3 Spine plot of patient satisfaction score out of PACU (Fig. 3a) and 24 h after the operation (Fig. 3b) in dexmedetomidine and control groups. Patient satisfaction score: 5 points, very satisfied; 4 points, satisfied; 3 points, relatively satisfied; 2 points, basically satisfied; 1 point, dissatisfied

including M2 and M3. The M3 receptor is mainly responsible for bladder contraction [29]. The catheter can stimulate the afferent nerves of the bladder to release acetylcholine, which leads to the contraction of detrusor mediated by muscarinic receptors. Therefore, muscarinic antagonists alleviate CRBD in different degrees [1]. Some studies showed that dexmedetomidine might reduce bladder contractility via α-2 receptor and M3 muscarinic receptor antagonism [16, 17]. On the other hand, catheter stimulation can cause inflammation and increase prostaglandin secretion, which is one of the plausible reasons for CRBD [30]. Therefore, some anti-inflammatory drugs can also alleviate CRBD. Another study showed that dexmedetomidine reduces the release of prostaglandins of inflammation, and hence, relieves CRBD [31]. In addition, dexmedetomidine exerts a sedative effect and relieves CRBD [10]. Another underlying mechanism is that after intravesical instillation, dexmedetomidine can be absorbed from bladder and play a systemically role of sedation, analgesia and anti-inflammatory, which need to be further verified.

In the current study, dexmedetomidine plays a role in intravesical instillation. The off-label method of dexmedetomidine is often used in clinical research, which has proved to be safe and effective. For example, dexmedetomidine is safely used in subarachnoid and epidural [32], neuraxial [33] and for children intranasal [34]. As a safe and widely used drug, intravesical dexmedetomidine instillation method has been approved by the Institutional Review Board and Hospital Research Ethics Committee. Several studies [23–25] showed that intravesical instillation is an effective way of administration of drugs, which had an obvious effect on the treatment of bladder-related diseases and reduce the systemic response. For instance, invasive immunotherapy, chemotherapy and chemohyperthermia for bladder cancer [35, 36], intragastric thermal gelatin matrix implantation for intractable hematuria [37], intragastric gentamicin for recurrent urinary tract infections treatment [38]. Dexmedetomidine is well absorbed through the mucous membrane. Iirola et al. [39] reported that peak plasma concentrations of dexmedetomidine were 38 min after intranasal administration, and the pharmacological effects were similar to the intravenous administration but with a later onset time. In the current study, dexmedetomidine was able to work through the bladder mucosa, with a significant effect at half an hour after administration. Even so, intravesical dexmedetomidine instillation has potential risk of bladder dysfunction such as urinary retention through a local α2-stimulating effect, which should be closely pay attention in clinical practice.

In this study, intravesical dexmedetomidine instillation alleviates the pain caused by catheter while in situ and on removal. The main causes of the pain during catheter in situ were as follows: the material and size of the catheter, the traction of the catheter drainage bag, the urethral discomfort, the stimulation of the bladder wall by the catheter, the obstruction of the catheter, catheter blockage, the hemorrhagic pseudopolyps, the fear of the catheter, and the psychological rejection [40]. In the present study, all patients were observed and nursed closely, and the material and size of the catheter were identical, and no catheter drainage bag traction, catheter obstruction, hemorrhagic pseudopolyps were observed. Therefore, we speculated that the main reason for the difference in the urethral pain between the two groups was the tolerance of catheter stimulation of the bladder wall and the difference in the fear and psychological rejection of the catheter. Dexmedetomidine is a solution to bladder irritation and psychological maladjustment of patients, thereby reducing the catheter-induced urethral pain. Systematic pain NRS score decreased at T4, and there was no significant change at other time points. The possible reason is that dextromethorphan was absorbed by bladder and played a systemic role, which need further study.

Patients' satisfaction at the time point out of PACU and 24 h after the operation was significantly improved after intravesical dexmedetomidine instillation because there were reductions in CRBD and catheter-induced urethral pain and patient satisfaction is closely related to the postoperative outcomes [41]. The improvement in the patients' satisfaction might reduce their CRBD and urethral pain.

No complications were detected in the control and experimental groups. Since the sample size of this study is small, and the patients selected are ASA I-II, their basic conditions are well. Clinically, we will encounter CRBD to aggravate the condition of patients with coronary heart disease, and dexmedetomidine might also lead to arrhythmia and other risks. What is more, intravesical dexmedetomidine instillation perhaps could prolong bladder dysfunction through a local α2-stimulating effect and dexmedetomidine still reduces CRBD after 24 h. There was no urinary retention or re-catheterisation complication in dexmedetomidine group. However, only 9 ureteral catheters were removed at 6 to 12 h after operation, and 38 catheters were removed at 12 to 24 h in this study. The safety of the intravesical dexmedetomidine instillation need further clinical validation.

Nevertheless, the present study has some limitations. The number of cases is small as only 167 patients were included in this single-center study. In the future, large sample and multi-center clinical verification is essential. The patients included in this study were male patients with catheter placement under general anesthesia. The type of operation is not uniform, and the duration of operation is varied. This study did not limit the factors such as midazolam and operation time, and did not make further subgroup analysis. Further subgroup study can be carried out after expanding the sample size in the future. Prolonged follow-up for bladder dysfunction was not implemented. The safety of intravesical dexmedetomidine instillation should be further studied. It is not sure if systemic dexmedetomidine has the same effect for CRBD, further research should include an arm with intravenous dose of dexmedetomidine. All the patients included in this study were ASA I-II patients with elective surgery, and the basic condition of the patients was good. Also, critical patients have not been analyzed previously. Moreover, the effect of different doses of dexmedetomidine on CRBD was not assessed in this study. Ten milliliter normal saline was injected into the cuff balloon of catheter for all paitents to prevent slippage in our research. This may also be a potential cause of bladder wall irritation. It is regretful that we did not follow up with further research on the effect of reducing the balloon volume for reducing CRBD.

Conclusions

Dexmedetomidine 0.5 μg/kg intravesical instillation reduces postoperative urinary discomfort and urethra pain caused by catheter in male patients under general anesthesia and improves patient satisfaction after the operation.

Abbreviations

CRBD: Catheter-related bladder discomfort; ASA: American Society of Anesthesiologists; NRS: Numerical rating scale; PACU: Post-anesthesia care unit; ECG: Electrocardiography; SpO_2: Peripheral oxygen saturation; NBP: Non-invasive blood pressure; RR: Respiratory rate; MAP: Mean arterial pressure; HR: Heart rate

Acknowledgements

We thank our colleagues at the Department of Anesthesiology and Perioperative Medicine, The Second Affiliated Hospital of Anhui Medical University for their help with the samples. In addition, we thank the patients who participated in this study.

Authors' contributions

Study design: HC, BW, RL, YZ. Study conduct: HC, QL, JZ. Data analysis: HC, BW, RL, YZ. Writing paper: HC, BW, QL, JZ, RL, YZ. All authors read and approved the final manuscript.

References

1. Bai Y, Wang X, Li X, Pu C, Yuan H, Tang Y, et al. Management of Catheter-Related Bladder Discomfort in patients who underwent elective surgery. J Endourol. 2015;29(6):640–9.
2. Park JY, Hong JH, Kim DH, Yu J, Hwang JH, Kim YK. Magnesium and bladder discomfort after transurethral resection of bladder tumor: a randomized, double-blind. Placebo-controlled Study Anesthesiology. 2020. https://doi.org/10.1097/ALN.0000000000003309.
3. Binhas M, Motamed C, Hawajri N, Yiou R, Marty J. Predictors of catheter-related bladder discomfort in the post-anaesthesia care unit. Annales francaises d'anesthesie et de reanimation. 2011;30(2):122–5.
4. Kim DH, Park JY, Yu J, Lee SA, Park S, Hwang JH, et al. Intravenous Lidocaine for the prevention of postoperative catheter-related bladder discomfort in male patients undergoing transurethral resection of bladder tumors: a randomized, double-blind, controlled trial. Anesth Analg. 2019. https://doi.org/10.1213/ANE.0000000000004405.
5. Agarwal A, Dhiraaj S, Singhal V, Kapoor R, Tandon M. Comparison of efficacy of oxybutynin and tolterodine for prevention of catheter related bladder discomfort: a prospective, randomized, placebo-controlled, double-blind study. Br J Anaesth. 2006;96(3):377–80.
6. Kim HC, Park HP, Lee J, Jeong MH, Lee KH. Sevoflurane vs. propofol in post-operative catheter-related bladder discomfort: a prospective randomized study. Acta Anaesthesiol Scand. 2017;61(7):773–80.
7. Li S, Song L, Ma Y, Lin X. Tramadol for the treatment of catheter-related bladder discomfort: a randomized controlled trial. BMC Anesthesiol. 2018; 18(1):194.
8. Maghsoudi R, Farhadi-Niaki S, Etemadian M, Kashi AH, Shadpour P, Shirani A, et al. Comparing the efficacy of Tolterodine and gabapentin versus placebo in catheter related bladder discomfort after percutaneous Nephrolithotomy: a randomized clinical trial. J Endourol. 2018;32(2):168–74.
9. Shin YS, Doo AR. Managing postoperative catheter-related bladder discomfort. J Anesth. 2019;33(2):347.
10. Kim JA, Ahn HJ, Yang M, Lee SH, Jeong H, Seong BG. Intraoperative use of dexmedetomidine for the prevention of emergence agitation and postoperative delirium in thoracic surgery: a randomized-controlled trial. Can J Anaesth. 2019;66(4):371–9.
11. Lee C, Lee CH, Lee G, Lee M, Hwang J. The effect of the timing and dose of dexmedetomidine on postoperative delirium in elderly patients after laparoscopic major non-cardiac surgery: a double blind randomized controlled study. J Clin Anesth. 2018;47:27–32.
12. Shin HJ, Koo BW, Bang SU, Kim JH, Hwang JW, Do SH, et al. Intraoperative dexmedetomidine sedation reduces the postoperative agitated behavior in elderly patients undergoing orthopedic surgery compared to the propofol sedation. Minerva Anestesiol. 2017;83(10):1042–50.

13. Su X, Meng ZT, Wu XH, Cui F, Li HL, Wang DX, et al. Dexmedetomidine for prevention of delirium in elderly patients after non-cardiac surgery: a randomised, double-blind, placebo-controlled trial. Lancet. 2016;388(10054): 1893–902.
14. Subramaniam B, Shankar P, Shaefi S, Mueller A, O'Gara B, Banner-Goodspeed V, et al. Effect of intravenous acetaminophen vs placebo combined with Propofol or Dexmedetomidine on postoperative delirium among older patients following cardiac surgery: the DEXACET randomized clinical trial. Jama. 2019;321(7):686–96.
15. Hegde SS. Muscarinic receptors in the bladder: from basic research to therapeutics. Br J Pharmacol. 2006;147(Suppl 2):S80–7.
16. Singh TK, Sahu S, Agarwal A, Gupta D, Mishra P. Dexmedetomidine for prevention of early postoperative catheter-related bladder discomfort in voluntary kidney donors: prospective, randomized, double-blind, placebo-controlled trial. J Anaesthesiol Clin Pharmacol. 2018;34(2):211–5.
17. Takizuka A, Minami K, Uezono Y, Horishita T, Yokoyama T, Shiraishi M, et al. Dexmedetomidine inhibits muscarinic type 3 receptors expressed in Xenopus oocytes and muscarine-induced intracellular Ca2+ elevation in cultured rat dorsal root ganglia cells. Naunyn Schmiedeberg's Arch Pharmacol. 2007;375(5):293–301.
18. Akca B, Aydogan-Eren E, Canbay O, Karagoz AH, Uzumcugil F, Ankay-Yilbas A, et al. Comparison of efficacy of prophylactic ketamine and dexmedetomidine on postoperative bladder catheter-related discomfort. Saudi Med J. 2016;37(1):55–9.
19. Kim HC, Lee YH, Jeon YT, Hwang JW, Lim YJ, Park JE, et al. The effect of intraoperative dexmedetomidine on postoperative catheter-related bladder discomfort in patients undergoing transurethral bladder tumour resection: a double-blind randomised study. Eur J Anaesthesiol. 2015;32(9):596–601.
20. Kwon Y, Jang JS, Hwang SM, Lee JJ, Tark H. Intraoperative administration of dexmedetomidine reduced the postoperative catheter-related bladder discomfort and pain in patients undergoing lumbar microdiscectomy. J Anesth. 2018;32(1):41–7.
21. Liu K, Chen J, Zhang K, Wang S, Li X. A diagnostic prediction model of acute symptomatic portal vein thrombosis. Ann Vasc Surg. 2019;61:394–9.
22. Wu M, Liang Y, Dai Z, Wang S. Perioperative dexmedetomidine reduces delirium after cardiac surgery: a meta-analysis of randomized controlled trials. J Clin Anesth. 2018;50:33–42.
23. Krhut J, Navratilova M, Sykora R, Jurakova M, Gartner M, Mika D, et al. Intravesical instillation of onabotulinum toxin a embedded in inert hydrogel in the treatment of idiopathic overactive bladder: a double-blind randomized pilot study. Scand J Urol. 2016;50(3):200–5.
24. Marttila T, Jarvinen R, Liukkonen T, Rintala E, Bostrom P, Seppanen M, et al. Intravesical Bacillus Calmette-Guerin versus combination of Epirubicin and interferon-alpha2a in reducing recurrence of non-muscle-invasive bladder carcinoma: FinnBladder-6 study. Eur Urol. 2016;70(2):341–7.
25. Tyagi P, Kashyap M, Hensley H, Yoshimura N. Advances in intravesical therapy for urinary tract disorders. Expert Opin Drug Deliv. 2016;13(1):71–84.
26. Ryu JH, Hwang JW, Lee JW, Seo JH, Park HP, Oh AY, et al. Efficacy of butylscopolamine for the treatment of catheter-related bladder discomfort: a prospective, randomized, placebo-controlled, double-blind study. Br J Anaesth. 2013;111(6):932–7.
27. Ishizuka O, Mattiasson A, Andersson KE. Role of spinal and peripheral alpha 2 adrenoceptors in micturition in normal conscious rats. J Urol. 1996;156(5): 1853–7.
28. Michel MC, Vrydag W. Alpha1-, alpha2- and beta-adrenoceptors in the urinary bladder, urethra and prostate. Br J Pharmacol. 2006;147(Suppl 2): S88–119.
29. Yamanishi T, Chapple CR, Chess-Williams R. Which muscarinic receptor is important in the bladder? World J Urol. 2001;19(5):299–306.
30. Andersson KE. Detrusor myocyte activity and afferent signaling. Neurourol Urodyn. 2010;29(1):97–106.
31. Liu Y, Liu W, Wang X, Wan Z, Liu Y, Leng Y. Dexmedetomidine relieves acute inflammatory visceral pain in rats through the ERK pathway, toll-like receptor signaling, and TRPV1 channel. J Mol Neurosci. 2018;66(2):279–90.
32. Li YZ, Jiang Y, Lin H, Yang XP. Subarachnoid and epidural dexmedetomidine for the prevention of post-anesthetic shivering: a meta-analysis and systematic review. Drug Design Dev Therapy. 2019;13:3785–98.
33. Abdallah FW, Brull R. Facilitatory effects of perineural dexmedetomidine on neuraxial and peripheral nerve block: a systematic review and meta-analysis. Br J Anaesth. 2013;110(6):915–25.
34. Ghai B, Jain K, Saxena AK, Bhatia N, Sodhi KS. Comparison of oral midazolam with intranasal dexmedetomidine premedication for children undergoing CT imaging: a randomized, double-blind, and controlled study. Paediatr Anaesth. 2017;27(1):37–44.
35. Biot C, Rentsch CA, Gsponer JR, Birkhauser FD, Jusforgues-Saklani H, Lemaitre F, et al. Preexisting BCG-specific T cells improve intravesical immunotherapy for bladder cancer. Sci Transl Med. 2012;4(137):137ra172.
36. Campodonico F, Di Stasi S, Lev GM, Terrone C, Bongiovanni L, Mattioli F, et al. Intravesical chemotherapy and Chemohyperthermia in non-muscle-invasive bladder Cancer; an overview on drug administration technologies and pharmacokinetics. Curr Drug Metab. 2017;18(7):657–65.
37. Margreiter M, Sharma V, Schauer I, Klingler HC. Intravesical hemostatic gelatin matrix instillation in the management of intractable hematuria. Urology. 2013;82(3):724–8.
38. Stalenhoef JE, van Nieuwkoop C, Menken PH, Bernards ST, Elzevier HW, van Dissel JT. Intravesical gentamicin treatment for recurrent urinary tract infections caused by multidrug resistant bacteria. J Urol. 2019;201(3):549–55.
39. Iirola T, Vilo S, Manner T, Aantaa R, Lahtinen M, Scheinin M, et al. Bioavailability of dexmedetomidine after intranasal administration. Eur J Clin Pharmacol. 2011;67(8):825–31.
40. Wilson M. Causes and management of indwelling urinary catheter-related pain. Br J Nurs. 2008;17(4):232–9.
41. Tevis SE, Kennedy GD, Kent KC. Is there a relationship between patient satisfaction and favorable surgical outcomes? Adv Surg. 2015;49:221–33.

The effects of anesthesia induction and positive pressure ventilation on right-ventricular function: An echocardiography-based prospective observational study

Harry Magunia[1*], Anne Jordanow[1], Marius Keller[1], Peter Rosenberger[1] and Martina Nowak-Machen[1,2]

Abstract

Background: General anesthesia induction with the initiation of positive pressure ventilation creates a vulnerable phase for patients. The impact of positive intrathoracic pressure on cardiac performance has been studied but remains controversial. 3D echocardiography is a valid and MRI-validated bed-side tool to evaluate the right ventricle (RV). The aim of this study was to assess the impact of anesthesia induction (using midazolam, sufentanil and rocuronium, followed by sevoflurane) with positive pressure ventilation (PEEP 5, tidal volume 6–8 ml/kg) on 2D and 3D echocardiography derived parameters of RV function.

Methods: A prospective observational study on fifty-three patients undergoing elective cardiac surgery in a tertiary care university hospital was designed. Transthoracic echocardiography exams were performed before and immediately after anesthesia induction and were recorded together with hemodynamic parameters and ventilator settings.

Results: After anesthesia induction TAPSE (mean difference − 1.6 mm (95% CI − 2.6 mm to − 0.7 mm; $p = 0.0013$) as well as the Tissue Doppler derived tricuspid annulus peak velocity (TDITVs') were significantly reduced (mean difference − 1.9% (95% CI: − 2.6 to − 1.2; $p < 0.0001$), but global right ventricular ejection fraction (RVEF; $p = 0.1607$) and right ventricular stroke volume (RVSV; $p = 0.1838$) did not change.

Conclusions: This data shows a preserved right ventricular ejection fraction and right ventricular stroke volume after anesthesia induction and initiation of positive pressure ventilation. However, the baso-apical right ventricular function is significantly reduced. Larger studies are needed in order to determine the clinical impact of these findings especially in patients presenting with impaired right ventricular function before anesthesia induction.

Keywords: Right ventricular function, Positive-pressure respiration, Anesthesiology, Echocardiography, Three-dimensional

* Correspondence: harry.magunia@med.uni-tuebingen.de
[1]Department of Anaesthesiology and Intensive Care Medicine, University Hospital Tübingen, Eberhard-Karls-University Tübingen, Hoppe-Seyler-Str. 3, 72076 Tübingen, Germany

Background

Anesthesia induction and initiation of intermittent positive pressure ventilation (IPPV) can lead to hemodynamic impairment due to several factors. IPPV is a key element of general anesthesia that is routinely used for major surgical procedures and as part of intensive care treatment provided to critically ill patients. The impact of positive intrathoracic pressure during IPPV and positive end expiratory pressure (PEEP) on the circulatory system has been studied and well described [1, 2]. The pathophysiological effects of IPPV with PEEP mainly consist of decreased venous return, decreased right ventricular (RV) output with a potential increase in RV end diastolic volume, increase in RV afterload and decreased pulmonary blood flow, which can disturb hemodynamic status in certain patients [3]. In addition, all anesthetic agents used for the induction and maintenance of general anesthesia have varying degrees of impact on systemic vascular resistance and cardiac contractility and can, hence, potentially impair right ventricular function [4]. However, the controversy of whether an increase in intrathoracic pressure during IPPV actually leads to an decreased right ventricular function and ejection fraction remains unclear, as some studies did not find a decrease in right ventricular filling pressures or RV function after the application of high PEEP levels [5, 6]. Other factors that contribute to hemodynamic changes during anesthesia induction are therapeutic measures, e.g. fluid administration and vasopressor therapy.

Two-dimensional (2D) transthoracic echocardiography has been used as a standard imaging modality to evaluate both cardiac dimensions and functions as well as inferior vena cava (IVC) diameters during varying levels of intrathoracic pressure in different clinical settings [7, 8]. Due to the complex anatomical shape and functional complexity of the right ventricle, 2D-echocardiography still relies on multiple surrogate parameters [9, 10]. Surrogate parameters used to estimate RV function are the tricuspid annular plane systolic excursion (TAPSE), the right ventricular fractional area change (RVFAC) or the tissue Doppler derived systolic movement of the lateral tricuspid annulus (TDITVs') [11]. In recent years, real-time 3-dimensional echocardiography (3DE) has become increasingly available as a bedside tool for clinicians worldwide [12, 13]. 3DE has been thoroughly validated against cardiac magnetic resonance imaging (CMRI) and offers the possibility to quantitatively assess right ventricular function and filling states based on volumetric models calculated from 3-dimensional volume datasets [14, 15]. This overcomes the problem of using surrogates while evaluating RV function.

To the best of our knowledge, this is the first study explicitly examining the effects of anesthesia induction and positive pressure ventilation on right ventricular function using 3D echocardiography. The specific aim of this prospective observational study was to examine the effects of anesthesia induction and IPPV on conventional 2D-echocardiography and 3D-echocardiography-derived determinants of right ventricular function in patients scheduled for cardiac surgery.

Methods

Study design

Approval of this prospective study (ClinicalTrials.gov Identifier NCT02820727) was given by the Institutional Review Board at the University Hospital Tübingen (IRB# 320/2015BO2). Sample size was calculated for comparing paired differences. The calculated sample size to achieve a power of 80% and a level of significance of 0.05 (two tailed), for detecting a 2 ± 5 mm change in TAPSE (effect size of 0.4) was $n = 52$. During the study period from 11/2015 to 11/2016, 554 adult patients above the age of 18 years who were scheduled for elective cardiac surgery at a tertiary care university hospital were screened for possible inclusion. The inclusion criteria were sinus rhythm and ability to give informed consent. Patients were only asked to give informed consent if an investigator capable of performing a comprehensive 3DE was available on the day of surgery. Right ventricular function was assessed by real time three-dimensional transthoracic echocardiography (TTE) immediately before anesthesia induction under spontaneous ventilation and as soon as possible after achieving hemodynamic stability after anesthesia induction and endotracheal intubation under controlled IPPV with constant PEEP. The study was performed according to the STROBE statement for observational studies [16].

Anesthesia management

Standardized monitoring was applied in all patients. The patients were not premedicated. All patients received an arterial cannula for blood pressure monitoring before anesthesia induction. Midazolam (0.1–0.15 mg/kg), sufentanil (0.3–0.5 μg/kg) and rocuronium (0.5–1 mg/kg) were applied intravenously (i.v.) for anesthesia induction and endotracheal intubation and were followed by sevoflurane (up to 1 minimal alveolar concentration (MAC)) for anesthesia maintenance. As per institutional standard, intravenous volume was administered restrictively using isotonic crystalloid solutions with a maximum of 15 ml/kg prior to initiation of cardiopulmonary bypass in all patients. A target mean arterial blood pressure (MBP) of > 65 mmHg was maintained during anesthesia induction using a continuous i.v. infusion of noradrenaline as a first line agent to counteract hypotension based on the clinical requirements. Pressure controlled positive pressure ventilation with a standardized PEEP of 5 cm H_2O and a peak inspiratory pressure (Pinsp) to receive a tidal volume of 6-8 ml/kg was initiated, and the inspiratory oxygen fraction was titrated to individual demands to maintain a SpO2 between 95 and 99%. End-tidal carbon dioxide levels were maintained between 35 and 37 mmHg by adjusting the ventilation frequency. All hemodynamic parameters were recorded during the echocardiography studies.

Echocardiography

A transthoracic real time 3DE study (Philips iE33-system, X5–1 Matrix transducer, Philips Healthcare Inc., Andover, USA) was performed in all patients by two experienced echocardiographers, trained in performing 3D imaging of the right ventricle. Echocardiography loops were recorded before and after anesthesia induction from transapical windows. The study protocol consisted of a 2D transapical 4-chamber view and 3D full volume acquisitions including the whole right and left ventricle. The 3D full volume datasets were acquired using an ECG-gated 4 heart beats-technique with a short apnoeic phase maintaining PEEP. Hemodynamic parameters were allowed to stabilize prior to the TTE exam. Tricuspid annular plane systolic excursion (TAPSE) was measured in an apical 4-chamber view using M-mode on the lateral tricuspid annulus. Systolic apical movement velocity of the lateral tricuspid annulus (TDITVs') was assessed using tissue Doppler imaging. All measurements were performed according to current ASE recommendations [11]. All 3D quantifications were performed offline. RV quantification was performed on a vendor independent platform (Tomtec Image Arena; Tomtec Imaging Systems GmbH, Unterschleissheim, Germany) by two trained echocardiographers blinded for each other's results. For quantification of the 3D datasets, software that had been validated against cardiac magnetic resonance imaging (CMRI) was used (Tomtec 4D RV-Function 2.0; Tomtec Imaging Systems GmbH, Unterschleissheim, Germany) [14, 15]. After adjustment of the 3D image in pre-defined axes, this software uses a speckle tracking based technique to identify right ventricular endocardial borders to generate a dynamic model of the right ventricular endocardial surface (Fig. 1). The RV end-diastolic (RVEDV) and end-systolic (RVESV) volumes were measured based on the generated RV model. RVEF was calculated as [(RVEDV-RVESV)/RVEDV] × 100%. To compare individual RV sizes, volumes were indexed to the body-surface area (RVEDVI and RVESVI). Based on the 3D RV model, the right ventricular free wall peak longitudinal strain (3D-RVLS-fw) and right ventricular septal-wall peak longitudinal strain (3D-RVLS-sw) was assessed as the difference

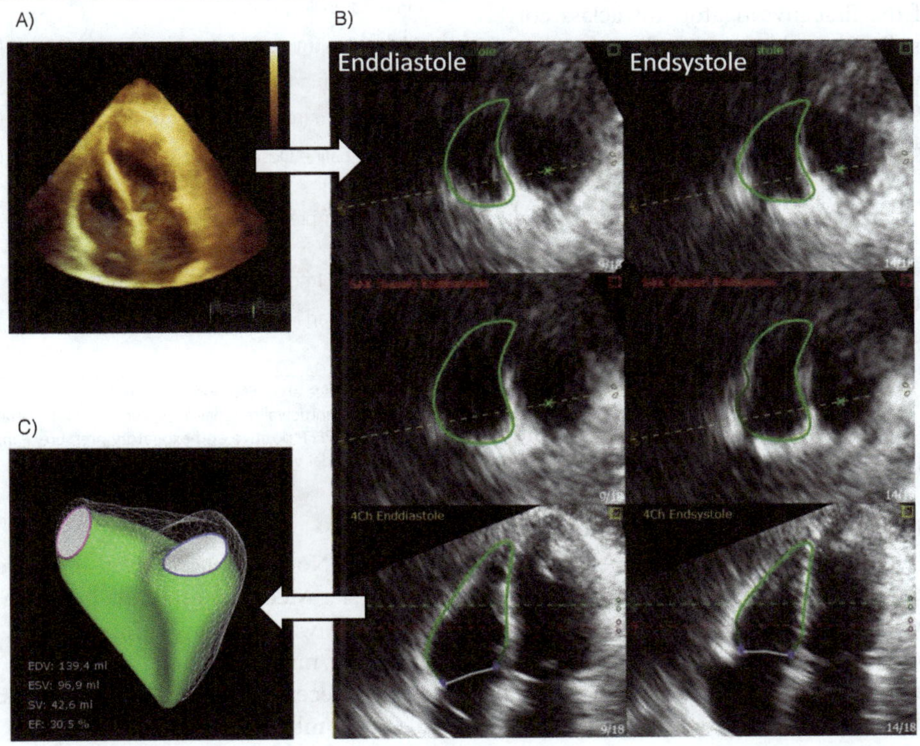

Fig. 1 **a** 3D full volume dataset of the left and right ventricle based on an apical 4-chamber view. **b** Endocardial border tracking by the Tomtec 4D RV-function package. The first column shows the enddiastolic frame, the second column shows the endsystolic frame. The First and second lines show medial and basal transversal planes of the RV. The third line shows the right ventricle in a reconstructed apical view. **c** Results of the Tomtec 4D RV-function package showing the volumetric model of the RV. The mesh grid shows the enddiastolic volume, the green inner model shows the endsystolic volume. Absolute values of volumes and the ejection fraction are also reported

in the measured distance of the curvature in systole and diastole of the free or septal RV wall: [(RV end-diastolic curvature (mm)-RV end-systolic curvature (mm))/RV end-diastolic curvature (mm))] × 100%. Stroke volume (SV) was calculated as SV = RVEDV * RVEF [17].

Statistical analysis

The normal distribution of the variables was assessed using skewness, kurtosis and the Shapiro-Wilk's tests. Continuous variables are reported as the mean values ± standard deviation. For echocardiographic and hemodynamic parameters, 95% confidence intervals of the mean are reported. Comparison of continuous variables between the different groups was performed using a Student's t test. Variables that were not normally distributed are reported as median and interquartile ranges (IQR). Comparison of these variables was performed using the Wilcoxon Rank-Sum test. The values of the different time points were compared using a two-tailed paired T-test. Categorical variables are reported as percentages. Differences in the variables were interpreted as significant at p values < 0.05.

To assess intra-observer reliability, 10 randomly selected datasets were analyzed by the initial investigator, blinded to the initial results, at a different time point. To calculate inter-observer reliability, 10 randomly selected datasets were assessed by a second investigator blinded for the results of the first investigator. Intraclass correlation coefficients (ICC) and corresponding 95% confidence intervals were calculated to assess intra-observer and inter-observer reliability.

All statistical analyses were performed using the SAS JMP software (ver. 14.0.0, SAS Institute Inc., Cary, USA) and IBM SPSS statistics (ver. 24, IBM, Armonk, USA).

Results

Fifty-nine patients gave informed consent to take part in this study. Three patients could not be studied due to changes in surgical planning, and three patients had a low imaging quality (stitching artefacts) insufficient for 3D volumetry. Fifty-three patients (44 male and 9 female) were included into the final analysis.

Table 1 Demographics, laboratory values, anesthesia induction agents and ventilator settings

Demographics and laboratory values	
Age [years]	64 (IQR 55 to 75)
Gender	
Male	44
Female	9
BMI [kg/m^2]	27 (SD 4)
BSA [m^2]	1.97 (SD 0.2)
Weight [kg]	82.5 (SD 14.8)
Height [cm]	174.5 (SD 8)
Planned cardiac surgeries	
CABG	16
AVR	13
MVR	6
Combination	15
Other	3
EuroSCORE II [%]	2.9 (IQR 1.9 to 7.5)
Creatinine [mg/dl]	0.9 (SD 0.2)
Prothrombin time (Quick's value) [%]	95 (SD 22)
Total Bilirubin [md/dl]	0.7 (IQR 0.5 to 0.9)
Anaesthesia induction agents and noradrenaline doses	
Midazolam [mg/kg]	0.14 (IQR 0.11 to 0.16)
Sufentanil [µg/kg]	0.56 (IQR 0.47 to 0.59)
Rocuronium [mg/kg]	0.79 (SD 0.26)
Noradrenaline Dose [µg/kg/min]	0.02 (IQR 0 to 0.05)
Parameters of pressure-controlled ventilation	
PEEP Level [mbar]	5
P insp [mbar]	15 (IQR 14 to 17)
TV [ml/kg]	7 (IQR 6 to 8)

BSA body-surface area, *BMI* body-mass index, *CABG* coronary artery bypass grafting, *AVR* aortic valve repair/replacement, *MVR* mitral valve repair/replacement, *PEEP* positive end-expiratory pressure, *P insp* inspiratory peak pressure, *TV* tidal volume

Patient characteristics

The median age of the patients was 64 years (IQR 55 to 75) having a median EuroSCORE II of 2.9% (IQR 1.9 to 7.5). Further demographic data as weight, height, body-surface-area, body-mass-index (BMI), preoperative laboratory values (creatinine, quick, total bilirubin) and the planned cardiac surgeries are given in Table 1.

Anesthesia induction and ventilator settings

The median level of the PEEP was 5 mbar, the median Pinsp was 15 (IQR 14 to 17) to obtain a TV of 7 ml/kg (IQR 6 to 8). Anesthesia induction agents are given in Table 1. No patient received noradrenaline prior to anesthesia. Median noradrenaline dose after anesthesia induction was 0.02 µg/kg/min (IQR 0 µg/kg/min to 0.05 µg/kg/min). During anesthesia induction the patients received a median dose of 330 ml (IQR 250 ml to 440 ml) of crystalloid fluids.

Hemodynamic data

Hemodynamic variables are given in Table 2. Patients experienced a significant reduction in heart rate (75 (SD

Table 2 Hemodynamic and echocardiographic parameters

	Pre	Post	Mean Difference (95% CI)	*p* value
Hemodynamic parameters				
HR [bpm]	75 (SD 15)	66 (SD 14)	−9 (−12 to −5)	< 0.0001
Systolic BP [mmHg]	136 (SD 24)	112 (SD 19)	−24 (−32 to − 17)	< 0.0001
Diastolic BP [mmHg]	70 (IQR 60 to 80)	57 (SD 11)	−13 (− 18 to −8)	< 0.0001 [a]
Mean BP [mmHg]	91 (IQR 80 to 104)	75 (SD 12)	−17 (− 22 to − 12)	< 0.0001 [a]
Echocardiographic parameters				
Right ventricle				
RVEDAI (cm^2/m^2) $n = 49$	13 (SD 3)	13 (SD 2)	−0.3 (−1 to 0.4)	0.3585
RVEDV (ml) $n = 53$	132 (SD 35)	132 (SD 36)	−0.0 (−8 to 8)	0.9996
RVESV (ml) $n = 53$	76 (SD 25)	78 (SD 27)	2.4 (−3.2 to 8.1)	0.3923
RVEDVI (ml/m^2) $n = 53$	67 (SD 17)	67 (SD 17)	−0.3 (−5.2 to 4.5)	0.9609
RVESVI (ml/m^2) $n = 53$	35 (IQR 32 to 44)	37 (IQR 30 to 45)	1.1 (−1.8 to 3.9)	0.4482
RVFAC (%) $n = 49$	38 (SD 9)	38 (SD 9)	−0.3 (−2.4 to 1.8)	0.7538
RVEF (%) $n = 53$	43 (SD 9)	42 (SD 8)	−1.4 (− 3.5 to 0.6)	0.1607
Stroke Volume (ml) $n = 53$	57 (SD 19)	54 (SD 16)	−3 (−7.5 to 1.5)	0.1838
TAPSE (mm) $n = 51$	18 (SD 4)	16 (SD 4)	−1.6 (−2.6 to −0.7)	0.0013
TDI TV s′ (cm/s) $n = 43$	13.2 (IQR 11.8 to 15.9)	11.8 (IQR 10.1 to 13.3)	−1.9 (−2.6 to − 1.2)	< 0.0001
3D-RVLS-fw (%) $n = 52$	−22.9 (SD 6)	− 21.4 (SD 5.9)	1.5 (0.1 to 2.9)	0.0366
3D-RVLS-sw (%) $n = 52$	−12.8 (SD 5.2)	− 12.3 (SD 3.9)	−0.3 (− 1.2 to 1.9)	0.5492
Tricuspid valve regurgitation (n=)				
None or trace	26			
Mild	25			
Moderate	2			
Severe	0			
Left ventricle				
LVEDVI (ml/m2) $n = 38$	80 (SD 24)	79 (SD 25)	−0.5 (−4.3 to 3.3)	0.7880
3D-LVEF (%) $n = 38$	53 (SD 16)	52 (SD 13)	−0.9 (−4.1 to 2.3)	0.5704

Pre: baseline values; Post: Post-anesthesia induction values; CI: confidence intervals (lower limit to upper limit); HR: heart rate; BP: blood pressure; RVEDAI: right ventricular end-diastolic area index to body surface area to RVEDVI: right ventricular end-diastolic volume indexed to body surface area to RVFAC: right ventricular fractional area change to 3D-RVEF: right ventricular ejection fraction derived by 3D volumetry to TAPSE: tricuspid plane systolic excursion to TDI TV s′: tissue Doppler derived peak systolic velocity of the lateral tricuspid annulus to 3D-RVLS-fw: right ventricular free wall peak longitudinal strain derived by 3D echocardiography to 3D-RVLS-sw: right ventricular septal wall peak longitudinal strain derived by 3D echocardiography to LVEDVI: left ventricular end-diastolic volume indexed to body surface area by 3D volumetry to LVEF: left ventricular ejection fraction derived by 3D volumetry

[a]Wilcoxon signed-rank test

15) bpm to 66 (SD 14) bpm, $p = < 0.0001$), systolic blood pressure (SBP; 136 (SD 24) mmHg to 112 (SD 19) mmHg; $p < 0.0001$), diastolic blood pressure (DBP; 70 (IQR 60 to 80) mmHg to 57 (SD 11) mmHg; $p < 0.0001$) and mean blood pressure (MBP; 91 (IQR 80 to 104) mmHg to 78 (SD 12) mmHg; $p < 0.0001$).

Echocardiographic data

A summary of the echocardiographic parameters is given in Table 2. No significant change in the RVEDV, RVEDVI, RVESV, RVESVI, RVEF, right ventricular end-diastolic area indexed to body surface area (RVEDAI), RVFAC, 3D-RVLS-sw or right ventricular stroke volume was recorded (Fig. 2 a).

After anesthesia induction and IPPV, the TAPSE was significantly reduced (18 (SD 4) mm to 16 (SD 4) mm; $p = 0.0013$) (Fig. 2 b). The TDITVs' was also significantly reduced (13.2 cm/s (IQR 12 to 15.9) to 11.8 cm/s (IQR 10.1 to 13.3), $p < 0.0001$). 3D-RVLS-fw also significantly decreased (– 22.9 (SD 6) % to – 21.4 (SD 5.9) %, $p = 0.0366$) (Fig. 2 c).

There was no significant correlation between the noradrenaline dose and the change in RVEF (r = 0.106, $p = 0.4451$), 3D-RVLS-fw (r = – 0.17, $p = 0.2284$), TAPSE (r = – 0.073, $p = 0.6129$) or TDITVs' (r = 0.07, $p = 0.6439$).

Subgroup analysis: patients with normal or impaired RVEF

For a subgroup analysis, patients were grouped based on their baseline RVEF. A baseline RVEF above 35% was considered normal, a baseline RVEF below or equal to 35% was considered depressed. Fourty-one patients with a median age of 64 years (IQR 53 to 74) were categorized into the group with a normal RVEF, twelve patients with a median age of 72 (IWR 63 to 77) were categorized into the group with depressed RVEF.

In both groups HR and MAP were significantly lower after anesthesia induction compared to the baseline values. RVEDV did not significantly change in either of the groups. In the group with a normal RVEF, all parameters reflecting RV function (RVEF, TAPSE, TDITVs' and 3D-RVLS-fw) worsened significantly (Table 3). The group with the depressed RVEF at baseline did not show a significant change of the RV functional parameters.

Observer variability

The ICC for the intra-observer reliability for the RVEDV was 0.924 (95% CI: 0.741–0.980), RVESV 0.847 (95% CI: 0.524–0.959), RVEF 0.984 (95% CI: 0.942–0.996), 3D-RVLS-fw 0.927 (95% CI: 0.749–0.981) and RVFAC 0.669 (95% CI: 0.143–0.905). The ICC for the inter-observer reliability for the RVEDV was 0.927 (95% CI: 0.737–0.981), RVESV 0.957 (95% CI: 0.839–0.989), RVEF 0.846 (95% CI: 0.497–0.959), 3D-RVLS-fw 0.834 (95% CI: 0.466–0.956) and RVFAC 0.662 (95% CI: 0.052–0.09.12).

Discussion

Anesthesia induction with endotracheal intubation and consecutive positive pressure ventilation constitutes a vulnerable phase for the right ventricle. Increased pulmonary vascular resistance due to the formation of atelectasis, hypercapnia or hypoxia can lead to right ventricular afterload increases. Additionally, positive pressure ventilation is known to alter right ventricular filling pressures. One of the first reports in 1948 showed that intrathoracic pressure was inversely correlated with right ventricular filling pressures [18]. Several subsequent studies have shown that positive pressure ventilation with high PEEP levels can lead to consecutive right heart dysfunction [19–21]. It is supposed that this is due to a reduction in venous return and increases in right ventricular afterload. Contrary to these studies an animal study by Luecke et al. showed that increasing levels of PEEP up to 21 cmH_2O did not alter RV function [22]. This finding is supported by a small study in cardiac surgery patients that applied the open-lung concept with PEEP levels of 17 cmH_2O [23].

In addition to the effect of mechanical ventilation, right ventricular function can be altered by hemodynamic changes, as well as the direct negative effects of anesthesia agents on right ventricular myocardial contractility. Propofol, for example, has been shown to alter systemic hemodynamic parameters without influencing the RVEDV or RVEF, measured by pulmonary artery catheter-based techniques [24, 25]. Midazolam, the sedative agent used in this study, is known to have little to no impact on pulmonary vascular resistance 5 min after anesthesia induction, but can reduce both the left- and right-ventricular stroke work indices [26, 27]. The impact of anesthetics on the left ventricular function has been previously investigated. In a study by Bhavsar et al. a bolus of 1.5-2 µg/kg sufentanil for anesthesia induction lead to a significantly decreased left ventricular global longitudinal strain whereas systemic hemodynamic parameters or stroke volume remained unchanged [28]. In a study during anesthesia induction in pediatric cardiac patients, left ventricular ejection fraction decreased after administration of sufentanil or fentanyl [29]. In an investigation by Frederiksen et al., these findings could not be confirmed [30]. The authors showed that sufentanil and remifentanil do not affect left ventricular global longitudinal strain [30]. Studies assessing the impact of opioids on the right ventricle are not available. There are controversial data in the literature regarding the effects of sevoflurane on right ventricular function. While the administration of 1–1.5 MAC of sevoflurane led to a significant decrease in right ventricular stroke work index (RVSWI) in anaesthetized pigs [31], pulmonary vascular resistance increased but RVSWI remained stable in another porcine study using a MAC of less than 1 [32]. Malan et al. studied the effects of sevoflurane on healthy volunteers and showed that systemic vascular resistance and mean pulmonary artery pressures are reduced [33]. Furthermore, they observed neither a change in left sided preload, measured by the

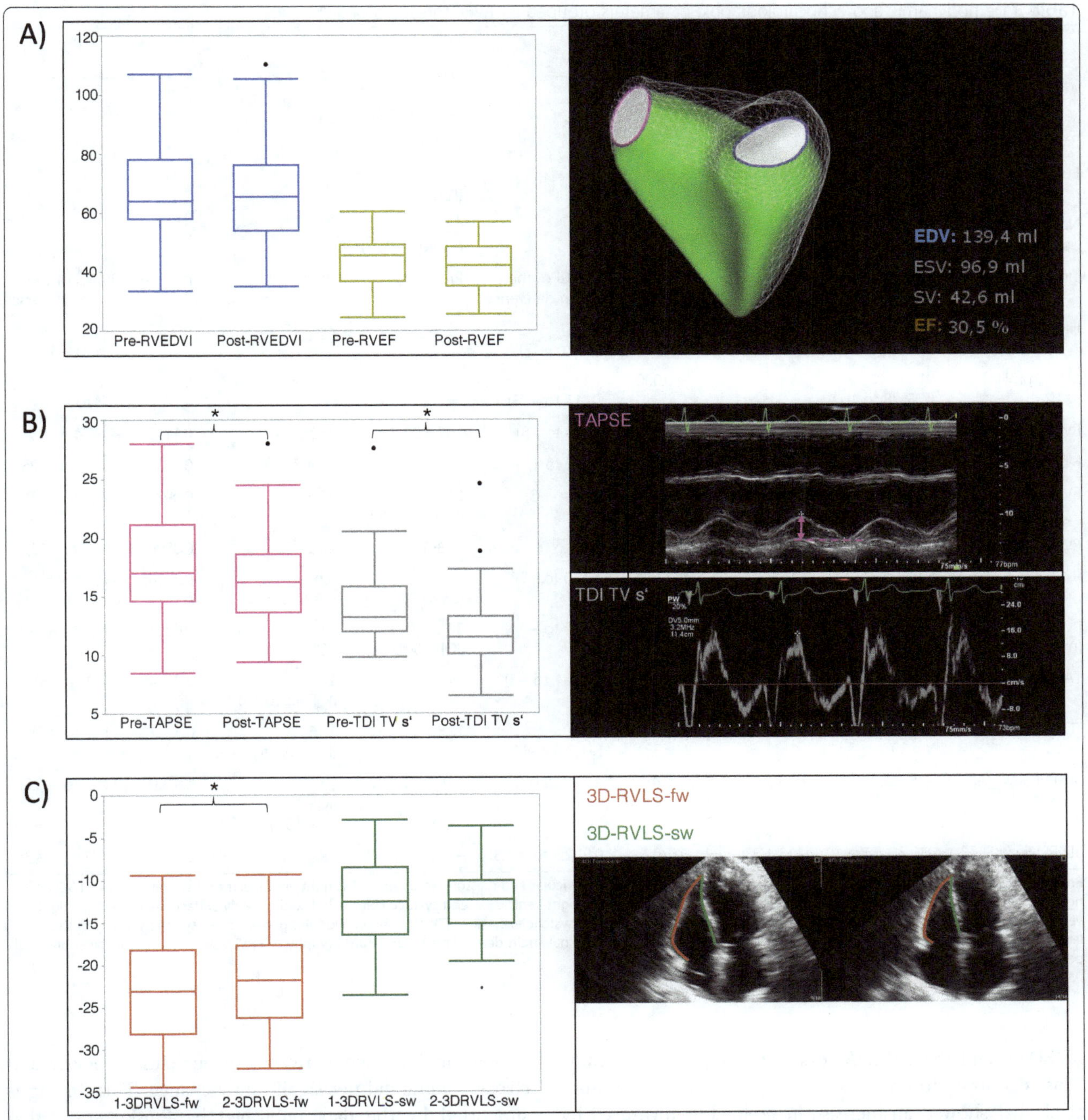

Fig. 2 a Bar graphs of the right ventricular end-diastolic volume indexed to body surface area (RVEDVI) and right ventricular ejection fraction (RVEF) before and after anesthesia induction are shown. No changes were observed regarding RVEDVI and RVEF. Right side shows an example of a volumetric model of the right ventricle together with an example of results given by the Tomtec 4D RV-function software. **b** Bar graphs of the tricuspid annular plane systolic excursion (TAPSE) and tissue Doppler-derived peak systolic velocity of the lateral tricuspid annulus (TDI TV s') before and after anesthesia induction are shown. Significant reductions were observed for the TAPSE and TDI TV s'. Right side shows examples of the TAPSE measurement in M-Mode and the measurement of the TDI TV s' in tissue spectral Doppler. **c** Bar graphs of the right ventricular peak systolic free wall strain (3DRVLS-fw) and septal wall strain (3DRVLS-sw) are shown. A significant decrease in 3DRVLS-fw was observed with no change in 3DRVLS-sw. Right side shows an example of the strain measurements in reconstructed 3D datasets

left ventricular end-diastolic area, nor in left ventricular fractional area change [33].

To date and to the best of our knowledge, no other study has comprehensively assessed established parameters of right ventricular mechanics and novel 3D echocardiographic parameters of right ventricular function during anesthesia induction and initiation of positive pressure ventilation. Right ventricular volume, quantified by the

Table 3 Hemodynamic and echocardiographic parameters grouped by RVEF threshold of 35%

	RVEF > 35% *N* = 41				RVEF ≤35% *N* = 12			
Age	64 (IQR 53 to 74)				72 (IQR 63 to 77)			
BMI (kg/m^2)	26 ± 4				29 ± 4			
EuroSCORE II [%]	2.8 (IQR 1.4 to 5.9)				7 (IQR 2.2 to 16.6)			
Noradrenaline dose [µg/kg/min]	0 (IQR 0 to 0.04)				0.03 (IQR 0 to 0.07)			
Time point	Pre	Post	*p* value	95%CI of the mean difference	Pre	Post	*p* value	95%CI of the mean difference
HR [bpm]	74 ± 15	66 ± 13	0.0005	−8 (−3 to −12)	77 ± 17	66 ± 15	0.0012	−11 (−6 to − 17)
MAP [mmHg]	91 (IQR 78 to 102)	75 ± 13	< 0.0001[a]	−17 (− 11 to −23)	91 (IQR 81 to 109)	78 ± 9	0.0005[a]	− 16 (−7 to − 26)
RVEDV [ml]	130 ± 35	133 ± 34	0.5479	4 (13 to −5)	145 ± 38	132 ± 44	0.1115	−14 (4 to −31)
RVESV [ml]	69 ± 19	75 ± 24	0.0253	7 (12 to 1)	102 ± 26	90 ± 36	0.0807	−12 (2 to −25)
RVEDVI [ml/m^2]	66 ± 16	68 ± 16	0.5416	2 (7 to −3)	64 (IQR 59 to 82)	65 ± 20	0.0923[a]	−7 (1 to −17)
RVESVI [ml/m^2]	35 ± 9	38 ± 11	0.0281	3 (6 to 0)	51 ± 14	44 ± 17	0.0594	−6 (0 to −13)
RVEF [%]	47 ± 6	43 (IQR 40 to 49)	0.0063[a]	−3 (0 to −5)	30 (26 to 34)	32 (28 to 37)	0.3394[a]	3 (8 to −2)
RV stroke volume [ml]	61 ± 19	57 ± 16	0.2001	−3 (2 to −9)	37 (IQR 35 to 54)	41 (IQR 32 to 54)	0.6221[a]	−1 (7 to −10)
TAPSE [mm]	19 ± 4	17 ± 4	0.0033 *N* = 39	−2 (−1 to −3)	14 ± 3	14 (IQR 11 to 15)	0.2334[a]	−1 (1 to −3)
TDI TV s'[cm/s]	14.5 ± 3.3 *N* = 33	12 ± 3.7	< 0.0001 *N* = 33	−2.3 (−1.5 to −3.1)	13.3 ± 3.5	11.6 (IQR 10.5 to 13.5)	0.5371[a]	−1 (1 to − 2)
3D-RVLS-fw [%]	−25 ± 4.9	− 22.9 ± 5.9	0.0143	2 (3.5 to 0.4)	−16 ± 3.2	−17.7 (IQR − 20.8 to − 10.5)	1.0000[a]	0 (3.3 to − 3.5)
3D-RVLS-sw [%]	−13.7 ± 5.3	− 13 ± 3.7	0.5709	0.5 (2.3 to − 1.3)	− 9.7 ± 3.5	−9.4 ± 3.3	0.8490	0.3 (3.6 to − 3)

Pre: baseline values; Post: post-anesthesia induction values; RVEDV: right ventricular end-diastolic volume; RVESV: right ventricular end-systolic volume; RVEDVI: right ventricular end-diastolic volume indexed to body surface area; RVESVI: right ventricular end-systolic volume indexed to body surface area; 3D-RVEF: right ventricular ejection fraction derived by 3D volumetry; TAPSE: tricuspid plane systolic excursion; TDI TV s': tissue Doppler derived peak systolic velocity of the lateral tricuspid annulus; 3D-RVLS-fw: right ventricular free wall peak longitudinal strain derived by 3D echocardiography; 3D-RVLS-sw: right ventricular septal wall peak longitudinal strain derived by 3D echocardiography

[a]Wilcoxon signed-rank test

RVEDVI, and the RVEDAI did not change in our study. This is contrary to previously published results by Couture et al. that showed an increase in preload as measured by the RVEDA after anesthesia induction [34]. PEEP and peak inspiratory pressure levels are not reported in the article of Couture et al. [34], thus making it difficult to compare their findings to our results. A potential reason for the different observations could be the different approach for the volumetric quantification, particularly the direct measurement of the RVEDVI in this study. The 3DE volumetric technique incorporates the whole right ventricle. This technique includes the right ventricular outflow tract in the volume calculation and overcomes the use of a single imaging plane used by Couture et al.. Foreshortened imaging planes in 2D echocardiography could be another potential reason for the different results. In our patients RVEF and stroke volume did not significantly change. This finding is supported by the data published by Pinsky et al. that showed no relevant change in ejection fraction during various PEEP levels [5]. Our data demonstrate that the longitudinal function of the right ventricle, as measured by indices that assess the movement of the lateral tricuspid annulus, namely, TAPSE and TDITVs', are significantly reduced after anesthesia induction and IPPV. This confirms the previous findings of Tousignant et al. that have shown a similar reduction in TAPSE [35]. But contrary to our results they did not experience a change in TDITVs' what could be due to the different patient population, the smaller number of included patients or different ventilator settings. The movement of the tricuspid annulus is not solely associated with right ventricular function and relies on the movement of the whole heart. Moreover, TAPSE has shown to be associated with left ventricular function [36, 37]. In addition, conflicting data exist about the lack of correlation of the TAPSE with cardiac MRI-derived RV ejection fraction [38, 39]. Imaging of longitudinal myocardial deformation does not only rely on the movement of the tricuspid annulus and directly assesses the longitudinal myocardial contractility. Right ventricular strain imaging is considered to detect even subtle changes in myocardial contractility [40]. In our patients we observed a significant but small decrease in right ventricular free wall strain. Due to the fact that the right ventricular myocardium has different contraction components, the reduction of the longitudinal contraction could have been compensated by the circumferential, antero-posterior or the twisting component leading to a stable RVEF and SV.

In a subgroup analysis we can show that patients with a normal RVEF at baseline experienced a significant decrease in the longitudinal myocardial contraction component accompanied by a small but significant reduction in RVEF. Interestingly, in the subgroup of patients with depressed RVEF (< 35%) no change of any of the RV parameters could be observed. This suggests that in patients with already reduced RVEF anesthesia and IPPV do not further worsen right ventricular myocardial function. Due to the small sample size of the subset (n = 12) additional larger studies in this specific patient collective are needed to confirm or falsify this finding.

In this prospective study, we showed the effects of anesthesia induction and initiation of positive pressure ventilation on right ventricular function. Our data clearly demonstrate that echocardiographic parameters assessing the tricuspid annular movement (TAPSE and TDITVs'), are significantly reduced despite stable loading conditions. The reduction in tricuspid annular movement might be directly associated with changes in intrathoracic pressures by the initiation of positive pressure ventilation. The longitudinal right ventricular myocardial contraction (3D-RVLS-fw) was also reduced in our patient population. In addition we showed that the ejection fraction assessed by 3DE also slightly decreased during anesthesia induction in a subgroup of patients presenting with a normal baseline RVEF but, however, stroke volume did not change.

Clinical implications

This study shows a decrease in longitudinal right ventricular function after anesthesia induction using sufentanil, midazolam and rocuronium and IPPV with currently recommended ventilator settings. In a group of patients with a normal baseline RVEF the RVEF also slightly decreased but RV stroke volume stayed stable. Despite the reduction in longitudinal function and the slight reduction in RVEF (mean – 3%) this effect seems not to be directly clinically relevant as the stroke volume remained stable. However, echocardiographers need to be aware that longitudinal RV function is depressed under anesthesia and intraoperative values should be cautiously compared to baseline measurements when judging RV function. Modern 3DE techniques especially 3D volumetry improve insights into right heart dimensions and function and enhance our understanding of anesthesia-related changes of ventricular function and physiology. Therefore, 3D echocardiography should be used to complement 2D echocardiographic examinations in the perioperative setting.

Study limitations

Our data have several limitations. The patients included in our single-center study do not represent a healthy collective but a cross section through patients presenting in cardiac anesthesia with various underlying diseases. Unfortunately, we cannot report on the changes in right ventricular afterload in our patients. The results for the 2D echocardiography measurements of RV longitudinal function could be biased because some values were missing during data collection. Although overall changes are small, the sample size might have been too small to reach significance for some of the 3D-based echocardiography parameters. The assessment of different right ventricular contraction components – such as longitudinal and circumferential shortening - could not be performed but might have given further insights into complex alterations of the myocardial contraction patterns. We do acknowledge that we can only report on the initial changes in right ventricular function and cannot address if this effect is reversible after emergence from anesthesia. In addition, the 3D technology that we used is not yet available in a broad clinical setting.

Conclusions

Our results suggest that tricuspid annular movement and longitudinal RV function decreases after anesthesia induction and positive pressure ventilation, while the stroke volume does not change. The latter finding questions the clinical relevance of the small changes seen. Further investigations are necessary to confirm this finding, especially in patients with a depressed baseline RVEF and during anesthesia induction with other anesthetics or different ventilator settings.

Abbreviations

2D: Two-dimensional; 3DE: 3-dimensional echocardiography; 3D-RVLS-fw: Right ventricular free wall peak longitudinal strain; 3D-RVLS-sw: Right ventricular septal-wall peak longitudinal strain; BMI: Body-mass-index; CMRI: Cardiac magnetic resonance imaging; DBP: Diastolic blood pressure; ICC: Intraclass correlation Coefficients; IPPV: Intermittent positive pressure ventilation; IQR: Interquartile ranges; IVC: Inferior vena cava; MAC: Minimal alveolar concentration; MBP: Mean blood pressure; PEEP: Positive end expiratory pressure; Pinsp: Peak inspiratory pressure; RV: Right ventricle; RVEDA: Right ventricular enddiastolic area; RVEDAI: Right ventricular enddiastolic area indexed to body surface area; RVEDV: Right ventricular end-diastolic volume; RVEDVI: Right ventricular end-diastolic volume indexed to body-surface area; RVEF: Right ventricular ejection fraction; RVESV: Right ventricular end-systolic volume; RVESVI: Right ventricular end-systolic volume indexed to body-surface area; RVESWI: Right ventricular stroke work index; RVFAC: Right ventricular fractional area change; SBP: Systolic blood pressure; SD: Standard deviation; SV: Stroke volume; TAPSE: Tricuspid annular plane systolic excursion; TDITVs': Tissue Doppler derived systolic movement of the lateral tricuspidannulus; TTE: Transthoracic echocardiography

Acknowledgements
We thank all of our colleagues in the cardiac anesthesiology division for supporting the data collection process.

Authors' contributions
HM and MN-M contributed substantially to all aspects of this manuscript, including study design, data collection, data analysis, data interpretation and draft of the first manuscript; AJ contributed substantially to data collection and data analysis; MK contributed substantially to data analysis; PR contributed substantially to data interpretation and revision of the manuscript. All authors approved the final manuscript.

Author details
[1]Department of Anaesthesiology and Intensive Care Medicine, University Hospital Tübingen, Eberhard-Karls-University Tübingen, Hoppe-Seyler-Str. 3, 72076 Tübingen, Germany. [2]Department of Anesthesia and Intensive Care Medicine, Klinikum Ingolstadt, Krumenauerstr. 25, 85049 Ingolstadt, Germany.

References

1. Fewell JE, Abendschein DR, Carlson CJ, Murray JF, Rapaport E. Continuous positive-pressure ventilation decreases right and left ventricular end-diastolic volumes in the dog. Circ Res. 1980;46:125–32.
2. Jardin F, Farcot JC, Boisante L, Curien N, Margairaz A, Bourdarias JP. Influence of positive end-expiratory pressure on left ventricular performance. N Engl J Med. 1981;304:387–92.
3. Soni N, Williams P. Positive pressure ventilation: what is the real cost? Br J Anaesth. 2008;101:446–57.
4. Forrest P. Anaesthesia and right ventricular failure. Anaesth Intensive Care. 2009;37:370–85.
5. Pinsky MR, Desmet JM, Vincent JL. Effect of positive end-expiratory pressure on right ventricular function in humans. Am Rev Respir Dis. 1992;146:681–7.
6. Pinsky MR. My paper 20 years later: effect of positive end-expiratory pressure on right ventricular function in humans. Intensive Care Med. 2014;40:935–41.
7. Mitaka C, Nagura T, Sakanishi N, Tsunoda Y, Amaha K. Two-dimensional echocardiographic evaluation of inferior vena cava, right ventricle, and left ventricle during positive-pressure ventilation with varying levels of positive end-expiratory pressure. Crit Care Med. 1989;17:205–10.
8. Eltzschig HK, Rosenberger P, Loffler M, Fox JA, Aranki SF, Shernan SK. Impact of intraoperative transesophageal echocardiography on surgical decisions in 12,566 patients undergoing cardiac surgery. Ann Thorac Surg. 2008;85:845–52.
9. Ling LF, Marwick TH. Echocardiographic assessment of right ventricular function: how to account for tricuspid regurgitation and pulmonary hypertension. JACC Cardiovasc Imaging. 2012;5:747–53.
10. Pleister A, Kahwash R, Haas G, Ghio S, Cittadini A, Baliga RR. Echocardiography and heart failure: a glimpse of the right heart. Echocardiography. 2015;32(Suppl 1):S95–107.
11. Lang RM, Badano LP, Mor-Avi V, et al. Recommendations for cardiac chamber quantification by echocardiography in adults: an update from the American Society of Echocardiography and the European Association of Cardiovascular Imaging. J Am Soc Echocardiogr. 2015;28:1–39 e14.
12. Magunia H, Rosenberger P. Application fields of intraoperative transesophageal 3D echocardiography. Anaesthesist. 2014;63:662–72 74-7.
13. Magunia H, Schibilsky D, Hilberath JN, Schlensak C, Rosenberger P, Nowak-Machen M. Echocardiographic features of the fully magnetically levitated LVAD. J Am Coll Cardiol Img. 2017;10:819–22.
14. Muraru D, Spadotto V, Cecchetto A, et al. New speckle-tracking algorithm for right ventricular volume analysis from three-dimensional echocardiographic data sets: validation with cardiac magnetic resonance and comparison with the previous analysis tool. Eur Heart J Cardiovasc Imaging. 2016;17:1279–89.
15. Medvedofsky D, Addetia K, Patel AR, et al. Novel approach to three-dimensional echocardiographic quantification of right ventricular volumes and function from focused views. J Am Soc Echocardiogr. 2015;28:1222–31.
16. von Elm E, Altman DG, Egger M, et al. The strengthening the reporting of observational studies in epidemiology (STROBE) statement: guidelines for reporting observational studies. J Clin Epidemiol. 2008;61:344–9.
17. Rudski LG, Lai WW, Afilalo J, et al. Guidelines for the echocardiographic assessment of the right heart in adults: a report from the American Society of Echocardiography endorsed by the European Association of Echocardiography, a registered branch of the European Society of Cardiology, and the Canadian Society of Echocardiography. J Am Soc Echocardiogr. 2010;23:685–713 quiz 86-8.
18. Cournand A, Motley HL, et al. Physiological studies of the effects of intermittent positive pressure breathing on cardiac output in man. Am J Phys. 1948;152:162–74.
19. Vieillard-Baron A, Charron C, Caille V, Belliard G, Page B, Jardin F. Prone positioning unloads the right ventricle in severe ARDS. Chest. 2007;132:1440–6.
20. Guervilly C, Forel JM, Hraiech S, et al. Right ventricular function during high-frequency oscillatory ventilation in adults with acute respiratory distress syndrome. Crit Care Med. 2012;40:1539–45.
21. Fougeres E, Teboul JL, Richard C, Osman D, Chemla D, Monnet X. Hemodynamic impact of a positive end-expiratory pressure setting in acute respiratory distress syndrome: importance of the volume status. Crit Care Med. 2010;38:802–7.
22. Luecke T, Roth H, Herrmann P, et al. Assessment of cardiac preload and left ventricular function under increasing levels of positive end-expiratory pressure. Intensive Care Med. 2004;30:119–26.
23. Reis Miranda D, Gommers D, Struijs A, et al. The open lung concept: effects on right ventricular afterload after cardiac surgery. Br J Anaesth. 2004;93:327–32.
24. Martin C, Perrin G, Saux P, Papazian L, Albanese J, Gouin F. Right ventricular end-systolic pressure-volume relation during propofol infusion. Acta Anaesthesiol Scand. 1994;38:223–8.
25. Sherry KM, Sartain J, Bell JH, Wilkinson GA. Comparison of the use of a propofol infusion in cardiac surgical patients with normal and low cardiac output states. J Cardiothorac Vasc Anesth. 1995;9:368–72.
26. Kawar P, Carson IW, Clarke RS, Dundee JW, Lyons SM. Haemodynamic changes during induction of anaesthesia with midazolam and diazepam (valium) in patients undergoing coronary artery bypass surgery. Anaesthesia. 1985;40:767–71.
27. Samuelson PN, Reves JG, Kouchoukos NT, Smith LR, Dole KM. Hemodynamic responses to anesthetic induction with midazolam or diazepam in patients with ischemic heart disease. Anesth Analg. 1981;60:802–9.
28. Bhavsar R, Sloth E, Folkersen L, Greisen JR, Jakobsen CJ. Sufentanil preserves hemodynamics and left ventricular function in patients with ischemic heart disease. Acta Anaesthesiol Scand. 2011;55:1002–9.
29. Glenski JA, Friesen RH, Hassanein RS, Henry DB. Comparison of the hemodynamic and echocardiographic effects of sufentanil, fentanyl, isoflurane, and halothane for pediatric cardiovascular surgery. J Cardiothorac Anesth. 1988;2:147–55.
30. Frederiksen CA, Juhl-Olsen P, Kremke M, Rasmussen LA, Lorenzen AG, Sloth E, Jakobsen C. Remifentanil and Sufentanil Preserve Left Ventricular Systolic and Diastolic Function in Patients with Ischemic Heart Disease-A Randomised Comparative Study. J Anesthesia Clin Res. 2014;5:437. https://doi.org/10.4172/2155-6148.1000437.
31. Kerbaul F, Bellezza M, Mekkaoui C, et al. Sevoflurane alters right ventricular performance but not pulmonary vascular resistance in acutely instrumented anesthetized pigs. J Cardiothorac Vasc Anesth. 2006;20:209–16.
32. Haraldsen P, Metzsch C, Lindstedt S, Algotsson L, Ingemansson R. Sevoflurane anesthesia during acute right ventricular ischemia in pigs preserves cardiac function better than propofol anesthesia. Perfusion. 2016; 31:495–502.
33. Malan TP Jr, DiNardo JA, Isner RJ, et al. Cardiovascular effects of sevoflurane compared with those of isoflurane in volunteers. Anesthesiology. 1995;83:918–28.
34. Couture P, Denault AY, Shi Y, et al. Effects of anesthetic induction in patients with diastolic dysfunction. Can J Anaesthesia. 2009;56:357–65.
35. Tousignant C, Bowry R, Cruz JD, Mazer CD. Induction of anesthesia does not

alter tricuspid annular velocities: a tissue Doppler assessment. Can J Anaesthesia. 2009;56:757–62.

36. Lopez-Candales A, Rajagopalan N, Saxena N, Gulyasy B, Edelman K, Bazaz R. Right ventricular systolic function is not the sole determinant of tricuspid annular motion. Am J Cardiol. 2006;98:973–7.
37. Giusca S, Dambrauskaite V, Scheurwegs C, et al. Deformation imaging describes right ventricular function better than longitudinal displacement of the tricuspid ring. Heart. 2010;96:281–8.
38. Anavekar NS, Gerson D, Skali H, Kwong RY, Yucel EK, Solomon SD. Two-dimensional assessment of right ventricular function: an echocardiographic-MRI correlative study. Echocardiography. 2007;24:452–6.
39. Park SJ, Park JH, Lee HS, et al. Impaired RV global longitudinal strain is associated with poor long-term clinical outcomes in patients with acute inferior STEMI. JACC Cardiovasc Imaging. 2015;8:161–9.
40. Morris DA, Krisper M, Nakatani S, et al. Normal range and usefulness of right ventricular systolic strain to detect subtle right ventricular systolic abnormalities in patients with heart failure: a multicentre study. Eur Heart J Cardiovasc Imaging. 2017;18:212–23.

18

Comparative efficacy of neuraxial and general anesthesia for hip fracture surgery

Xinxun Zheng, Yuming Tan, Yuan Gao and Zhiheng Liu*

Abstract

Background: The choice of anesthesia technique remains debatable in patients undergoing surgical repair of hip fracture. This meta-analysis was performed to compare the effect of neuraxial (epidural/spinal) versus general anesthesia on perioperative outcomes in patients undergoing hip fracture surgery.

Methods: Medline, Cochrane Library, Science-Direct, and EMBASE databases were searched to identify eligible studies focused on the comparison between neuraxial and general anesthesia in hip fracture patients between January 2000 and May 2019. Perioperative outcomes were extracted for systemic analysis. Sensitivity analyses were conducted using a Bonferroni correction and the leave-one-out method. The evidence quality for each outcome was evaluated by the Grading of Recommendations Assessment, Development and Evaluation (GRADE) system.

Results: Nine randomized controlled trials (RCTs) including 1084 patients fulfilled our selection criteria. The outcomes for the meta-analysis showed that there were no significant differences in the 30-day mortality (OR = 1.34, 95% CI 0.56, 3.21; $P = 0.51$), length of stay (MD = − 0.65, 95% CI -0.32, 0.02; $P = 0.06$), and the prevalence of delirium (OR = 1.05, 95% CI 0.27, 4.00; $P = 0.95$), acute myocardial infarction (OR = 0.88, 95% CI 0.17, 4.65; $P = 0.88$), deep venous thrombosis (OR = 0.48, 95% CI 0.09, 2.72; $P = 0.41$), and pneumonia (OR = 1.04, 95% CI 0.23, 4.61; $P = 0.96$) for neuraxial anesthesia compared to general anesthesia, and there was a significant difference in blood loss between the two groups (MD = − 137.8, 95% CI -241.49, − 34.12; $p = 0.009$). However, after applying the Bonferroni correction for multiple testing, all the adjusted *p*-values were above the significant threshold of 0.05. The evidence quality for each outcome evaluated by the GRADE system was low.

Conclusions: In summary, our present study demonstrated that there might be a difference in blood loss between patients receiving neuraxial and general anaesthesia, however, this analysis was not robust to adjustment for multiple testing and therefore at high risk for a type I error. Due to small sample size and enormous inconsistency in the choice of outcome measures, more high-quality studies with large sample size are needed to clarify this issue.

Keywords: Neuraxial anesthesia, General anesthesia, Hip fracture

* Correspondence: zhiheng_liu_tongji@163.com
Department of Anesthesiology, Shenzhen Second People's Hospital, The First Affiliated Hospital of Shenzhen University, Shenzhen 518000, China

Background

Hip fracture is one of the most common injuries that occurs in about 1.6 million people around the world each year; the number is estimated to reach more than six million by 2050 [1]. Moreover, there are a range of comorbidities in elderly patients with hip fracture, which are associated with an increased risk of morbidity and mortality [2]. Most hip fractures should be treated surgically that requires some type of anesthesia [3].

Thus far, the ideal choice between neuraxial and general anesthesia has not been identified. Several studies demonstrated that compared with general anesthesia, neuraxial anesthesia has some advantages such as airway management avoidance, no intubation requirement, and prolonged postoperative analgesia [4]. Furthermore, neuraxial anesthesia could decrease blood loss, potentially reduce risk of postoperative nausea and vomitting (PONV), as well as deep venous thrombosis [4–6]. Conversely, general anesthesia is reported to provide a more stable hemodynamic state, faster induction, and avoid some complications such as pneumonia, epidural haematoma and infection [7, 8]. However, the effect of the two anesthesia techniques on patients with hip fracture is controversial regarding postoperative outcomes. A recent systematic review including 15 studies revealed that neuraxial anesthesia was only associated with a shorter length of hospital stay in patients undergoing hip fracture surgery. This review emphasized that sensitivity analyses showed marginal statistical significance for length of stay favoring spinal anaesthesia, and the definitions of reported outcomes varied widely or were unclear, making evaluation in a standardized manner very difficult [9]. Another systematic review reported a reduced in-hospital mortality in the neuraxial anaesthesia group, but no definitive conclusion can be drawn for longer-term mortality [10]. Both of them have recommended that further high-quality studies be performed.

To date, several most recent randomized controlled trials (RCTs) have been published, which assessed the effect of the two anesthesia techniques for hip fracture surgery. Through including these RCTs, our study aimed to systematically evaluate perioperative outcomes of patients with hip fracture surgery, and provide more reliable evidence to identify the optimal technique.

Methods

This meta-analysis was conducted in accordance with Preferred Reporting Items for Systematic Reviews and Meta-analyses (PRISMA) guidelines. It was registered in the international prospective register of systematic reviews (Prospero: CRD42020143172).

Search strategy

Medline, Cochrane Library, Science-Direct, and EMBASE databases were searched by two independent reviewers

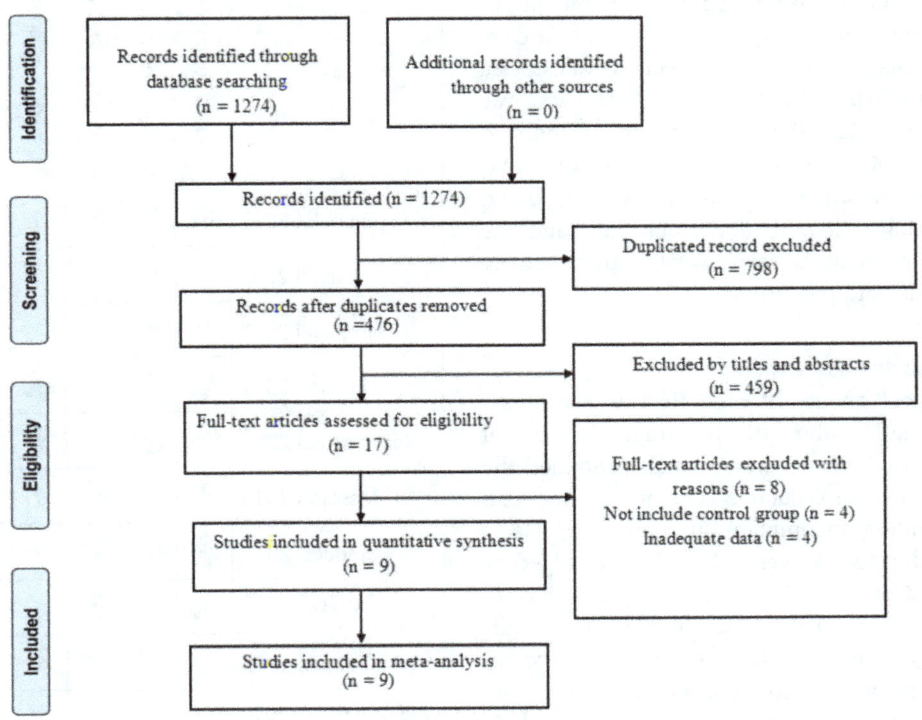

Fig. 1 The flow diagram of study selection

between January 2000 and May 2019. We selected studies of neuraxial anesthesia compared with general anesthesia in patients undergoing hip fracture surgery. Following iterms were searched for both alone and in various combinations, "hip fracture" or "femur fracture" or "intertrochanteric" or "femoral neck" AND "regional anesthesia" or "spinal anesthesia" or "neuraxial anesthesia" or "epidural anesthesia". The "related articles" function in Medline was performed to expand the search. Reference lists were also hand-searched for relevant studies. No language restriction was placed on our search.

Inclusion and exclusion criteria

Two independent reviewers screened article titles and abstracts based on the following inclusion criteria: (1) randomized controlled trials (RCTs) with no language restriction; (2) studies comparing general anesthesia with neuraxial anesthesia (epidural or spinal) in patients undergoing hip fracture surgery; (3) studies provided numerical data. The following exclusion criteria was used: (1) studies that did not meet the inclusion criteria; (2) unpublished data or repeated data; (3) abstracts, case reports, comments, conference papers, or animal studies, meta-analysis and systematic reviews.

Data extraction

Two independent reviewers designed a structured table and collected all the relevant data into a database. The following information was extracted from each study that met the inclusion criteria: first author's name, publication year, country, sample size, age, American Society of Anesthesiologists (ASA) physical status, anesthesia technique, surgery type, study outcome measures. We also attempted to contact the corresponding authors to verify the accuracy of the data and to obtain further analytical data. We performed a meta-analysis for blood loss, 30-day mortality, length of hospital stay, and the prevalence of delirium, acute myocardial infarction, deep venous thrombosis, and pneumonia.

Methodological quality assessment

The methodological quality of each RCT was assessed using the Cochrane Handbook for Systematic Reviews of Interventions 5.1 by two reviewers, which contained the following items: random sequence generation, allocation concealment, blinding, incomplete outcome data, selective reporting, and other sources of bias. It was judged by answering a question, with "yes" indicating low risk of bias, "no" indicating high risk of bias, and "unclear" indicating unclear or unknown risk of bias [11]. The corresponding author was also consulted when any disagreement exists, and a consensus was reached by discussion.

Statistical analysis

The statistical analysis of the pooled data were performed using Review Manager software (version 5.1, The Cochrane Collaboration, Oxford, England). For continuous variables, standardized mean difference (SMD) or weighted mean (WMD) difference was calculated with the 95% confidence intervals (CIs) as a summary statistic. For dichotomous variables, relative risk (RR) and 95% CIs were used. The combined effect was considered significant at a 2-sided $P < 0.05$. The p-value with the Cochrane Q-test was texted, and the I^2 statistic was used to judge inconsistency of treatment effects across studies. A random effect model was used if high heterogeneity was detected ($p < 0.10$, $I^2 > 50\%$); otherwise, a fixed effect model was used if low heterogeneity existed ($p > 0.10$, $I^2 < 50\%$). Sensitivity analyses included a

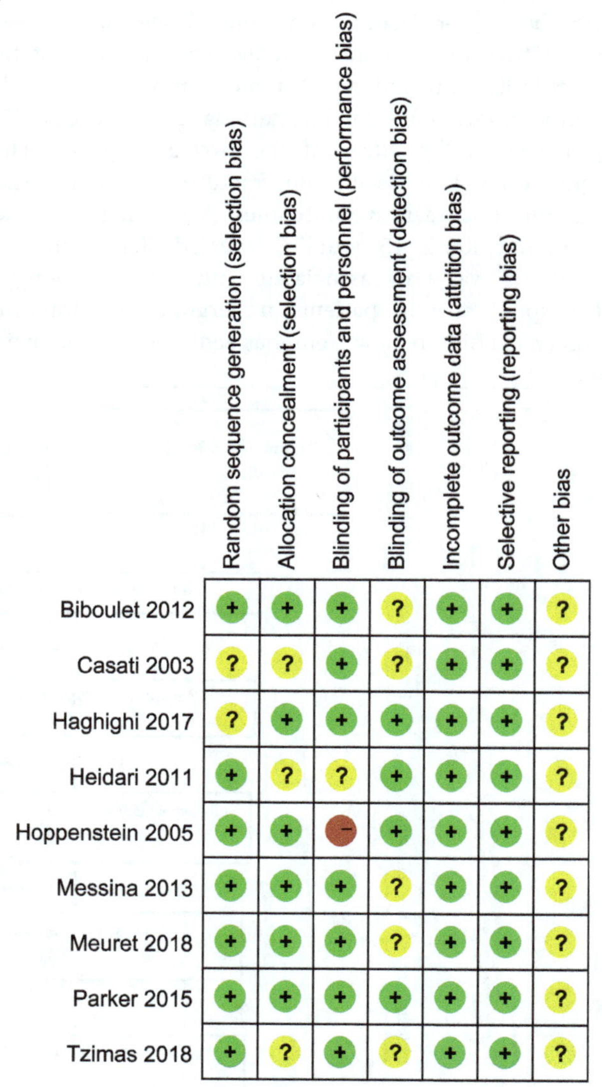

Fig. 2 Summary of risk bias assessment. "+" = low risk of bias; "?" = unclear risk of bias; and "-" = high risk of bias

Table 1 The descriptive characteristics of included studies

Study	Country	Sample size (male/female)	Age in years	ASA status	anesthesia	surgery type	Study outcome measures
Casati et al. (2003) [13]	Italy	30 (7/23)	84	II-III	GA vs Spinal	Hemiarthroplasty	Delirium; MMSE
Hoppensteinet al. (2005) [14]	Israel	60	> 65	I-III	GA vs Spinal	Hemiarthroplasty	Hemodynamic change; Delirium
Heidariet al. (2011) [15]	Iran	387 (257/130)	> 60	I-III	GA vs NA	–	Length of stay; 30-day mortality; Acute myocardial infarction; Pneumonia; Blood loss
Biboulet et al. (2012) [16]	France	45 (14/31)	> 75	III-IV	GA vs Spinal	Hemiarthroplasty Intramedullary nail	30-day mortality; Acute myocardial infarction
Messina et al. (2013) [17]	Italy	20 (7/13)	> 75	III	GA vs Spinal	–	Blood loss; Hemodynamic change
Parker et al. (2015) [18]	UK	322 (87/235)	> 49	I-III	GA vs Spinal	Arthroplasty Sliding hip screw Intramedullary nail	Delirium; 30-day mortality Acute myocardial Infarction; Pneumonia; Length of stay; DVT
Haghighi et al. (2017) [19]	Iran	100 (80/20)	> 60	I-III	GA vs Spinal	–	Blood loss; PONV
Meuret et al. (2018) [20]	France	40 (8/32)	> 75	I-III	GA vs HUSA	Arthroplasty Dynamic hip screw Intramedullary nail	PONV; DVT
Tzimas et al. (2018) [21]	Greece	70 (33/37)	76	I-III	GA vs Spinal	–	Delirium; MMSE

MMSE mini mental state examination, *PONV* post operative nausea and vomitting, *GA* general anesthesia, *NA* neuraxial anesthesia, *ASA* American Society of Anesthesiologists, *HUSA* hypobaric unilateral spinal anesthesia, *DVT* deep venous thrombosis

Bonferroni correction to adjust for multiple testing as well as the leave-one-out method. Publication bias was evaluated by funnel plot, if our meta-analysis included more than 10 studies [12].

Evidence synthesis

The evidence grade for the main outcomes are assessed using the guidelines of the (GRADE) system working group including the following items: risk of bias, inconsistency, indirectness, imprecision and publication bias. The recommendation level of evidence is classified into the following categories: (1) high, which means that further research is unlikely to change confidence in the effect estimate; (2) moderate, which means that further research is likely to significantly change confidence in the effect estimate but may change the estimate; (3) low, which means that further research is likely to significantly change confidence in the effect estimate and to change the estimate; and (4) very low, which means that any effect estimate is uncertain. The evidence quality is graded using the GRADEpro Version 3.6 software. The evidence quality was graded using the GRADEpro

Study or Subgroup	Neuraxial Events	Neuraxial Total	General Events	General Total	Weight	Odds Ratio M-H, Random, 95% CI
Casati 2003	1	15	3	15	18.0%	0.29 [0.03, 3.12]
Heidari 2011	12	190	26	197	37.7%	0.44 [0.22, 0.91]
Parker 2015	3	158	0	164	13.7%	7.41 [0.38, 144.53]
Tzimas 2018	10	37	4	33	30.6%	2.69 [0.75, 9.59]
Total (95% CI)		**400**		**409**	**100.0%**	**1.05 [0.27, 4.00]**
Total events	26		33			

Heterogeneity: Tau² = 1.11; Chi² = 8.87, df = 3 (P = 0.03); I² = 66%
Test for overall effect: Z = 0.07 (P = 0.95)

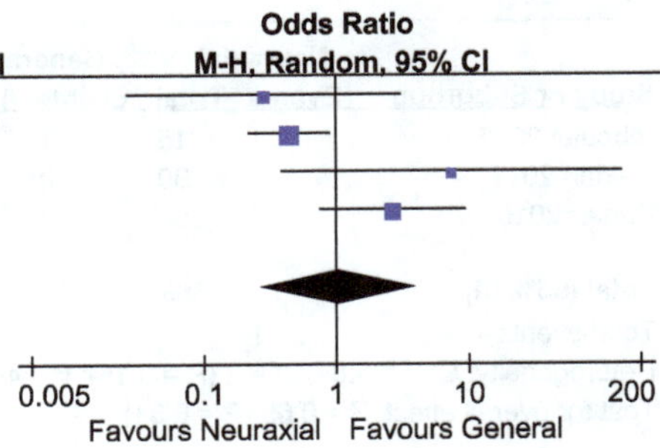

Fig. 3 Forest plot of delirium rate for neuraxial anesthesia versus general anesthesia

Study or Subgroup	Neuraxial Mean	Neuraxial SD	Neuraxial Total	General Mean	General SD	General Total	Weight	Mean Difference IV, Random, 95% CI
Haghighi 2017	365	62.99	50	513.7	151.19	50	35.7%	-148.70 [-194.10, -103.30]
Heidari 2011	458.8	335	190	696.8	432.5	197	31.6%	-238.00 [-314.92, -161.08]
Messina 2013	161	91	10	190	65	10	32.7%	-29.00 [-98.31, 40.31]
Total (95% CI)			**250**			**257**	**100.0%**	**-137.80 [-241.49, -34.12]**

Heterogeneity: Tau² = 7307.67; Chi² = 16.20, df = 2 (P = 0.0003); I² = 88%
Test for overall effect: Z = 2.61 (P = 0.009)

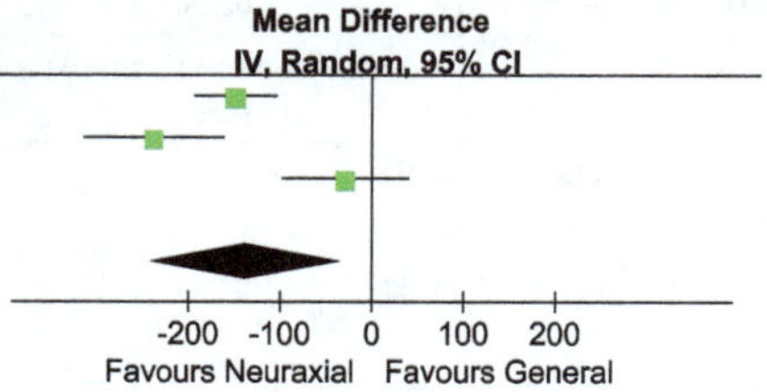

Fig. 4 Forest plot of blood loss for neuraxial anesthesia versus general anesthesia

Version 3.6 software. The strengths of the recommendations were based on the quality of the evidence.

Results

Study identification and selection

A total of 1274 relevant studies were identified according to the search strategy. However, 798 publications were excluded after checking for duplicates. Among the 476 remaining articles, 359 articles were excluded after reviewing the titles and abstracts. Then we assessed 17 studies with full texts for eligibility. Eight studies were excluded because four of them included no control groups, and others provided inadequate data. Finally, nine RCTs with a total of 1084 patients between 2003 and 2018 met our inclusion criteria, and were included in the meta-analysis [13–21]. The flow diagram of study selection is shown in Fig. 1.

Study characteristics

All the included studies were written in English, which examined perioperative outcomes between hip fracture patients who receive neuraxial or general anesthesia undergoing surgical repair. There were a total of 1084 patients, whose ages were older than 49 years-old. Seven studies looked at outcomes relating to spinal anesthesia compared with general anesthesia [13, 14, 16–19, 21], one study examed outcomes for hypobaric unilateral spinal anesthesia and general anesthesia [20], and the other study compared general versus neuraxial anesthesia that encompassed spinal and epidural anesthesia [15]. In the terms of surgery type, two studies performed arthroplasty, hip screw and intramedullary nail [18, 20]; two studies included hemiarthroplasty only [13, 14], and one study performed hemiarthroplasty and Intramedullary nail [16]. Only one study was at a high risk of performance bias [14], and the other studies were all at low risk or unclear (Fig. 2). The characteristics of the included studies is shown in Table 1.

Outcomes for meta-analysis

Delirium rate was reported in four studies with 400 patients in the neuraxial anesthesia group and 409 patients in the general anesthesia group [13, 15, 18, 21]. The *P* value with the Cochran's Q test was 0.03, and the I^2 statistic was 66%, which indicated high heterogeneity among these studies. Thus a random effect model was used to analyze the results. The pooled data showed no significant difference in delirium rate between the two groups (OR = 1.05, 95% CI 0.27, 4.00; $P = 0.95$, Fig. 3).

Three studies examed blood loss during hip fracture surgery with 250 patients in the neuraxial anesthesia group and 257 patients in the general anesthesia group [15, 17, 19]. The *P* value with the Cochran's Q test was 0.0003, and the I^2 statistic was 88%, which indicated high heterogeneity among these studies. Thus a random effect model was used to analyze the results. The pooled data showed a significant difference between the two groups (MD = − 137.8, 95% CI -241.49, − 34.12; $p = 0.009$, Fig. 4).

Three studies were included in the meta-analysis for 30-day mortality, involving 363 patients in the neuraxial anesthesia group and 389 patients in the general anesthesia group [15, 16, 18]. The *P* value with the Cochran's Q test was 0.21, and the I^2 statistic was 48%,

Study or Subgroup	Neuraxial Events	Neuraxial Total	General Events	General Total	Weight	Odds Ratio M-H, Fixed, 95% CI
Biboulet 2012	1	15	1	28	7.5%	1.93 [0.11, 33.21]
Heidari 2011	5	190	0	197	5.5%	11.71 [0.64, 213.27]
Parker 2015	5	158	8	164	87.1%	0.64 [0.20, 1.99]
Total (95% CI)		**363**		**389**	**100.0%**	**1.34 [0.56, 3.21]**
Total events	11		9			

Heterogeneity: Chi² = 3.84, df = 2 (P = 0.15); I² = 48%
Test for overall effect: Z = 0.65 (P = 0.51)

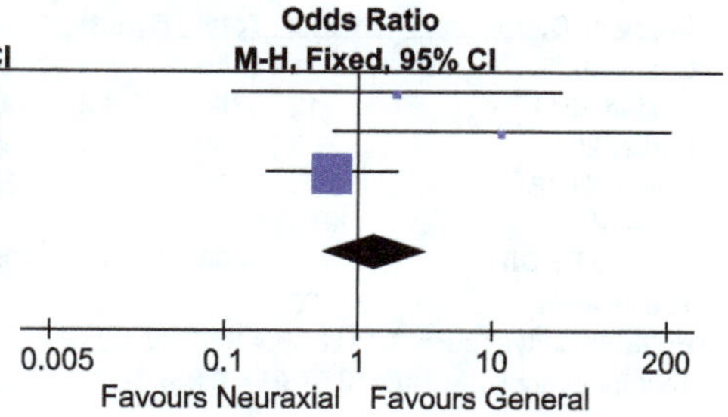

Fig. 5 Forest plot of 30-day mortality for neuraxial anesthesia versus general anesthesia

Study or Subgroup	Neuraxial Events	Neuraxial Total	General Events	General Total	Weight	Odds Ratio M-H, Fixed, 95% CI
Biboulet 2012	0	15	1	28	34.6%	0.59 [0.02, 15.41]
Heidari 2011	1	190	1	197	32.7%	1.04 [0.06, 16.70]
Parker 2015	1	158	1	164	32.7%	1.04 [0.06, 16.74]
Total (95% CI)		**363**		**389**	**100.0%**	**0.88 [0.17, 4.65]**
Total events	2		3			

Heterogeneity: Chi² = 0.08, df = 2 (P = 0.96); I² = 0%

Test for overall effect: Z = 0.15 (P = 0.88)

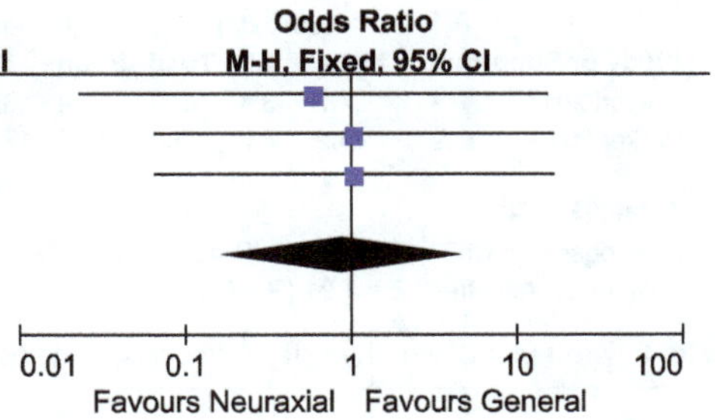

Fig. 6 Forest plot of acute myocardial infarction rate for neuraxial anesthesia versus general anesthesia

which indicated low heterogeneity among these studies. Thus a fixed effect model was used to analyze the results. The pooled data revealed that there was no significant difference in 30-day mortality between the two groups (OR = 1.34, 95% CI 0.56, 3.21; *P* = 0.51, Fig. 5).

Acute myocardial infarction rate was reported in three studies with 363 patients in the neuraxial anesthesia group and 376 patients in the general anesthesia group [15, 16, 18]. The *P* value with the Cochran's Q test was 0.96, and the I^2 statistic was 0%, which indicated low heterogeneity among these studies. Thus a fixed effect model was used to analyze the results. The pooled data showed no significant difference in the acute myocardial infarction rate between the two groups (OR = 0.88, 95% CI 0.17, 4.65; *P* = 0.88, Fig. 6).

Two studies provided the outcome of pneumonia rate, which involved 363 patients in the neuraxial anesthesia group and 389 patients in the general anesthesia group [15, 18]. The *P* value with the Cochran's Q test was 0.42, and the I^2 statistic was 0%, which indicated low heterogeneity among these studies. Thus a fixed effect model was used to analyze the results. The pooled data showed no significant difference in pneumonia rate between the two groups (OR = 1.04, 95% CI 0.23, 4.61; *P* = 0.96, Fig. 7).

Two studies reported length of stay in a way that could be comparable by meta-analysis, including 348 patients in the neuraxial anesthesia group and 361 patients in the general anesthesia group [15, 18]. The *P* value with the Cochran's Q test was 0.54, and the I^2 statistic was 0%, which indicated low heterogeneity among these studies. Thus a fixed effect model was used to analyze the results. The pooled data revealed that no significant difference was detected in the length of stay between the two groups (MD = – 0.65, 95% CI -0.32, 0.02; *P* = 0.06, Fig. 8).

Two studies were included in the meta-analysis for deep venous thrombosis rate, involving 179 patients in the neuraxial anesthesia group and 183 patients in the general anesthesia group [18, 20]. The *P* value with the Cochran's Q test was 0.60, and the I^2 statistic was 0%, which indicated low heterogeneity among these studies. Thus a fixed effect model was used to analyze the results. The pooled data revealed that there was no significant difference in deep venous thrombosis rate between the two groups (OR = 0.48, 95% CI 0.09, 2.72; *P* = 0.41, Fig. 9).

Sensitivity analysis

Sensitivity analyses were performed by the leave-one-out approach in the comparison of blood loss. No difference was detected in the direction of the outcome with each study removed in turn, which showed that this result had good reliability (Fig. 10).

After adjustment for multiple testing using the Bonferroni correction, adjusted *p*-values were 0.054 for the comparison of blood loss, 0.36 for the comparison of length of stay and 1.0 for the other outcomes. All of them were above the significant threshold of 0.05, thus there was no significant difference in each comparison.

Study or Subgroup	Neuraxial Events	Neuraxial Total	General Events	General Total	Weight	Odds Ratio M-H, Fixed, 95% CI
Heidari 2011	1	190	0	197	14.4%	3.13 [0.13, 77.23]
Parker 2015	2	158	3	164	85.6%	0.69 [0.11, 4.17]
Total (95% CI)		**348**		**361**	**100.0%**	**1.04 [0.23, 4.61]**
Total events	3		3			

Heterogeneity: Chi² = 0.65, df = 1 (P = 0.42); I² = 0%

Test for overall effect: Z = 0.05 (P = 0.96)

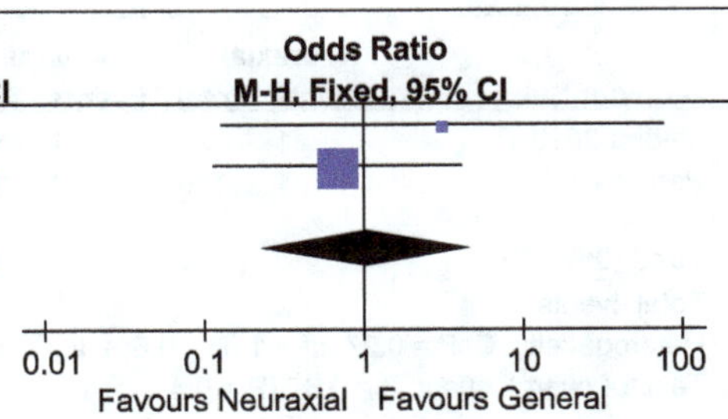

Fig. 7 Forest plot of pneumonia rate for neuraxial anesthesia versus general anesthesia

Study or Subgroup	Neuraxial Mean	Neuraxial SD	Neuraxial Total	General Mean	General SD	General Total	Weight	Mean Difference IV, Fixed, 95% CI
Heidari 2011	7.7	3.4	190	8.4	3.5	197	95.3%	-0.70 [-1.39, -0.01]
Parker 2015	16.2	14.6	158	15.9	13.7	164	4.7%	0.30 [-2.79, 3.39]
Total (95% CI)			**348**			**361**	**100.0%**	**-0.65 [-1.32, 0.02]**

Heterogeneity: Chi² = 0.38, df = 1 (P = 0.54); I² = 0%
Test for overall effect: Z = 1.91 (P = 0.06)

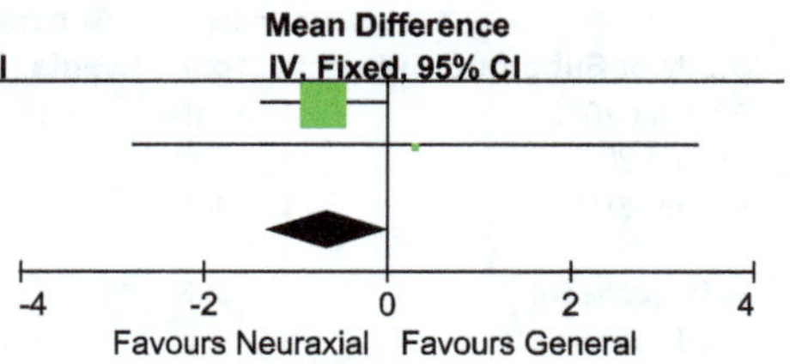

Fig. 8 Forest plot of length of stay for neuraxial anesthesia versus general anesthesia

Quality of the evidence and recommendation strengths

A total of seven outcomes in this meta-analysis were evaluated using the GRADE system (Table 2). The evidence quality for each outcome was low. Therefore, we demonstrate that the overall evidence quality is low, which means that further research is likely to significantly change confidence in the effect estimate and may change the estimate.

Discussion

In our study, a total of nine RCTs with 1084 patients were included to make an updated meta-analysis. However, no significant difference was detected in the 30-day mortality, length of stay, and the prevalence of delirium, acute myocardial infarction, and pneumonia in patients undergoing hip fracture surgery where either neuraxial or general anesthesia was used. We first focused on the comparison of blood loss between the two anesthesia techniques. The leave-one-out method showed that the result had good reliability. However, after applying the Bonferroni correction, the adjusted p-value for this comparison was above the significance threshold ($p = 0.054$), which revealed there was no significant difference. The sample size was also small, and the overall evidence was low, indicating that further research is likely to significantly change confidence in the effect estimate and may change the estimate. Based on the current available evidence, more high-quality RCTs are required for further investigation.

According to methodological quality assessment, eight out of nine RCTs in our study were assessed as high-quality. Moreover, our study included several RCTs, in which the results were published after the most recent systematic review of this topic, making our results more dependable. Of note, all of the RCTs showed low risk of attrition bias and reporting bias that may contribute to reducing systematic bias. Another strength of our study is low heterogeneity, detected in five out of six outcome measures assessed using I^2 statistic, demonstrating consistent outcomes across the comparisons. In addition, the adjustment was made by the Bonferroni correction to decrease the risk of type I error caused by multiple statistical tests in our study. Also, some data of previous reviews dated back to the 1980s [9, 10], in which the type of anaesthetic techniques may not reflect current clinical practice, and it may restrain us from finding clinically relevant differences between the two techniques [9, 22], while our study included most recent RCTs.

According to pharmacology, neuraxial anesthesia could lead to lower heart rate, and blood pressure than general anesthesia by blocking alpha and beta adrenergic receptors. Consequently, controlled blood pressure resulted in intraoperative less blood loss in neuraxial anesthesia patients [16, 23]. Current practice revealed that the number of patients who needed blood transfusion was larger in general anesthesia group, which means patients receiving spinal anesthesia had less blood loss than those receiving general anesthesia [19, 24, 25]. In consistency with this result, a systematic review by Richman et al. Including 66 articles demonstrated that the use of neuraxial anesthesia resulted in a significant decrease in estimated blood loss [26]. However, a meta-

Study or Subgroup	Neuraxial Events	Neuraxial Total	General Events	General Total	Weight	Odds Ratio M-H, Fixed, 95% CI
Meuret 2018	1	21	1	19	25.5%	0.90 [0.05, 15.47]
Parker 2015	1	158	3	164	74.5%	0.34 [0.04, 3.32]
Total (95% CI)		**179**		**183**	**100.0%**	**0.48 [0.09, 2.72]**
Total events	2		4			

Heterogeneity: Chi² = 0.27, df = 1 (P = 0.60); I² = 0%
Test for overall effect: Z = 0.82 (P = 0.41)

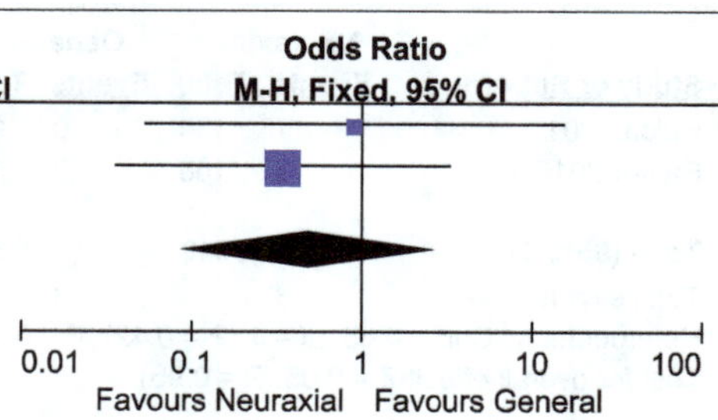

Fig. 9 Forest plot of deep venous thrombosis rate for neuraxial anesthesia versus general anesthesia

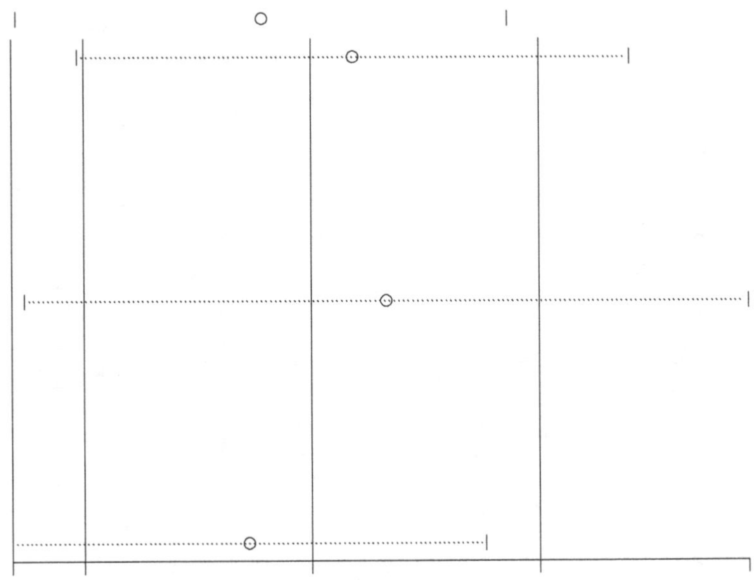

Fig. 10 Sensitivity analysis of blood loss for neuraxial anesthesia versus general anesthesia

analysis by Hu er al. including 21 RCTs stated that there was insufficient evidence to support the use of neuraxial anesthesia in decreasing intraoperative blood loss [27]. In our study, only three RCTs involving 507 patients have been summarised. Two of them showed the neuraxial anesthesia was assosiated with statistically significant decrease in blood loss, the other showed no significant difference between the two anesthesia techniques. However, the results from our meta-analysis indicating decreased blood loss with neuraxial anesthesia are limited by a high degree of heterogeneity (88%) and low-quality evidence for this outcome. Also, we did not investigate whether this resulted in a clinically meaningful difference in perioperative blood transfusions.

Delirium is a very common postoperative complication, which leads to lasting cognitive and functional decline, and increasing length of stay [18, 28]. There are many precipitating factors in developing delirium, including infection, myocardial and cerebral ischaemia, urinary retention, pain, constipation as well as electrolyte abnormalities [29]. Furthermore, several studies have investigated the incidence of delirium in elderly patients, who were admitted to be hospitalized for a variety of reasons, and the prevalence amongst medical wards was estimated to range from 29 to 64% [29–31]. Additionally, the development of delirium is thought to be multifactorial process. Certain patient characteristics are also easy to cause delirium, including pre-existing cognitive impairment, sleep deprivation, medical immobilities, visual impairment, hearing impairment and poly pharmacy [32, 33]. Our study detected no significant difference in delirium rate between general and neuraxial anesthesia. It is noteworthy that none of the included studies represented relative characteristics and potential risk factors that causing delirium in hip fracture patients perioperatively. Thus the result may be unconvincing.

Our study detect comparable outcomes in the incidence of 30-day mortality between the two groups. In line with this result, a retrospective study reported that the anesthesia technique has little effect on postoperative mortality, and the type of anesthesia given by the anesthesiologist should be selected based on the individual physical condition [34]. The study of Lienhart et al. including 425 patients indicated that their coexisting disease has great influence on 30-day mortality in old patients such as diabetes, cardiovascular disease, etc [35]. Delay of surgery for more than 24 h was a main factor affecting postoperative mortality in geriatric hip fracture patients [36]. The retrospective cohort study of Pincus et al. Investigated 42,230 patients undergoing hip fracture surgery, and demonstrate that a preoperative waiting time of more than 24 h was associated with a greater risk of 30-day mortality and other complications [37].

In our study, the incidence of myocardial infarction and pneumonia were similar in both groups. Zuo et al. detected the same result, and suggested that the neuraxial anesthesia might be a better choice in hip fracture surgery [38]. However, Urwin et al. proposed that the incidence of myocardial infarction and pneumonia was lower in patients receiving neuraxial anesthesia, and a significant lower incidence of intraoperative hypotension was detected in patients receiving general anesthesia [39]. It should be noted that Urwin et al. evaluated 2161 patients retrospectively. Moreover, all of the included

Table 2 The GRADE evidence quality for main outcome

Quality assessment							No of patients		Effect		Quality	Importance
No of studies	Design	Risk of bias	Inconsistency	Indirectness	Imprecision	Other considerations	Experim-ental	Control	Relative (95% CI)	Absolute		
Delirium rate												
4	randomised trials	serious	no serious inconsistency	serious	no serious imprecision	none	26/400 (6.5%)	33/409 (8.1%)	OR 1.05 (0.27 to 4)	4 more per 1000 (from 58 fewer to 179 more)	⊕⊕LOW	IMPORTANT
								12.7%		6 more per 1000 (from 89 fewer to 241 more)		
Acute myocardial infarction rate												
3	randomised trials	no serious risk of bias	serious	serious	no serious imprecision	none	2/363 (0.55%)	3/376 (0.8%)	OR 0.73 (0.14 to 3.74)	2 fewer per 1000 (from 7 fewer to 21 more)	⊕⊕LOW	IMPORTANT
								0.6%		2 fewer per 1000 (from 5 fewer to 16 more)		
30-day Mortality												
3	randomised trials	serious	no serious inconsistency	no serious indirectness	serious	none	11/331 (3.3%)	16/343 (4.7%)	OR 0.71 (0.33 to 1.53)	13 fewer per 1000 (from 31 fewer to 23 more)	⊕⊕ LOW	IMPORTANT
								4.9%		14 fewer per 1000 (from 32 fewer to 24 more)		
Blood loss (Better indicated by lower values)												
3	randomised trials	serious	serious	no serious indirectness	no serious imprecision	none	250	257	–	MD −137.80 lower (−241.49 lower to −34.12 higher)	⊕⊕ LOW	IMPORTANT
Pneumonia rate												
2	randomised trials	serious	serious	no serious indirectness	no serious imprecision	reporting bias	3/348 (0.9%)	3/361 (0.8%)	OR 1.04 (0.23 to 4.61)	0 more per 1000 (from 6 fewer to 29 more)	⊕ VERY LOW	NOT IMPORTANT
								0.9%		0 more per 1000 (from 7 fewer to 31 more)		
Length of stay												
2	randomised trials	serious	no serious inconsistency	serious	no serious imprecision	reporting bias	348	361	–	MD −0.65 lower (−1.32 lower to 0.02 higher)	⊕ VERY LOW	NOT IMPORTANT
Deep venous thrombosis rate												
2	randomised trials	serious	no serious inconsistency	serious	no serious imprecision	None	2/179 (1.1%)	4/183 (2.2%)	OR 0.48 (0.09 to 2.72)	0 more per 1000 (from 2 fewer to 19 more)	⊕ VERY LOW	NOT IMPORTANT
								2.3%		0 more per 1000 (from 6 fewer to 32 more)		

studies were performed more than 20 years ago, which are now somewhat dated, since many drugs used for anesthesia techniques and health care systems have been improved a lot. Thus their findings could not provide worthy references to some extent.

There was no significant difference regarding the length of stay between the two anesthesia techniques. Sutcliffe et al. surveyed 1333 volunteers of hip surgery, and found no difference in factors of hospitalization in both groups [40]. Neverthless, Neuman et al. conducted a matched retrospective cohort study involving 56,729 patients, and found a modestly shorter length of stay in the neuraxial anesthesia group. The authors also proposed that the fracture type and performed surgery procedure were important factors; minimally invasive approaches and optimal quality of fracture reduction may decrease the length of stay [41]. In addition, Grant et al. declared that the pain severity was lower in patients receiving general anesthesia, resuting in shorter length of stay [42]. A notable point is that waiting time prior to surgery extended the length of stay [43]. In our meta-analysis, one study reported the overall length of stay [18] while the other documented the length of stay before and after the surgery [15]. It is difficult to draw a definite conclusion due to the existence of aforementioned multiple factors. Also, the small sample size in our study should be taken into consideration.

Perioperative deep venous thrombosis is common in hip fracture patients. Several studies concluded that neuraxial anaesthesia was associated with fewer incidents of deep venous thrombosis when compared to general anaesthesia [39, 44, 45]. It was thought that in neuraxial anaesthesia sympathetic block could lead to vasodilatation of the lower limbs, and then the increased blood flow to the lower limbs was likely to reduce the coagulability and viscosity of blood [46]. A Cochrane review published in 2016 by pooling the results from 31 RCTs showed a reduced risk of deep venous thrombosis in the neuraxial group without potent thromboprophylaxis. Nevertheless, the level of evidence was very low for this outcome [22]. Another Cochrane review concluded that there was a marginal advantage for neuraxial anaesthesia regarding the incidence of deep venous thrombosis [47]. Our study included only two RCTs, and detected no significant difference in the incidence of deep venous thrombosis between the two groups.

Objectively speaking, several limitations of our study should be mentioned. A major limitation is that the sample size was relatively small, and the sample size varied widely among the included studies. Another notable limitation is that most of the included studies did not describe whether additional sedation was used in hip fracture patients receiving neuraxial anesthesia, for instance, the use of propofol sedation could influence the prevalence of postoperative delirium [48]. Also, no information is available in the terms of the dosage of the anesthesia used. In addition, the inconsistent definition of length of stay and delirium may account for the wide prevalence range for these outcomes. There are numerous confounding factors such as the diversity of patient groups, health care systems, surgical and anesthetic techniques that may affect the perioperative outcomes, leading to potential biases. This issue would be possibly considered as a weakness. Last but not least, the outcome measures were not identical in each trial, thus we did not have sufficient data to perform other meta-analyses, which potentially affects the current findings of our study. Therefore, more high-quality RCTs with large sample size are required for a firm conclusion.

Conclusion

In summary, our present study demonstrated that there might be a difference in blood loss between patients receiving neuraxial and general anaesthesia, however, this analysis was not robust to adjustment for multiple testing and therefore at high risk for a type I error. We suggest that the choice of anaesthesia (neuraxial or general) should be made by the anaesthesiologist based on the individual patient's requirements, comorbidities, potential postoperative complications, consultation of geriatrician and orthopaedic surgeon, and the clinical experience of the anaesthesiologist. Due to small sample size and enormous inconsistency in the choice of outcome measures, more high-quality studies with large sample size are needed to to clarify this issue.

Abbreviations

ASA: American Society of Anesthesiologists; CI: Confidence interval; GRADE: The grading of recommendations, assessment, development, and evaluation methodology; GA: General anesthesia; HUSA: Hypobaric unilateral spinal anesthesia; MMSE: Mini mental state examination; NA: Neuraxial anesthesia; PONV: Postoperative nausea and vomiting; PRISMA: Preferred reporting items for systematic reviews and meta-analyses; RCT: Randomized controlled trial; RR: Risk ratio; SMD: Standardized mean difference; WMD: Weighted mean difference; DVT: Deep venous thrombosis

Acknowledgements

Not applicable.

Authors' contributions

XZ and ZL designed and conceived the study, performed the statistical analysis, and drafted the manuscript. YG participated in the interpretation of data, analysis, and drafting of the manuscript. YT participated in the study design and coordination, and helped to draft the manuscript. All authors read and approved the final manuscript.

References

1. Dhanwal DK, Dennison EM, Harvey NC, Cooper C. Epidemiology of hip fracture: worldwide geographic variation. Indian J Orthop. 2011;45:15–22.
2. Hickson LJ, Farah WH, Johnson RL, et al. Death and postoperative complications after hip fracture repair: Dialysis effect. Kidney Int Rep. 2018;3: 1294–303.
3. White SM. Anaesthesia type and cement reactions in hip fracture surgery. Anaesthesia. 2019;74(4):543–4.

4. White SM. Foss NB.Anesthesia aspects in the treatment of fragility fracture patients. Injury. 2018;49:1403–8.
5. Radić N, Radinović K, Ille M, et al. The selection of best anesthesiological technique for hip fracture surgery in older high-risk patients. Acta Chir Iugosl. 2012;59:113–5.
6. Kowark A, Rossaint R. General versus spinal anesthesia for the elderly hip fractured patient. Curr Opin Anaesthesiol. 2019;32:116–9.
7. Rivas E. Geriatric patients undergoing non-elective surgery for hip fracture: can management be optimized? J Clin Anesth. 2019;59:112–3.
8. Zhong H, Wang Y, Wang Y. Comparison of the effect and clinical value in general anesthesia and combined spinal-epidural anesthesia in elderly patients undergoing hip arthroplasty. Exp Ther Med. 2019;17:4421–6.
9. O'Donnell CM, McLoughlin L, Patterson CC, et al. Perioperative outcomes in the context of mode of anesthesia for patients undergoing hip fracture surgery: systematic review and meta-analysis. Br J Anaesth. 2018;120:37–50.
10. Waesberghe JV, Stevanovic A, Rossaint R, et al. General vs. neuraxial anaesthesia in hip fracture patients: a systematic review and meta-analysis. BMC Anesthesiol. 2017;17(1):87.
11. Higgins J, Green S. Cochrane handbook for systematic reviews of interventions version 5.1.0. The Cochrane Collaboration. 2011. Available from: http://handbook-5-1.cochrane.org/..
12. Sterne JA, Higgins JP. Recommendations for examining and interpreting funnel plot asymmetry in meta-analyses of randomised controlled trials. BMJ. 2011;343(5):d4002.
13. Casati A, Aldegheri G, Vinciguerra E, et al. Randomized comparison between sevoflurane anesthesia and unilateral spinal anesthesia in elderly patients undergoing orthopaedic surgery. Eur J Anaesthesiol. 2003;20(8):640–6.
14. Hoppenstein D, Zohar E, Ramaty E, et al. The effects of general vs spinal anesthesia on frontal cerebral oxygen saturation in geriatric patients undergoing emergency surgical fixation of the neck of femur. J Clin Anesth. 2005;17(6):431–8.
15. Heidari SM, Soltani H, Hashemi SJ, et al. Comparative study of two anesthesia methods according to postoperative complications and one month mortality rate in the candidates of hip surgery. J Res Med Sci. 2011; 16(3):323–30.
16. Biboulet P, Jourdan A, Van Haevre V, et al. Hemodynamic profile of target-controlled spinal anesthesia compared with 2 target-controlled general anesthesia techniques in elderly patients with cardiac comorbidities. Reg Anesth Pain Med. 2012;37(4):433–40.
17. Messina A, Frassanito L, Colombo D, et al. Hemodynamic changes associated with spinal and general anesthesia for hip fracture surgery in severe ASA III elderly population: a pilot trial. Minerva Anestesiol. 2013;79(9): 1021–9.
18. Parker MJ, Griffiths R. General versus regional anesthesia for hip fractures. A pilot randomised controlled trial of 322 patients. Injury. 2015;46(8):1562–6.
19. Haghighi M, Sedighinejad A, Nabi BN, et al. Is spinal anesthesia with low dose lidocaine better than sevoflorane anesthesia in patients undergoing hip fracture surgery. Arch Bone Jt Surg. 2017;5(4):226–30.
20. Meuret P, Bouvet L, Villet B, et al. Hypobaric unilateral spinal anesthesia versus general anesthesia in elderly patients undergoing hip fracture surgical repair: a prospective randomised open trial. Turk J Anaesthesiol Reanim. 2018;46(2):121–30.
21. Tzimas P, Samara E, Petrou A, et al. The influence of anesthetic techniques on postoperative cognitive function in elderly patients undergoing hip fracture surgery: general vs spinal anesthesia. Injury. 2018;49(12):2221–6.
22. Guay J, Parker MJ, Gajendragadkar PR, Kopp S. Anaesthesia for hip fracture surgery in adults. Cochrane Database Syst Rev. 2016;2:CD000521.
23. Ing C, Sun L S, Friend AF, et al. Differences in intraoperative hemodynamics between spinal and general anesthesia in infants undergoing pyloromyotomy. Paediatr Anaesth. 2017;27(7):733-41.
24. Liu JL, Xiao LW, Mao WG, et al. Comparative outcomes of peripheral nerve blocks versus general anesthesia for hip fractures in geriatric Chinese patients. Patient Prefer Adherence. 2014;8:651–9.
25. Rosberg B, Fredin H, Gustafson C. Anesthetic techniques and surgical blood loss in total hip arthroplasty.[J]. Acta Anaesthesiol Scand. 2010;26(3):189–93.
26. Richman JM, Rowlingson AJ, Maine DN, et al. Does neuraxial anesthesia reduce intraoperative blood loss?: a meta-analysis. J Clin Anesth. 2006;18(6): 427–35.
27. Hu S, Zhang ZY, Hua YQ, et al. A comparison of regional and general anesthesia for total replacement of the hip or knee: a meta-analysis. J Bone Joint Surg Br. 2009;91(7):935–42.
28. Schubert M, Schürch R, Boettger S, et al. A hospital-wide evaluation of delirium prevalence and outcomes in acute care patients - a cohort study. BMC Health Serv Res. 2018;18(1):550.
29. Elie M, Cole MG, Primeau FJ, et al. Delirium risk factors in elderly hospitalized patients. J Gen Intern Med. 2010;13(3):204–12.
30. Holt R, Young J, Heseltine D. Effectiveness of a multi-component intervention to reduce delirium incidence in elderly care wards. Age Ageing. 2013;42(6):721–7.
31. Hernandez BA, Lindroth H, Rowley P, et al. Post-anesthesia care unit delirium: incidence, risk factors and associated adverse outcomes. Br J Anaesth. 2017;119(2):288–90.
32. Smith TO, Cooper A, Peryer G, et al. Factors predicting incidence of post-operative delirium in older people following hip fracture surgery: a systematic review and meta-analysis. Int J Geriatr Psychiatry. 2017;32(4):386–96.
33. Pessoa RF, Nácul FE. Delirium in the critically ill patient. Rev Bras Ter Intensiva. 2006;18(2):190–5.
34. Chu CL, Chiou HY, Chou WH, et al. Leading comorbidity associated with 30-day post-anesthetic mortality in geriatric surgical patients in Taiwan: a retrospective study from the health insurance data. BMC Geriatr. 2017;17(1):245.
35. Lienhart A, Auroy Y, Péquignot F, et al. Survey of anesthesia-related mortality in France. Anesthesiology. 2006;105(6):1087–97.
36. Carretta E, Bochicchio V, Rucci P, et al. Hip fracture: effectiveness of early surgery to prevent 30-day mortality. Int Orthop. 2011;35(3):419.
37. Pincus D, Ravi B, Wasserstein D, et al. Association between wait time and 30-day mortality in adults undergoing hip fracture surgery. JAMA. 2017; 318(20):1994.
38. Zuo D, Jin C, Shan M, et al. A comparison of general versus regional anesthesia for hip fracture surgery: a meta-analysis. Int J Clin Exp Med. 2015; 8(11):20295–301.
39. Urwin SC, Parker MJ, Griffiths R. General versus regional anesthesia for hip fracture surgery: a meta- analysis of randomized trials. Br J Anaesth. 2000; 84(4):450–5.
40. Sutcliffe AJ, Parker M. Mortality after spinal and general anesthesia for surgical fixation of hip fractures. Anaesthesia. 1994;49(3):237–40.
41. Neuman MD, Rosenbaum PR, Ludwig JM, et al. Anesthesia technique, mortality, and length of stay after hip fracture surgery. JAMA. 2014;311(24): 2508–17.
42. Grant MC, Pio Roda CM, Canner JK, et al. The impact of anesthesia-influenced process measure compliance on length of stay: results from an enhanced recovery after surgery for colorectal surgery cohort. Anesth Analg. 2019;128(1):68–74.
43. Shetty V, Vowlar S, Villar R. The role of anesthesia and the anesthetist in reducing the length of stay after primary Total hip Arthroplasty. J Arthroplast. 2007;22(2):305.
44. Macario A, Dexter F. What are the most important risk factors for a patient's developing intraoperative hypothermia? Anesth Analg. 2002;94(1):215–20.
45. Breen P, Park KW. General anesthesia versus regional anesthesia. Int Anesthesiol Clin. 2002;40(1):61–71.
46. Davis FM, Quince M, Laurenson VG. Deep vein thrombosis and anaesthetic technique in emergency hip surgery. BMJ. 1980;281(6254):1528–9.
47. Parker MJ, Handoll HHG, Griffiths R. Anaesthesia for hip fracture surgery in adults. Cochrane Database Syst Rev. 2004;4:CD000521.
48. Sieber FE, Zakriya KJ, Gottschalk A, et al. Sedation depth during spinal anesthesia and the development of postoperative delirium in elderly patients undergoing hip fracture repair. Mayo Clin Proc. 2010; 85:18–26.

19

Ketorolac tromethamine pretreatment suppresses sufentanil-induced cough during general anesthesia induction

Zhen Tian[1,2], Bei Hu[1,2*], Min Miao[1,2], Lulu Zhang[1,2], Lin Wang[1,2] and Bin Chen[1,2]

Abstract

Background: To observe the effect of pretreatment with ketorolac tromethamine on sufentanil-induced cough in general anesthesia patients.

Methods: A total of 102 patients were screened, and 90 patients were scheduled for elective surgery under general anesthesia. The 90 patients were randomly divided into two groups: the control group (C group) and the observation group (KT group). Five minutes before anesthesia induction, the observation group was given ketorolac tromethamine 0.5 mg/kg intravenously within 3 s, while the control group was given the same amount of normal saline intravenously. All patients were given a sufentanil bolus of 0.5 μg/kg (within 3 s) intravenously. One minute later, propofol 2.5 mg/kg and vecuronium 0.15 mg/kg were injected intravenously, and endotracheal intubation was guided by laryngoscopy. The number of coughs that occurred within 1 min after sufentanil injection was recorded. The mean arterial pressure (MAP), heart rate (HR) and pulse oxygen saturation (SpO_2) were recorded at T0 (immediately before pretreatment), T1 (5 min after pretreatment), T2 (before intubation), T3 (1 min after intubation) and T4 (5 min after intubation). The incidence of adverse reactions, including nausea and vomiting, dizziness, drowsiness, delay of recovery, restlessness in the recovery period, respiratory depression and postoperative incision pain, was analyzed.

Results: Within 1 min after sufentanil injection, the incidence and severity of cough in the KT group was significantly lower than that in the C group ($P < 0.05$). At T0, T1, T2, T3 and T4, there were no significant differences in MAP, HR and SpO2 between the two groups ($P > 0.05$). There was no significant difference in the dosage of sufentanil, propofol, remifentanil and vecuronium, the incidence of nausea and vomiting, the delay of recovery, dizziness, drowsiness or respiratory depression between the two groups ($P > 0.05$). However, the incidence of restlessness and the number of patients with VAS scores > 3 in the KT group were significantly lower than those in the C group ($P < 0.05$).

(Continued on next page)

* Correspondence: sqrmyyhb@163.com
[1]Department of Anesthesiology, Suqian People's Hospital of Nanjing Drum-tower Hospital Group, Suqian 223800, China
[2]Department of Anesthesiology, The Affiliated Suqian Hospital of Xuzhou Medical University, Suqian 223800, China

(Continued from previous page)

Conclusion: Pretreatment with intravenous ketorolac tromethamine can significantly reduce the incidence of sufentanil-induced cough during induction of general anesthesia, which can also significantly reduce postoperative incision pain and restlessness during the recovery period.

Keywords: Ketorolac tromethamine, Sufentanil, Cough response, General anesthesia

Background

Sufentanil, commonly used in general anesthesia for its strong analgesic properties, can produce an irritating cough during intravenous induction [1, 2]. Studies have shown that 25 to 42% of patients experience this kind of cough reaction after intravenous injection of sufentanil [2, 3]. Sometimes, the cough reaction will be explosive or spasmodic, which will cause a sharp rise in blood pressure, intracranial pressure, intraocular pressure, intrapulmonary pressure and abdominal pressure. Therefore, for patients with hypertension, intracranial hypertension, pulmonary bullae, hemangioma and high intra-abdominal pressure, the risks of anesthesia induction are significantly increased when using sufentanil [4].

Various agents, such as remifentanil, dexmedetomidine, magnesium sulfate, lidocaine, and dezocine, have been used to suppress cough during the induction of general anesthesia [5, 6]. However, their clinical application was somewhat limited due to their potential additional side effects, including sharp decreases in heart rate and blood pressure, myocardial inhibition, respiratory depression, long onset time, long duration and low effective rate [7, 8]. Therefore, it is a challenge for anesthesiologists to find a safe and effective drug with fewer adverse reactions to inhibit the sufentanil-induced cough response during the induction of general anesthesia.

Aspirin is a common nonsteroidal anti-inflammatory and analgesic drug. Alexander T et al. reported that a moderate dose of aspirin (500 mg/day) could reduce angiotensin converting enzyme inhibitor-induced cough [9]. Ketorolac tromethamine is a new nonsteroidal anti-inflammatory and analgesic drug that is widely used in the short-term treatment of acute moderate and severe pain, including postoperative incision pain [10, 11]. At present, the clinical effect and safety of ketorolac tromethamine for suppressing sufentanil-induced cough during the induction of general anesthesia remain unclear.

The purpose of this study was to investigate the effectiveness of ketorolac tromethamine for treating the sufentanil-induced cough response by intravenous injection prior to general anesthesia induction.

Materials and methods

This study was approved by the Institutional Research Ethics Committee of the Suqian People's Hospital of Nanjing Drum-Tower Hospital Group, Suqian, Jiangsu, China. The trial was registered in the Chinese Clinical Trial Registry (No. Chi CTR2000030287). Written informed consent was obtained from each patient following the principles of the Helsinki Declaration. And This study is adhered to CONSORT guidelines.

A total of 102 adult patients with ASA physical status I or II, aged 18–65 years, weighing 45 to 89 kg, with BMIs between 18.0 and 30.0 kg/m^2, were enrolled in this study. The patients were scheduled for elective surgery under general anesthesia in Suqian People's Hospital of Nanjing Drum-Tower Hospital Group from February 2020 to March 2020. The exclusion criteria were a history of asthma, chronic cough, and upper respiratory tract infection within 2 weeks. Patients with a history of peptic ulcer or bleeding, heart disease, aneurysm, liver disease, kidney disease, or participation in other clinical trials or who the researchers considered inappropriate to participate in this experiment were also excluded. Ninety patients were randomly divided into two groups via a computer-generated random number list: the control group (C Group, $n = 45$) and the observation group (KT Group, $n = 45$).

No patient received premedication in this study. In the operating room, noninvasive blood pressure (NBP), pulse oxygen saturation (SpO_2), and electrocardiograms (ECGs) were routinely monitored. Patients were cannulated through the median cubital vein of the forearm with a 20G venous trocar needle. 5 min before general anesthesia induction, KT group patients were given ketorolac tromethamine 0.5 mg/kg (diluted to 5 ml using normal saline) intravenously within 3 s, while those in the C group were given 5 ml of normal saline only. The ketorolac tromethamine or normal saline was prepared by a nurse anesthetist and administered by an experienced anesthesiologist who was blind to the procedure. All patients were given 100% oxygen via a face mask with an oxygen flow rate of 5 L/min for 3 min. General anesthesia was induced with a bolus of sufentanil 0.5 μg/kg administered within 3 s intravenously, and 1 min later, propofol 2.5 mg/kg and vecuronium 0.15 mg/kg were infused sequentially. Endotracheal intubation was performed using a Macintosh laryngoscope. The depth of general anesthesia was maintained under propofol 5 mg/kg/h, remifentanil 10 μg/kg/h and vecuronium 0.05 mg/kg/h and was adjusted based on the vital signs of the patients.

The frequency of cough within 1 min following sufentanil injection was recorded, and the severity was graded depending on the cough frequency (mild, 1–2; moderate, 3–4; severe, ≥ 5, [12, 13]).

The mean arterial pressure (MAP), heart rate (HR) and S_PO_2 were recorded at the following time-points: T0, before pretreatment of ketorolac tromethamine or normal saline, i.e., the baseline value; T1, 5 min after pretreatment; T2, before intubation; T3, 1 min after intubation; and T4, 5 min after intubation.

The incidence of adverse reactions, including nausea and vomiting, dizziness, drowsiness, delay of recovery, restlessness in the recovery period and respiratory depression, was analyzed. In brief, the adverse reactions of the two groups were evaluated by professional anesthesiologists according to the following unified criteria: because nausea and dizziness are subjective assessments, for the evaluation of nausea and dizziness, the patients (who had recovered from the anesthesia) were questioned by the anesthesiologist and were recorded as having nausea and/or dizziness if the answer was "Yes". The vomiting judgment was performed according to the patient's self-report and the anesthesiologist's observation. Drowsiness was defined as sleeping again within 120 s of waking up without external interference. Recovery delay referred to the patient's consciousness not being recovered and the patient being unable to make correct responses to external stimulation and language instruction 120 min after general anesthesia. Restlessness in the recovery period was defined as the patients mood being more excited in the recovery period, even crying and being restless, and the patients making strong movements that could not be comforted. Respiratory inhibition referred to respiratory arrest time greater than 15 s or S_PO_2 less than 90% for more than 15 s when patients without oxygen inhaled during the recovery period. The postoperative incision pain of the patients was evaluated by the VAS scoring method, with a score of 0–10. The number of patients with VAS scores > 3 was recorded.

Sample size determination

In our preliminary study, the incidence of cough elicited by 0.5 μg/kg sufentanil infused within 3 s was 31.8% (7/22), which was reduced to 4.5% (1/22) when ketorolac tromethamine pretreatment was performed. To achieve 80% statistical power with $\alpha = 0.05$, each group would require no less than 33 cases. Considering that there may be a dropout rate of 20%, we recruited 51 patients for each group to allow for missing data.

Statistical analysis

SPSS 22.0 software (IBM Corp, Armonk, NY, USA) was used for statistical analysis. The presented data were evaluated for normal distributions by the Kolmogorov–Smirnov test. Measurement data are presented as the mean ± standard deviation, and Student's t test was used to assess the differences between two groups. The differences in ranked data were analyzed by the Mann–Whitney U test. The chi-square test or Fisher's exact test was adopted to assess the difference in categorical data presented as absolute or relative effect sizes. A P-value < 0.05 was considered significant.

Results

Among 102 patients, 5 patients refused to participate in the study, 4 patients had a history of hypertension, and 3 patients underwent a change in anesthesia protocol (Fig. 1); therefore, 90 patients were enrolled for further study. There were no significant differences in sex, age, weight, BMI, ASA physical status or anesthesia time between the two groups ($P > 0.05$) (Table 1).

The incidence and severity of cough within 1 min after sufentanil injection in the KT group was significantly lower than that in the C group ($P < 0.05$) (Table 2).

There were no significant differences in MAP, HR or S_PO_2 between the two groups at T0, T1, T2, T3 and T4 ($P > 0.05$) (Table 3).

There was no significant difference in the dosage of sufentanil, propofol, remifentanil and vecuronium between the two groups ($P > 0.05$) (Table 4).

The incidences of restlessness and the number of patients with VAS scores > 3 in the anesthesia recovery period in the KT group were significantly lower than those in the C group ($P < 0.05$). There were no significant differences in the incidences of nausea and vomiting, delay of recovery, dizziness, drowsiness or respiratory depression between the two groups ($P > 0.05$) (Table 5).

Discussion

At present, sufentanil, fentanyl and other opioid analgesics injected intravenously during the induction period of clinical anesthesia show strong analgesic effects and little influence on hemodynamic indexes [14, 15], and they can effectively inhibit tracheal intubation responses (such as increased heart rate and increased blood pressure) [16, 17]. However, it is easy to cause coughing reactions of different degrees within 1 min of intravenous injection [18]. For patients with hypertension, pulmonary bullae, hemangioma and intracranial hypertension, this may have severe consequences.

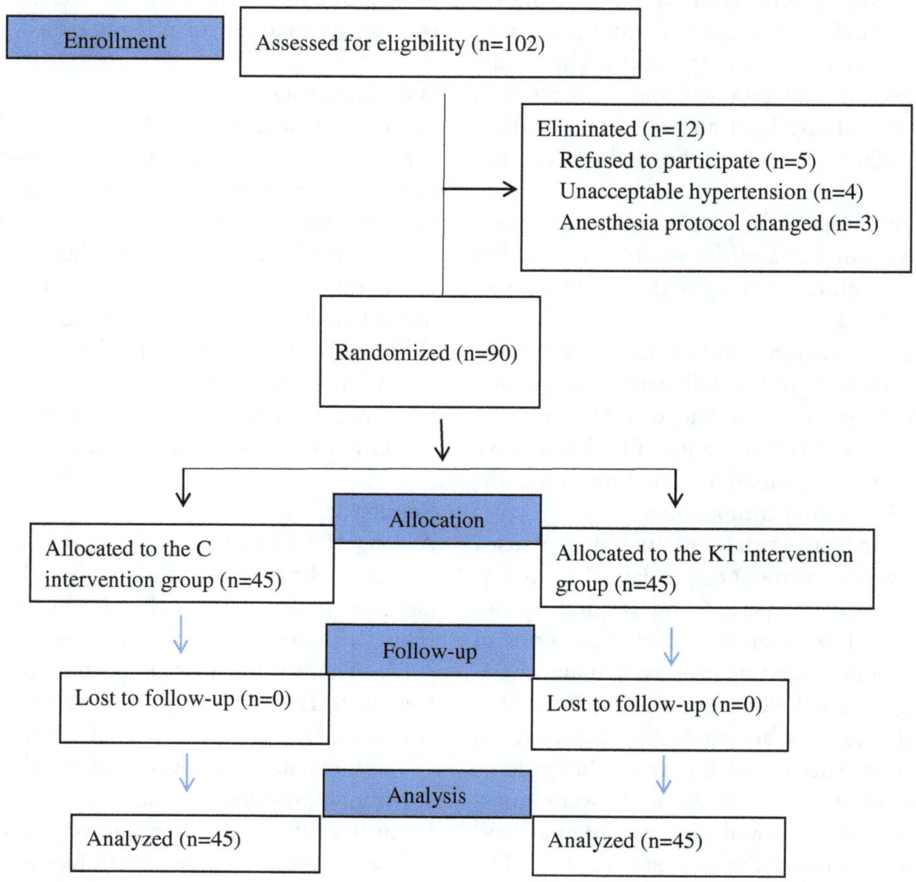

Fig. 1 Flow chart of patients participating in this study

The various incidence rates among different studies might be due to the different doses of sufentanil used and differences in concentration, administration rate, race and age [19]. In a study by Agarwal et al., sufentanil 0.3 μg/kg injected over 5 s elicited cough in 15.8% of patients, while in another study by Li et al., the incidence of cough was 37% after the injection of sufentanil 0.5 μg/kg within 3 s, and with a high dose of sufentanil (1 μg/kg), the incidence of sufentanil-induced cough could be up to 45.8% [20, 21]. In our study, we administered sufentanil 0.5 μg/kg intravenously within 3 s before the operation in the C group. Within 1 min, the incidence of sufentanil-induced cough was 31.1%, which is similar to the conclusions of relevant research.

Five minutes before anesthesia induction, intravenous ketorolac tromethamine 0.5 mg/kg pretreatment can significantly reduce the incidence of coughing reactions during the induction period in general anesthesia patients and can significantly reduce restlessness in the recovery period of patients, which increases safety.

Many studies have been performed on the mechanism of the sufentanil-induced cough response, but the relevant mechanism is still not very clear [3–5]. It may be related to sufentanil activating the C-fiber receptor of

Table 1 Demographic data and basic clinical characteristics of the patients in the two groups

	C Group	KT Group	*P* value
Sex (male/female)	19/26	21/24	> 0.05
Age (year)	47.8 ± 8.9	48.1 ± 9.1	> 0.05
ASA (I/II)	28/17	30/15	> 0.05
Weight (kg)	69.8 ± 10.2	69.4 ± 9.9	> 0.05
BMI (kg/m^2)	24.6 ± 3.4	24.9 ± 3.1	> 0.05
Anesthesia time (min)	95.9 ± 20.8	97.0 ± 21.0	> 0.05

Values are expressed as the mean ± standard deviation

Table 2 Incidence and severity of cough in the two groups

Groups	Incidence of cough (n(%))	Severity of cough (n(%))			
		None	Mild	Moderate	Severe
C group	14(31.1)	31(68.9)	3(6.7)	11(24.4)	0(0.0)
KT group	3(6.7)	42(93.3)	2(4.4)	1(2.2)	0(0.0)
P value	< 0.05	< 0.05			

Table 3 Comparison of MAP, HR and SpO2 values at different time points

Groups		T0	T1	T2	T3	T4
C group	MAP (mmHg)	94.7 ± 11.2	94.0 ± 9.8	84.3 ± 10.5	90.9 ± 10.9	82.7 ± 9.5
	HR (bpm)	76.3 ± 7.5	75.8 ± 6.2	69.2 ± 7.4	79.1 ± 7.1	68.7 ± 6.4
	SpO_2 (%)	98.1 ± 1.2	97.8 ± 0.9	99.0 ± 0.7	99.0 ± 0.8	99.0 ± 1.0
KT group	MAP (mmHg)	93.9 ± 11.5	93.4 ± 9.6	83.9 ± 10.2	89.2 ± 10.3	81.9 ± 9.3
	HR (bpm)	75.9 ± 7.3	75.2 ± 6.0	68.9 ± 7.6	78.8 ± 7.0	68.4 ± 6.6
	SpO_2 (%)	97.9 ± 1.0	97.7 ± 0.8	98.8 ± 0.7	99.0 ± 1.0	99.2 ± 0.5

Values are expressed as the mean ± standard deviation

the bronchus, adapting the pulmonary stretch receptors (RARs), inducing airway hyperresponsiveness, inhibiting the efferent impulse of the sympathetic nerve, increasing the comparative advantage of the vagus nerve, and finally leading to the occurrence of the cough response [5, 6]. At present, there are few reports about ketorolac tromethamine reducing the sufentanil-induced cough response. It has been reported that intravenous injection of dezocine before anesthesia induction can inhibit the cough response induced by sufentanil or fentanyl to some extent by activating the *K* receptor and inhibiting histamine release [5]. Considering that ketorolac tromethamine is a nonsteroidal anti-inflammatory drug, the mechanism of a ketorolac tromethamine injection reducing the cough response may be related to the reduction of histamine release and other reasons [10].

Ketorolac tromethamine is a new nonsteroidal anti-inflammatory drug (NSAID). Motov S et al. found that intravenous infusion of 30 mg ketorolac tromethamine can significantly improve moderate to severe pain in emergency patients [22]. Studies by Yang HL et al. suggested that injection of ketorolac tromethamine before tracheal intubation can reduce the incidence of sore throat caused by endotracheal intubation from 71.6 to 21.1% [23]. Compared with other NSAIDs, ketorolac tromethamine has a weaker anti-inflammatory effect and stronger analgesic effect and has been widely used in the clinic [10, 24]. In this study, ketorolac tromethamine significantly reduced the number of patients with VAS scores greater than 3. Pretreatment with a ketorolac tromethamine injection also played a role in the recovery period of anesthesia, significantly reducing the postoperative incision pain of patients, and the incidence of restlessness caused by pain and other adverse stimulation naturally decreased significantly. To a certain extent, it provided patients with a comfortable medical experience and humane care.

To evaluate the possible adverse reactions and safety of ketorolac tromethamine injection pretreatment, we compared the mean arterial pressure, heart rate and blood oxygen saturation values of the two groups of patients at different time points. The results suggest that pretreatment with ketorolac tromethamine injection does not have adverse effects on the vital signs of patients. Additionally, the results showed that the incidence of nausea, delayed recovery, dizziness, drowsiness and respiratory depression was not significantly increased when ketorolac tromethamine was used in advance, making it safe for patients. However, it is undeniable that one of the main risks of NSAIDs, such as ketorolac tromethamine, is that they may affect bleeding during and after the operation by inhibiting platelet function. However, the dosage of drugs used in this study was not large and was within the scope of reasonable use in the instructions. In addition, this study has limited the research subjects; for example, patients who had a history of peptic ulcer or bleeding, liver or kidney disease, or blood system diseases before operation were excluded. Under these premises, ketorolac tromethamine will not have a significant impact on the operation or postoperative bleeding.

There are also some deficiencies in our research. First, due to the limitation of objective conditions, we have

Table 4 Comparison of anesthetic dosages between the two groups

Groups	C group	KT group	*P* value
Sufentanil (μg)	39.2 ± 8.0	38.7 ± 7.8	> 0.05
Propofol (mg)	640.4 ± 85.4	629.3 ± 84.5	>0.05
Vecuronium (mg)	17.0 ± 3.8	16.5 ± 3.6	> 0.05
Remifentanil (mg)	1.2 ± 0.3	1.1 ± 0.2	> 0.05

Values are expressed as the mean ± standard deviation

Table 5 Comparison of adverse reactions during the recovery period (n(%))

Groups	C group	KT group	*P* value
Nausea and vomiting	3 (6.7)	4 (8.9)	> 0.05
Delay of recovery	1 (2.2)	2 (4.4)	> 0.05
Dizziness	3 (6.7)	3 (6.7)	> 0.05
Drowsiness	2 (4.4)	3 (6.7)	> 0.05
Restlessness in the recovery period	7 (15.6)	1 (2.2)	< 0.05
Depressed respiration	0 (0.0)	1 (2.2)	> 0.05
VAS score > 3	8 (17.8)	1 (2.2)	< 0.05

not studied the mechanism of ketorolac tromethamine in inhibition of the cough response and cannot give more reasonable inferences about the relevant mechanisms. We describe the relevant effects objectively because there is no relevant report about ketorolac tromethamine injection or other nonsteroidal drugs inhibiting sufentanil-induced cough. Second, the pretreatment dose of ketorolac tromethamine that was used (0.5 mg/kg) may not be the most appropriate dose for ketorolac tromethamine to inhibit the sufentanil-induced cough response, but it was given according to the early postoperative analgesic dose recommended in the drug instructions [10]. Third, our study was a single center study with a small sample size. To determine whether pretreatment with ketorolac tromethamine injection can reduce the sufentanil-induced cough response, we still need a large sample and multicenter study.

Conclusion

Pretreatment with intravenous ketorolac tromethamine 0.5 mg/kg can significantly reduce the incidence and severity of sufentanil-induced cough during induction of general anesthesia, which can also significantly and safely reduce postoperative incision pain and restlessness in the recovery period. To a certain extent, it provided a comfortable medical experience and humane care, which is worth popularizing.

Abbreviations

NBP: Noninvasive blood pressure; SpO_2: Pulse oxygen saturation; ECG: Electrocardiogram; MAP: Mean arterial pressure; HR: Heart rate

Acknowledgments

We would like to thank Bei Hu from Suqian People's Hospital of Nanjing Drum-Tower Hospital Group for assistance with the article.

Authors' contributions

ZT, BH designed the study, performed the statistical analysis, and drafted the manuscript. BC, MM, and LLZ interpreted the data, revised the manuscript, collected the data and assisted in drafting the manuscript. LW and BH revised the manuscript and approved the version to be published. All authors read and approved the final submitted version of the manuscript.

References

1. Ambesh SP, Singh N, Srivastava K. Fentanyl induced coughing caused life-threatening airway obstruction in a patient with arteriovenous malformation of tongue and hypopharynx. Internet J Anesthesiology. 2009; 20(1):7–10.
2. Tang Q, Qian Y, Zhang Q, Yang J, Wang Z. Effects of different priming doses of propofol on fentanyl-induced cough during anesthesia induction: a preliminary randomized controlled study. Ups J Med Sci. 2010;115(2):121–4.
3. Shen JC, Xu JG, Zhou ZQ, Liu HJ, Yang JJ. Effect of equivalent doses of fentanyl, sufentanil, and remifentanil on the incidence and severity of cough in patients undergoing abdominal surgery: a prospective, randomized, double-blind study. Curr Ther Res Clin Experimental. 2008; 69(6):480–7.
4. Yoo YC, Na S, Jeong JJ, Choi EM, Moon BE, Lee JR. Dose-dependent attenuation by fentanyl on cough during emergence from general anesthesia. Acta Anaesthesiol Scand. 2011;55(10):1215–20.
5. Xu Y, Zhu Y, Wang S, Ren Y, Miao C. Dezocine attenuates fentanyl-induced cough in a dose-dependent manner-a randomized controlled trial. Int J Clin Exp Med. 2015;8(4):6091–6.
6. Sridharan K, Sivaramakrishnan G. Comparison of fentanyl, Remifentanil, Sufentanil and Alfentanil in combination with Propofol for general anesthesia: a systematic review and meta-analysis of randomized controlled trials. Curr Clin Pharmacol. 2019;14(2):116–24.
7. Liu XS, Xu GH, Shen QY, Zhao Q, Cheng XQ, Zhang J, Gu EW. Dezocine prevents sufentanil-induced cough during general anesthesia induction: a randomized controlled trial. Pharmacol Rep. 2015;67(1):52–5.
8. Sun S, Huang SQ. Effects of pretreatment with a small dose of dexmedetomidine on sufentanil-induced cough during anesthetic induction. J Anesth. 2013;27(1):25–8.
9. Tenenbaum A, Grossman E, Shemesh J, Fisman EZ, Nosrati I, Motro M. Intermediate but not low doses of aspirin can suppress angiotensin-converting enzyme inhibitor-induced cough. Am J Hypertens. 2000; 13(7):776–82.
10. Gurunathan U, Parker SL, Maguire R, Ramdath D, Bijoor M, Wallis SC, Roberts JA. Population pharmacokinetics of Periarticular ketorolac in adult patients undergoing Total hip or Total knee replacement surgery. Anesth Analg. 2019;129(3):701–8.
11. Vadivelu N, Gowda AM, Urman RD, Jolly S, Kodumudi V, Maria M, Taylor R, Pergolizzi JV. Ketorolac tromethamine - routes and clinical implications. Pain Pract. 2015;15(2):175–93.
12. Lin W, Sun J, Fu S. A small dose of remifentanil pretreatment suppresses sufentanil-induced cough during general anesthesia induction: a randomized, double-blind, placebo-controlled trial. BMC Anesthesiol. 2019; 19(1):164.
13. Zhou W, Zhang D, Tian S, Yang Y, Xing Z, Ma R, Zhou T, Bao T, Sun J, Zhang Z. Optimal dose of pretreated-dexmedetomidine in fentanyl-induced cough suppression: a prospective randomized controlled trial. BMC Anesthesiol. 2019;19(1):89.
14. Pandey CK, Raza M, Ranjan R, Lakra A, Agarwal A, Singh U, Singh RB, Singh PK. Intravenous lidocaine suppresses fentanyl-induced coughing: a double-blind, prospective, randomized placebo-controlled study. Anesth Analg. 2004;99(6):1696–8.
15. Firouzian A, Emadi SA, Baradari AG, Mousavi R, Kiasari AZ. Can low dose of propofol effectively suppress fentanyl-induced cough during induction of anaesthesia? A double blind randomized controlled trial. J Anaesthesiol Clin Pharmacol. 2015;31(4):522–5.
16. Li Y, Wang B, Zhang LL, He SF, Hu XW, Wong GT, Zhang Y. Dexmedetomidine combined with general anesthesia provides similar intraoperative stress response reduction when compared with a combined general and epidural anesthetic technique. Anesth Analg. 2016;122(4):1202–10.
17. Sun ZT, Yang CY, Cui Z, Zhang J, Han XP. Effect of intravenous dezocine on fentanyl-induced cough during general anesthesia induction: a double-blinded, prospective, randomized, controlled trial. J Anesth. 2011;25(6):860–3.
18. Shrestha SK, Bhattarai B, Shah RS. Preemptive use of small dose fentanyl suppresses fentanyl induced cough. Kathmandu Univ Med J (KUMJ). 2012; 10(40):16–9.
19. An LJ, Gui B, Su Z, Zhang Y, Liu HL. Magnesium sulfate inhibits sufentanil-induced cough during anesthetic induction. Int J Clin Exp Med. 2015;8(8): 13864–8.
20. Agarwal A, Gautam S, Nath SS, Gupta D, Singh U. Comparison of the incidence and severity of cough induced by sufentanil and fentanyl: a prospective, randomised, double-blind study. Anaesthesia. 2007;62(12):1230–2.
21. Li J, Li K. Effects of pre-inhalation of salbutamol on cough reflex induced by Sufentanil. In: Sadeghian SH, Mehta U, Rajbongshi P, editors. AER-Advances in Engineering Research; 2016. p. 237–9.
22. Motov S, Yasavolian M, Likourezos A, Pushkar I, Hossain R, Drapkin J, Cohen V, Filk N, Smith A, Huang F, et al. Comparison of intravenous ketorolac at three single-dose regimens for treating acute pain in the emergency department: a randomized controlled trial. Ann Emerg Med. 2017;70(2):177–84.
23. Yang HL, Liu FC, Tsai SC, Tsay PK, Lin HT, Liu HE. Ketorolac Tromethamine spray prevents Postendotracheal-intubation-induced sore throat after general anesthesia. Biomed Res Int. 2016;2016:4582439.
24. Almeida DR, Johnson D, Hollands H, Smallman D, Baxter S, Eng KT, Kratky V, ten Hove MW, Sharma S, El-Defrawy S. Effect of prophylactic nonsteroidal antiinflammatory drugs on cystoid macular edema assessed using optical coherence tomography quantification of total macular volume after cataract surgery. J Cataract Refract Surg. 2008;34(1):64–9.

Volume kinetic analysis of fluid retention after induction of general anesthesia

Robert G. Hahn[1,2*] and Janis Nemme[3,4]

Abstract

Background: Induction of general anesthesia increases the hemodilution resulting from infusion of crystalloid fluid, which is believed to be due to slower distribution caused by arterial hypotension. When normal distribution returns is not known.

Methods: An intravenous infusion of 25 mL kg^{-1} of Ringer's lactate was infused over 30 min to 25 volunteers just after induction of general anesthesia for open abdominal hysterectomy. A two-volume model was fitted to the repeated measurements of the blood hemoglobin concentration and the urinary excretion using mixed-effects modelling software. Individual-specific covariates were added in sequence.

Results: Distribution of infused fluid was interrupted during the first 20 min of the infusions. During this time 16.6 mL kg^{-1} of lactated Ringer's had been infused, of which virtually all remained in the circulating blood. Thereafter, the fluid kinetics was similar to that previously been found in awake volunteers except for the elimination rate constant (k_{10}), which remained to be very low (0.86×10^{-3} min^{-1}). Redistribution of infused fluid from the interstitium to the plasma occurred faster (higher k_{21}) when the arterial pressure was low. No covariance was found between the fixed parameters and preoperatively concentrated urine, the use of sevoflurane or propofol to maintain the anesthesia, or the plasma concentrations of two degradation products of the endothelial glycocalyx, syndecan-1 and heparan sulfate.

Conclusions: Induction of general anesthesia interrupted the distribution of lactated Ringer's solution up to when 16.6 mL kg^{-1} of crystalloid fluid had been infused. Plasma volume expansion during this period of time was pronounced.

Keywords: Ringer's lactate, Brain natriuretic peptide, Heparan sulfate, Syndecan-1, Pharmacokinetics

Background

Pharmacokinetic methods can be applied to fluid volumes, which is of interest in anesthesia and surgery where large amounts are given by intravenous infusion. The most commonly used approach is volume kinetics, which uses the hemodilution and the urinary excretion as input in the calculations [1, 2]. The hemodilution is the inverse of the blood water concentration and, therefore, shows how the infused volume is distributed; as per volume, the blood contains little more than hemoglobin and water [2, 3]. So far, volume kinetics has dealt with anesthesia and surgery where fluid is given to ensure adequate organ perfusion. The volume of infused fluid is critical because the elimination efficacy is strongly impaired during general anesthesia [4–6]. However, certain issues still remain to be resolved with regard to the kinetics of crystalloid fluid in this setting.

* Correspondence: r.hahn@telia.com; robert.hahn@sll.se
[1]Research Unit, Södertälje Hospital, 152 86 Södertälje, Sweden
[2]Karolinska Institutet at Danderyds Hospital (KIDS), Stockholm, Sweden

One such issue is why excessive hemodilution from infused fluid develops when induction of general epidural, spinal or anesthesia is associated with hypotension [7–10] but not when the arterial pressure is unchanged [7, 11]. A reasonable interpretation of this relationship is that anesthesia-induced vasodilatation lowers the arterial pressure and, in turn, increases the intravascular retention of infused fluid by reducing the capillary filtration. However, the exchange of fluid between the plasma to the interstitial fluid space occurs at a fairly normal rate during ongoing surgery even when the arterial pressure is low [12]. Molecular mechanisms, such as a rise of the plasma concentrations of brain natriuretic peptide (BNP) and glycocalyx degradation products [13–15], may also have a role in this process.

Another issue was to examine whether the urinary concentration of metabolic waste products before the operation reduces rate of subsequent elimination of infused fluid, which has been shown in conscious patients [16, 17]. For this purpose, fluid volume kinetic analysis was performed on a crystalloid fluid load of 25 mL kg^{-1} given before open hysterectomy.

The primary hypothesis was that the excessive intravascular fluid retention after induction of general anesthesia is caused by a reduction of the capillary leakage, as given by the kinetic model. The secondary hypothesis was that a mathematical link exists between volume kinetic parameters and the plasma concentrations of BNP, glycocalyx degradation products and the urinary concentration of metabolic waste products. The kinetic analysis served as primary outcome measure and the measurements of metabolic waste products and their associations with the kinetics as secondary outcome measures.

Methods

A total of 25 clinical patients scheduled for elective abdominal hysterectomy were recruited to an open label randomized parallel clinical trial with the primary aim to compare two anesthesia methods, sevoflurane and intravenous propofol, with regard to their influence the degradation of the endothelial glycocalyx layer [18]. Ethical approval (No. 270116-17 L) was provided by the Ethics Committee of Riga Stradins University (Chairperson P. Stradins) on January 27, 2016, and registered at controlled-trials.com as ISRCTN81005631 on May 17, 2016 (retrospectively, first patient studied on March 22, 2016). All patients gave us their written informed consent to participate. Patients were included if being aged 25–55 years, free from cardiopulmonary or renal disease, and complicated surgery was not expected. The study adheres to the CONSORT Guidelines. After fasting overnight, patients were given general anesthesia induced with propofol but maintained with either sevoflurane as inhaled anesthetic (N = 13) or an intravenous propofol infusion (N = 12). The result of that comparison is described elsewhere [18].

Volume loading, blood sampling, and analysis

At the start of surgery, an intravenous infusion of Ringer's lactate (25 mL kg^{-1}) was administered over 30 min. No more fluids were given except for the anesthesia drugs. No vasopressor or inotrophic agent was used. Blood (3 mL) was taken from a cubital vein for measurement of the blood hemoglobin (Hb) concentration on a Coulter HMx 5-diff (Beckman Coulter Inc., Brea, CA) with a coefficient of variation (CV) of 0.7% was taken every 10 min during the 30-min infusions and then every 15 min up to the end of surgery.

Blood (3 mL) and urine were also sampled at baseline, after anesthesia induction, and then at 30, 60, and 90 min later after the fluid infusion had been initiated, and 2 h after the anesthesia had been terminated. These samples were used to measure the plasma concentration of brain natriuretic peptide (BNP) on an Architect i2000, Abbott Park, Illinois, USA with a CV of 5.6%. The normal range is < 100 ng L^{-1}. Results below the limit of detection (10 ng L^{-1}) were set to that value. Moreover, the plasma concentrations of two endothelial shedding products, syndecan-1 and heparan sulfate, were analyzed using enzyme-linked immunosorbent assay (ELISA) kits from Diaclone, France, and Amsbio, Abingdon, UK, with CV% values of 6.2, and < 10%, respectively. The normal value of syndecan-1 for humans is 32 ng/mL (manufacturer data) and for heparan sulfate it is 5.9 μg mL^{-1} [14].

Urinary creatinine concentration was measured within 36 h on a Cobas Integra 400 Plus instrument (Roche Diagnostics, Switzerland) with a CV of 2%. The urine osmolality was measured with an Osmomat 3000 (Gonotech, Berlin, Germany) and the urine-specific weight on a Urisys 2400 (Roche Diagnostics, Switzerland) with CVs being 3 and 0.1%, respectively.

Population volume kinetics

Volume kinetics is a method for analyzing the distribution and elimination of infusion fluids [1, 2]. The approach has similarities to drug pharmacokinetics but uses the excreted urine volume and the plasma dilution derived from serial analyses of the blood Hb concentration as inputs in the calculations.

All included patients are analyzed in a single run, and then the influence of various covariates on the model parameters is tested sequentially. The model is built to agree with physiological data where isotonic infusion fluids distribute between two compartments: the plasma and the interstitial fluid space. Several models have been attempted to characterize fluid kinetics during surgery, but the one shown in Fig. 1a has been found to be most

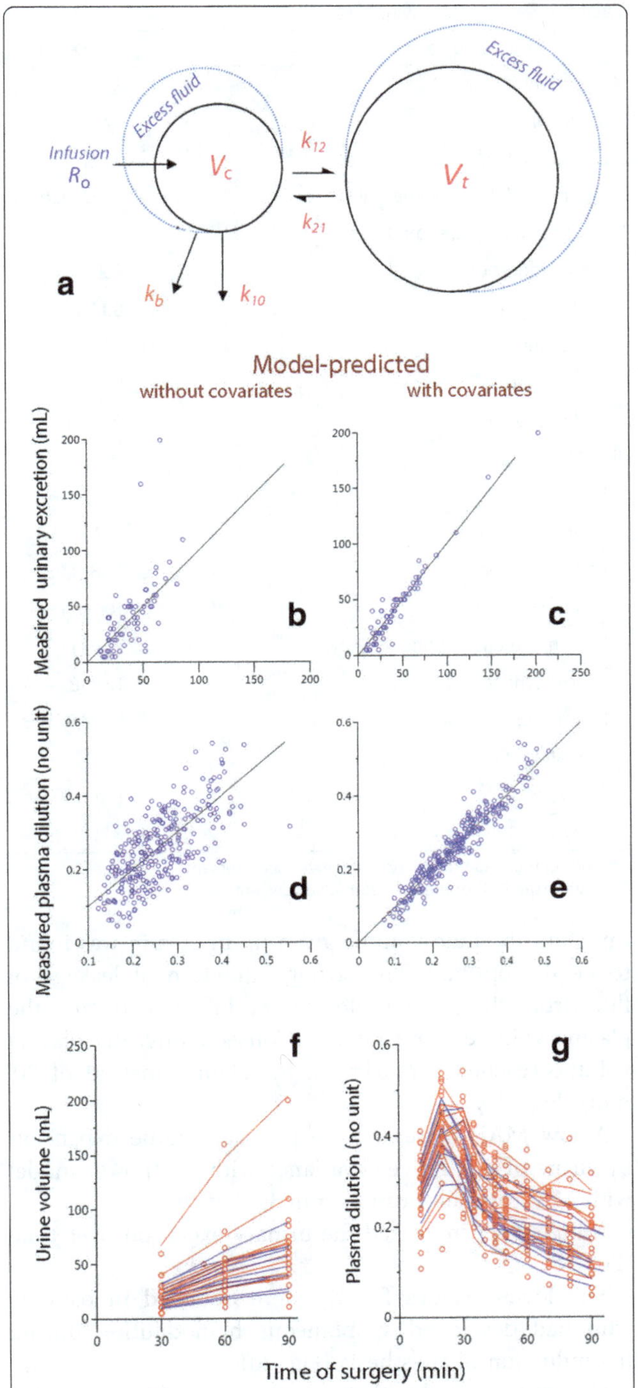

Fig. 1 The kinetic model (a), residual plots (b-e) and final curve fits (f and g)

appropriate: fluid is infused into an expandable central (V_c) space and becomes distributed to the peripheral (V_t) fluid space. Fluid is translocated from V_c to V_t in proportion by a rate constant k_{12} to the central volume expansion, which is written as ($v_c - V_c$). Fluid is returned from V_t to V_c via another rate constant, k_{21}. Elimination occurs from V_c by one or two routes (k_{10} and k_b) in proportion to ($v_c - V_c$). The rate constant k_{10} represents fluid that is collected as urine while k_b governs fluid filtered from V_c that does not equilibrate with V_c or V_t during the period of the study [5, 6, 19, 20].

The differential equations for the single-elimination route model are:

$$dv_c/dt = R_o - k_{12}(v_c - V_c) + k_{21}(v_t - V_t) - k_{10}(v_c - V_c) - k_b(v_c - V_c) \quad (1)$$

$$dv_t/dt = k_{12}(v_c - V_c) - k_{21}(v_t - V_t) \quad (2)$$

where R_o is the rate of infusion, v_c and v_t are the constantly changing volumes of distribution for newly infused fluid, and V_c and V_t are the baseline volumes.

The Hb-derived fractional plasma dilution was used to indicate the volume expansion of V_c resulting from the infusion. Hence:

$$(v_c - V_c)/V_c = [(\text{Hb}/\text{hb})-1)]/(1-\text{baseline hematocrit}) \quad (3)$$

Symbols in capital letters denote baseline values. A minor correction was made for the effects of surgical hemorrhage and blood sampling on the plasma dilution [1, 12]. The measured urinary excretion during 30-min intervals was then used to estimate k_{10} as follows (AUC = area under the curve):

$$k_{10} = \text{urinary excretion}/\text{AUC for}(v_c - V_c) \quad (4)$$

Covariate analysis

Twenty individual-specific covariates were evaluated in a forward stepwise fashion, as guided by plots of random effects ("eta" plots). The routine for identifying statistically justified covariates is described in detail elsewhere [4]. In short, a covariate was included if it decreased the residual error of the model (expressed as − 2 log likelihood by 3.8, which corresponds to $P < 0.05$), the 95% confidence interval of the parameter estimate did not include zero, and the CV% for the inter-individual variability was < 50%.

Continuous covariates assessed only once were age, body weight, surgical blood loss, C-reactive protein, the use of sevoflurane or propofol for maintaining the anesthesia, the syndecan-1 and heparan sulfate concentrations before and 2 h after the surgery, and the preoperative urinary specific gravity, osmolality, and the urinary creatinine concentration. The plasma concentrations of syndecan-1 and heparan sulfate served as time-varying covariates and were included four times per operation, while heart rate and the systolic, diastolic, and mean arterial pressure (MAP) were assessed at every blood sampling time point. The time period before and after 10, 20, and 30 min were evaluated as categorical covariates in an exponential covariate model, as fluid was infused at a rate of 0.833 mL kg^{-1} min^{-1} and our belief was that the fluid kinetics would change depending on the infused volume. In the last situation, all time points up to 30 min were set to 1 and all time points after 30 min were given the value 0.

The kinetic program used was Phoenix software for nonlinear mixed effects (NLME), version 1.3 (Certara, St. Louis, MO). The goodness-of-fit of the model was illustrated by residual plots and the performance of the model by predictive checks.

The study was powered to detect a doubling of the plasma BNP concentration as a result of the volume loading, as described previously [18]. An effect size of 1.0 and power 90% at the $P < 0.01$ level yielded $N = 20$. Data with a normal distribution are presented as the mean (SD), data with a skewed distribution as the median (25th–75th percentiles) and kinetic output as the mean (CI). $P < 0.05$ was statistically significant.

Results

Kinetic analysis of Hb changes

The kinetic analysis was based on 298 time points during the 25 operations. All data are given in the Additonal file 1 and the model used is illustrated in Fig. 1a. Selected key characteristics of the operations are shown in Table 1.

The search strategy used to find the optimal parameter estimates is shown in Table 2. The final base model with the fixed model parameters is shown in the upper part of Table 3 and the covariate effects in the lower part of Table 3. Two routes of elimination were optimal; one of these (k_{10}) corresponded to the measured urinary excretion.

Comparisons between the measured and predicted urinary excretion and the plasma dilution based on the fixed parameters alone are shown in Fig. 1b and c. The corresponding plots that also consider the covariates are presented in Fig. 1d and e, and the final curve fits for each individual are displayed in Fig. 1f and h.

Predictive check and covariates

A predictive check the kinetic model, based on 1000 simulations, is given in Fig. 2a. The close agreement between the percentiles for the predicted and the observed data indicates good model performance and that the model is robust.

The most important covariate was "Time ≤ 20 min," which means that k_{12}, k_b, and V_c showed lower values during the first 20 min of the infusion, when 2/3 of 25 mL kg^{-1} = 16.6 mL kg^{-1} (mean 1245 mL) of lactated Ringer's was infused. An exponential covariate model was used to examine if a more precise prediction could be obtained by placing the cut-off at other points in time, but the fluid volume given up to 20 min was found to be the optimal. The strong inhibition of leakage of fluid from the plasma allowed the infusion to raise the plasma volume more rapidly. Consequently, the plasma volume reached a maximum by 20 min (instead of 30 min) (Fig. 2b).

Table 1 Key surgical variables

Measured Variable	Result
N	25
Age (years)	47 (5)
Body weight (kg)	75 (14)
Infused fluid volume (mL)	1869 (336)
Mean arterial pressure (mmHg)	
Before induction	100 (15)
After induction	80 (10)
End of infusion	92 (17)
During surgery[a]	85 (14)
End of study (90 min)	91 (18)
Blood Hb (g/L)	
Before induction	119.5 (16.3)
After induction	117.1 (15.9)
End of infusion	95.8 (14.2)
End of study (90 min)	104.6 (15.8)
Brain natriuretic peptide (BNP; ng/L)[a]	20.9 (11.2)
Plasma syndecan-1 (ng/mL)[a]	12.8 (8.6–20.9)
Plasma heparan sulfate[a]	6.5 (4.9–10.3)
Operating time (min)	91 (10)
Blood loss (mL)	150 (100–162)
Urinary excretion (mL)	50 (39–70)

[a] based on the mean for all intraoperative measurements
Data are mean (SD) or median (25th–75th percentile)

A low MAP increased the plasma volume expansion by virtue of a negative covariance with k_{21} (power model with MAP overall mean 85 mmHg; Fig. 2b).

A high BNP increased the urinary excretion over time (Fig. 2c).

The lowest values for k_{12} were obtained in patients who had developed spontaneous hemodilution during the induction of anesthesia (Fig. 2d).

V_c also increased with the body weight (power model, mean 74.8 kg; Fig. 2e) and k_{10} with the plasma concentration of BNP (power model; mean 20.9 ng L^{-1}; Fig. 2f).

Factors that did not serve as statistically significant covariates to any of the fixed parameters included age, the preoperative biomarkers of concentrated urine, the use of sevoflurane or propofol, and the plasma concentrations of levels of C-reactive protein and the two shedding substances that reflect glycocalyx degradation.

Additonal file 2 is a list of all potential covariates and their associations with the fixed parameters.

Table 2 Key features of the search protocol used to find the final population kinetic model

Optimization routine	Added covariate	Target parameter	LL	-2(LL)	AIC
Naive			−72	152	165
FOCE LB			57	−113	−93
+ 2 elimination routes			67	−134	−110
	Time ≤ 20 min	k_{12}	111	−219	−193
	Time ≤ 20 min	k_b	113	−227	−200
	Time ≤ 20 min	V_c	128	−256	−227
	Body weight	V_c	140	−280	−248
	BNP	k_{10}	143	−285	−251
FOCE ELS	MAP	k_{21}	159	−318	−282

A reduction −2(LL) by 3.8 is significant by $P < 0.05$ and > 6.6 points by $P < 0.01$)
FOCE LB First-Order Conditional Estimation according to Lindstrom-Bates, *FOCE ELS* FOCE Extended Least Squares, *LL* Log likelihood, *AIC* Akaike Criterion

Concentrated urine

The three markers of concentrated urine (urine-specific gravity, creatinine, and osmolality) correlated closely (Fig. 3a and b). None of them served as statistically significant covariate to the fluid kinetics.

The urine became more concentrated during the surgery ($P < 0.001$ repeated-measures ANOVA) and remained most concentrated in the propofol group at 2 h ($P < 0.04$; Fig. 3c). The overall low urine flow rate promoted further concentration, particularly if the urine flow was less than 1 mL min^{-1} during 30 min (Fig. 3d).

Discussion

The pharmacokinetic approach used here, volume kinetics, uses the inverse of the hemodilution and the urinary excretion as input in pharmacokinetic calculations [1, 2]. The calculations distinguish a "wall" between a central (V_c) and an extravascular compartment (V_t), which probably represents the difficulty for fluid to expand the interstitial fluid space. The hemodilution pattern, and not the magnitude of the hemodilution, determines how much fluid is allocated to each one of the two spaces. In the present study, the V_c volume was 3.2 L, which is the volume with which the infused fluid quickly equilibrates. It also corresponds closely to the expected plasma volume.

The present study shows that induction of general anesthesia transiently changes the kinetics of infused crystalloid fluid. The most striking finding was a strong inhibition of the distribution of fluid during the first 20 min of the infusion, up to when 16.6 mL kg^{-1} body weight had been infused. The rate constant k_{12} was then reduced to a small fraction of the normal value found during the remainder of the experiment. Figure 2b illustrates that the amount of fluid residing in the central compartment V_c at 20 min closely agrees with the total

Table 3 Population kinetic parameters in the final model

	Covariate	Best estimate	2.5% CI	97.5% CI	CV%
Fixed parameter					
tvV_c (mL)	–	3205	2906	3504	4.8
tvk_{12} (10^{-3} min^{-1})	–	69.0	46.3	91.7	16.7
tvk_{21} (10^{-3} min^{-1})	–	93.5	67.8	119.5	14.1
tvk_{10} (10^{-3} min^{-1})	–	0.86	0.72	1.00	8.4
tvk_b (10^{-3} min^{-1})	–	15.8	12.0	19.6	12.1
Covariate effect					
k_{12}	Time ≤ 20 min	−16.5	− 19.0	−14.0	−7.8
k_b	Time ≤ 20 min	− 16.5	−7.9	−19.0	− 7.9
V_c	Time ≤ 20 min	−0.35	− 0.44	− 0.26	− 13.3
V_c	Body weight	1.49	0.96	2.03	18.2
k_{10}	BNP	0.37	0.12	0.62	33.9
k_{21}	MAP	−1.47	−1.99	−0.94	− 18.1

The three "Time" covariates are exponential models, the others are power models
BNP Brain natriuretic peptide, *MAP* Mean arterial pressure, *tv* Typical value, *CI* Confidence interval, *CV* Coefficient of variation (inter-individual)

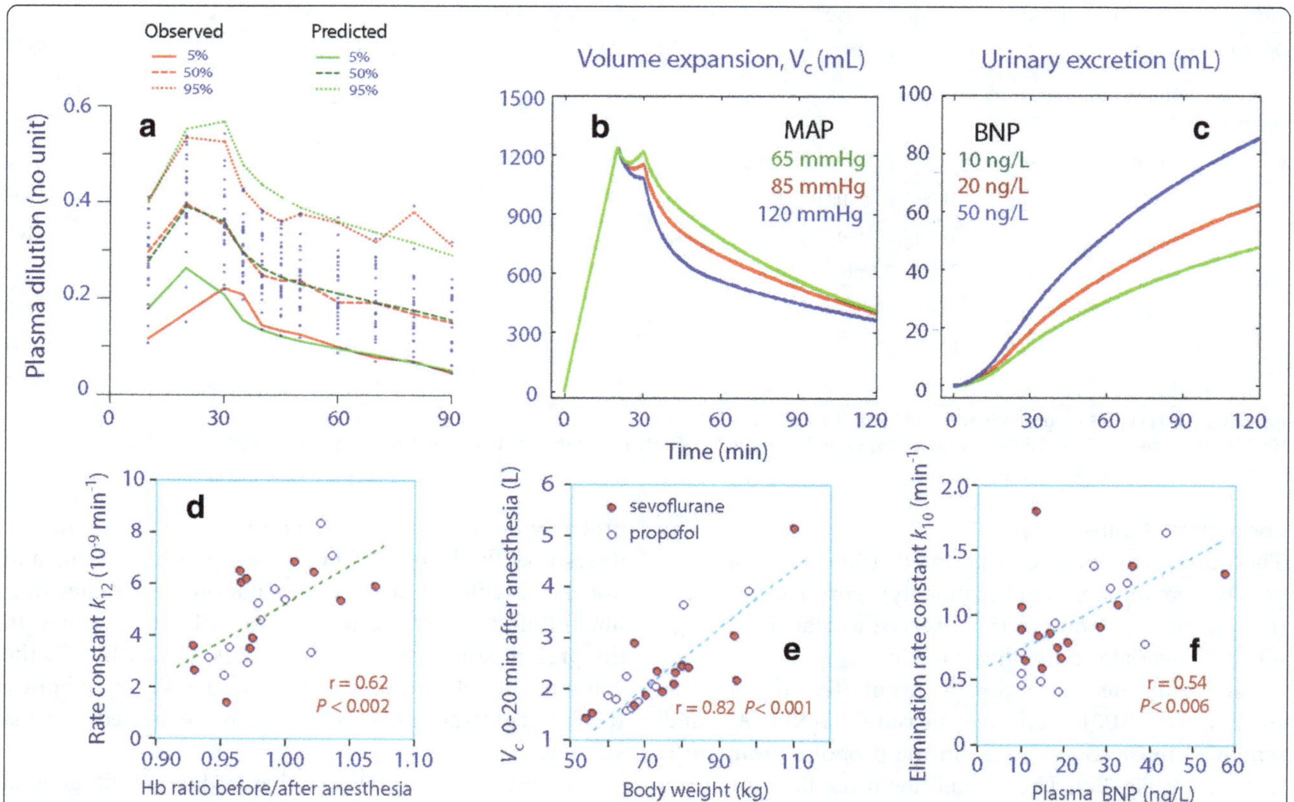

Fig. 2 Predictive check of the kinetic analysis (a). Computer-based simulations (b and c). Correlations between measured parameters and kinetic constants (d, e and f)

amount of fluid that had been infused at that time. The anesthesia-induced vasodilatation and the resulting drop in the MAP by 20 mmHg are sufficient to explain the almost complete "shut-off" of the distribution [4]. However, the present study shows, for the first time, when fluid filtration begins again, and that is when approximately 1.25 L of fluid has been infused and the plasma volume has increased by the same volume.

The results would be quite different if anesthesia had not been induced. The hypotension-associated interruption of capillary filtration doubled the maximum plasma dilution in response to 25 mL kg^{-1} of crystalloid fluid from the expected 20% [21, 22] to 40% (Fig. 1 g and Fig. 2 a). In the absence of hemorrhage, these figures can the transposed into the relative (%) increase of the plasma volume.

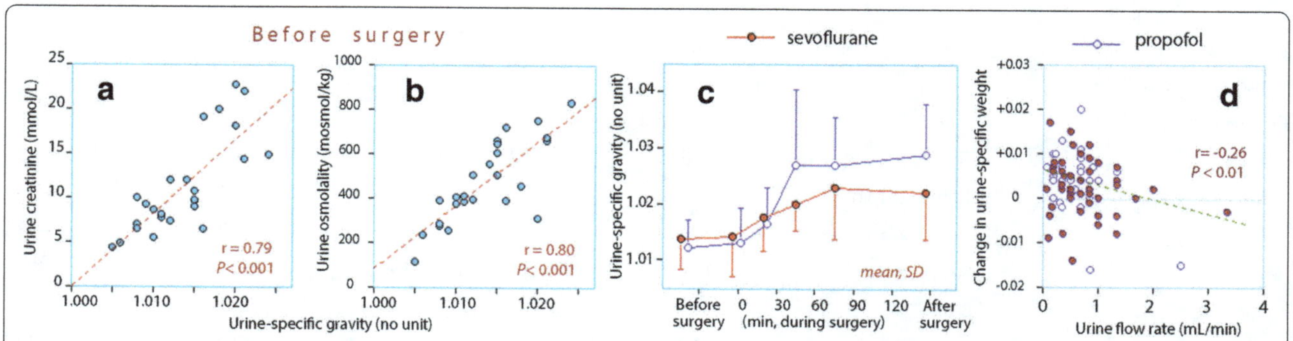

Fig. 3 Concentrated urine. One extreme outlier was omitted in the subplot in D, which shows the change in urine-specific weight over a period of 30 min versus the urine flow rate

Spontaneous hemodilution, which averaged 2% but occasionally reached 7–8%, occurred during the induction of anesthesia. i.e. before any fluid had been infused, which degree correlated with the very low k_{12} that prevailed until 16.6 mL kg^{-1} of lactated Ringer's had been infused (Fig. 2d). There was also a temporarily smaller V_c, which suggests that the fluid infused early primarily became enriched in the central circulation. The restoration of V_c and k_{12} after 16.6 mL kg^{-1} had been infused accounts for the unexpected observation that the greatest plasma volume expansion occurred before the end of the infusion.

The diuretic response to infused fluid is reduced by approximately 90% during general anesthesia, which is strongly associated with the reduction of MAP [4–7]. In the present study, all patients underwent general anesthesia, but covariance between MAP and k_{10} was difficult to demonstrate due to the very low overall k_{10}; the parameter value was only 0.00086 (i.e. half-life of 13 h) while the corresponding value in cohorts of conscious volunteers has varied between 0.015 and 0.028 (half-life 25–50 min) [19, 20]. Interestingly, most of the infused fluid was not eliminated as urine but in proportion by the rate constant k_b to the expansion of V_c at any given time. The fluid that was eliminated from the kinetic system by this mechanism remained in the body but did not equilibrate with the plasma during the period of the study. A higher k_b than k_{10} has previously been reported only during general anesthesia [2, 23, 24].

The poor diuretic response to infused fluid might also explain the lack of covariance between fluid kinetics and concentrated urine, which is index of low habitual intake of water and/or overt dehydration [25, 26]. An inhibitory effect of preoperatively concentrated urine on the diuretic response to volume loading with crystalloid fluid [16] and 20% albumin [17] has previously been found in conscious patients. In the present study, the process of further concentrating the urine during the surgery was followed in a step-wise fashion. The urine became gradually more concentrated (Fig. 3c) and was most likely to occur whenever the urine flow rate fell below 1 mL min^{-1} (Fig. 3c). The theoretical importance of this process of is that patients with a low habitual intake of water might have their urine so much more concentrated during the surgery that the concentrating capacity of the kidneys is exceeded, which causes a postoperative rise in plasma creatinine [27–29]. Unfortunately, plasma creatinine was not measured after the surgery.

Although the diuresis was very small, an elevated BNP was associated with slightly increased urine volumes (Fig. 2c, f). This biomarker of ventricular distention doubles in response to volume loading with 25 mL min^{-1} of crystalloid fluid in awake volunteers [30] but apparently to a smaller degree during general anesthesia.

A currently popular view is that surgical trauma and hypervolemia cause degradation of the endothelial glycocalyx layer whereby the capillary leakage of macromolecules and fluid would increase [13–15]. The degree of acute glycocalyx degradation can be evaluated by measuring the plasma concentrations of, for example, syndecan-1 and heparan sulfate. The present data did not disclose any marked elevations of these biomarkers (Table 1). Their plasma concentrations actually followed the hemodilution pattern quite well and showed no covariance with k_{12} or k_b, which are else the relevant parameters to indicate increased capillary leakage.

Limitations include that capillary filtration was regained only after having administrated a fairly large bolus volume of Ringer's. When a Starling equilibrium adequate for general anesthesia has developed after infusion of smaller amounts of fluid, such as 500 mL, is unknown. Slow capillary refill of the same kind as during induction of anesthesia would probably continue but, in any event, equilibrium would certainly occur later than the 20 min found here.

The cut-off points for changed fluid kinetics were evaluated only at 10-min intervals. A higher resolution could have been obtained by sampling blood at shorter intervals. Not only the infused fluid volume, but also the time from the anesthesia induction, might contribute to restoration of the distribution function. No massive elevations of the biomarkers for cardiac strain and glycocalyx degradation were found, which limits the possibilities to identify them as covariates. Finally, the kinetic model is constructed to reasonably well agree with known body physiology, but what the fixed kinetic parameters represent is still not finally proven.

Conclusions

A fluid volume kinetic method shows the excessive hemodilution occurring when crystalloid fluid is infused after induction of general anesthesia corresponds to a nearly complete interruption of the capillary filtration up to the point in time when 16.6 mL kg^{-1} of lactated Ringer's has been infused. The small urinary excretion did not cause intravascular overload as fluid could be filtered to extravascular tissues both with and without being in equilibrium with the plasma.

Abbreviations

ANOVA: Analysis of variance; BNP: Brain natriuretic peptide; AUC: Area under the curve; Hb: Hemoglobin; LL: Log likelihood; h: Hour; L: Liter; mL: Milliliter; k_{12}: Rate constant for fluid passing from v_c to v_t; k_{21}: Rate constant for fluid passing from v_t to v_c; k_{10}: Rate constant for fluid leaving the kinetic system as urine; k_b: Rate constant for fluid leaving the kinetic system but not as urine; MAP: Mean arterial pressure; R_o: Rate of infusion; V_c and v_c: Size of central body fluid space at baseline and during fluid therapy, respectively; V_t and v_t: Size of peripheral body fluid space at baseline and during fluid therapy, respectively

Acknowledgements
The authors are grateful to the staff of the operations department at Paul Stradins Clinical University Hospital, Riga, Latvia, for their help in collecting the data.

Author details
Robert G. Hahn: Researcher at Södertälje Hospital, Södertälje, Sweden: Professor of Anesthesia and Intensive care at Karolinska Institutet at Danderyds Hospital (KIDS), Stockholm, Sweden.
Janis Nemme: Specialist in Anesthesia and Intensive care, Department of Anaesthesiology and Intensive Care, Riga Stradins University and Paul Stradins Clinical University Hospital, Riga, Latvia.

Authors' contributions
RGH planned the study, performed the kinetic analysis, and wrote the manuscript. JN helped planning the study, wrote all applications, and collected the data. The authors read and approved the final manuscript.

Author details
[1]Research Unit, Södertälje Hospital, 152 86 Södertälje, Sweden. [2]Karolinska Institutet at Danderyds Hospital (KIDS), Stockholm, Sweden. [3]Department of Anesthesiology and Intensive Care, Riga Stradins University, Riga, Latvia. [4]Paul Stradins Clinical University Hospital, Riga, Latvia.

References

1. Hahn RG. Volume kinetics for infusion fluids (review). Anesthesiology. 2010; 113(2):470–81. https://doi.org/10.1097/ALN.0b013e3181dcd88f.
2. Hahn RG. Understanding volume kinetics. Acta Anaesthesiol Scand 2020; 64(5): 570–8.
3. Lijnema TH, Huizenga JR, Jager J, Mackor AJ, Gips CH. Gravimetric determination of the water concentration in whole blood, plasma and erythrocytes and correlations with hematological and clinico-chemical parameters. Clin Chim Acta. 1993;214(2):129–38.
4. Hahn RG, Lyons G. The half-life of infusion fluids: an educational review. Eur J Anesthesiol. 2016;33(7):475–82. https://doi.org/10.1097/EJA.0000000000000436.
5. Hahn RG. Arterial pressure and the rate of elimination of crystalloid fluid: a population-based study. Anesth Analg. 2017;124(6):1824–33. https://doi.org/10.1213/ANE.0000000000002075.
6. Li Y, Yi S, Zhu Y, Hahn RG. Volume kinetics of Ringer's lactate solution in acute inflammatory disease. Br J Anesth. 2018;121(3):574–80. https://doi.org/10.1016/j.bja.2018.04.023.
7. Hahn RG. Hemoglobin dilution from epidural-induced hypotension with and without fluid loading. Acta Anaesthesiol Scand. 1992;36(3):241–4.
8. Hahn RG. Increased hemodilution in hypotension induced by epidural anesthesia. Acta Aneasthesiol Scand. 1993;37(4):357–60.
9. Drobin D, Hahn RG. Time course of increased hemodilution in hypotension induced by extradural anaesthesia. Br J Anaesth. 1996;77(2):223–6.
10. Li Y, Zhu S, Hahn RG. The kinetics of Ringer's solution in young and elderly patients during induction of general anesthesia with propofol and epidural anesthesia with bupivacaine. Acta Anaesthesiol Scand. 2007;51(7):880–7.
11. Hahn RG, Lindahl C, Drobin D. Volume kinetics of acetated Ringer's solution during experimental spinal anesthesia. Acta Anesthesiol Scand. 2011;55(8): 987–94. https://doi.org/10.1111/j.1399-6576.2011.02493.x.12.
12. Ewaldsson CA, Hahn RG. Kinetics and extravascular retention of acetated Ringer's solution during isoflurane and propofol anesthesia for thyroid surgery. Anesthesiology. 2005;103:460–9. https://doi.org/10.1097/00000542-200509000-00006.
13. Rehm M, Haller M, Orth V, Kreimeier U, Jacob M, Dressel H, et al. Changes in blood volume and hematocrit during acute perioperative volume loading with 5% albumin or 6% hetastarch solutions in patients before radical hysterectomy. Anesthesiology. 2001;95(4):849–56.
14. Rehm M, Bruegger D, Christ F, Conzen P, Thiel M, Jacob M, et al. Shedding of the endothelial glycocalyx in patients undergoing major vascular surgery with global and regional ischemia. Circulation. 2007;116(17):1896–906.
15. Chappell D, Bruegger D, Potzel J, Jacob M, Brettner F, Vogeser M, et al. Hypervolemia increases release of atrial natriuretic peptide and shedding of the endothelial glycocalyx. Crit Care. 2014;18(5):538.
16. Hahn RG, Isacson MN, Fagerström T, Rosvall J, Nyman CR. Isotonic saline in elderly men: an open-labelled controlled infusion study of electrolyte balance, urine flow and kidney function. Anaesthesia. 2016;71(2):155–62. https://doi.org/10.1111/anae.13301.
17. Hahn RG, Zdolsek M, Hasselgren E, Zdolsek J, Björne H. Fluid volume kinetics of 20% albumin. Br J Clin Pharmacol. 2019;85(6):1303–11. https://doi.org/10.1111/bcp.13897.
18. Nemme J, Hahn RG, Krizhanovskii C, Ntika S, Sabelnikovs O, Vanags I. Hypervolemia does not cause degradation of the endothelial glycocalyx layer during open hysterectomy performed under sevoflurane or propofol anesthesia. Acta Anesthesiol Scand. 2020;64(4):538–45. https://doi.org/10.1111/aas.13511.
19. Hahn RG. The elimination half-life of crystalloid fluid is shorter in female than in male volunteers; a retrospective population kinetic analysis. Biol Sex Differ. 2016;7:54. https://doi.org/10.1186/s13293-016-0105-7.
20. Hahn RG. Influences of the red blood cell count on the distribution and elimination of crystalloid fluid. Medicina (Kaunas). 2017;53(4):233–41. https://doi.org/10.1016/j.medici.2017.07.005.
21. Drobin D, Hahn RG. Volume kinetics of Ringer's solution in hypovolemic volunteers. Anesthesiology. 1999;90(1):81–91. 9915316.
22. Drobin D, Hahn RG. Kinetics of isotonic and hypertonic plasma volume expanders. Anesthesiology. 2002;96(6):1371–80. 12170049.
23. Brauer KI, Svensén C, Hahn RG, Traber L, Prough D. Volume kinetic analysis of the distribution of 0.9% saline in conscious versus isoflurane-anesthetized sheep. Anesthesiology. 2002;96(2):442–9. 11818780.
24. Connolly CM, Kramer GC, Hahn RG, Chaisson NF, Svensén C, Kirschner RA, et al. Isoflurane but not mechanical ventilation promotes extravascular fluid accumulation during crystalloid volume loading. Anesthesiology. 2003;98(3): 670–81. https://doi.org/10.1097/00000542-200303000-00015.
25. Perrier E, Vergne S, Klein A, Poupin M, Rondeau P, Le Bellego L, et al. Hydration biomarkers in free-living adults with different levels of habitual fluid consumption. Br J Nutr. 2013;109(9):1678–87. https://doi.org/10.1038/ejcn.2013.93.
26. Armstrong LE, Soto JA, Hacker FT Jr, Casa DJ, Kavouras SA, Maresh CM. Urinary indices during dehydration, exercise and rehydration. Int J Sport Nutr. 1998;8:345–55.
27. Hahn RG, Li Y, He R. Fluid retention is alleviated by crystalloid but not by colloid fluid after induction of general anesthesia: an open-labelled clinical trial. J Anesth Clin Res. 2016;7:1. https://doi.org/10.4172/2155-6148.1000597.
28. Hahn RG. Renal injury during hip fracture surgery: an exploratory study. Anesthesiol Intensive Ther. 2015;47(4):284–90. https://doi.org/10.5603/AIT.a2015.0029.
29. Ellis RJ, Del Vecchio SJ, Kalma B, Ng KL, Morais C, Francis RS, et al. Association between preoperative hydration status and acute kidney injury in patients managed surgically for kidney tumours. Int Urol Nephrol. 2018; 50(7):1211–7. https://doi.org/10.1007/s11255-018-1901-2.
30. Norberg Å, Hahn RG, Li H, Olsson J, Prough DS, Börsheim E, et al. Population volume kinetics predicts retention of 0.9% saline infused in awake and isoflurane-anesthetized volunteers. Anesthesiology. 2007;107(1): 24–32. https://doi.org/10.1097/01-anes.0000268387.34758.6d.

Comparison of preemptive paracetamol, paracetamol-diclofenac and paracetamol-tramadol combination on postoperative pain after elective abdominal surgery under general anesthesia, ethiopia

Zemedu Aweke[1], Fetene Seyoum[1], Tewoderos Shitemaw[2*] and Derartu Neme Doba[1]

Abstract

Background: In the practice of postoperative pain management, pain is still poorly managed in low resource setting where the practice of epidural and opioid free analgesia is impractical. There has been a recent trend of combining different drugs and concept of preemptive analgesia but the therapeutic superiority remains understudied for postoperative pain management. The aim of this study is to assess postoperative analgesic effect of preemptive Paracetamol, Paracetamol-diclofenac and Paracetamol-tramadol combination in patients undergoing laparotomy surgery.

Methods: Three-arm, randomized control trial study conducted on 63 patients undergone laparotomy surgery; group-P (paracetamol 1 g), group-PD (1 g + diclofenac 75 mg) and group-PT (paracetamol 1 g + tramadol 100 mg). The Numerical Rating Scale (NRS) pain rating system was used for this study. The primary endpoint of the study was total amount of analgesia consumption. Post-operative analgesic therapy [intravenous tramadol, 50 mg] were provided when patients complain of pain (request medication) or a numeric rating scale ≥4 was recorded. Secondary endpoint of the study were the time of first analgesic request and the intensity of the pain during 24 h post-op follow up period. Parametric data were analyzed using (ANOVA) and nonparametric data analyzed by Kuruska-Wallis H rank test. Chi-square test used for categorical variable. Statistical significance were sated at *p* value < 0.05 with a power of 80%.

(Continued on next page)

* Correspondence: tewoderosshitemaw@gmail.com
[2]Department of Anesthesia, Kotebe Metropolitan University, Menelik II Medical & Health Science College, Addis Ababa, Ethiopia

(Continued from previous page)

Results: The mean total tramadol consumption was significant higher in paracetamol group 250 ± 79.06 mg compared to paracetamol-diclofenac (173.81 ± 87.49 mg $p = 0.008$) and paracetamol-tramadol (154.76 ± 70.54 mg $p = 0.001$) group. Time to first analgesic request was significantly shorter within paracetamol group (87.62 ± 20.95 min) compared to paracetamol-diclofenac (103.01 ± 23.53 min $p = 0.029$) and paracetamol-tramadol (144.05 ± 14.72 min $p < 0.001$) group. There was statistically significant difference at 4th, 6th and 8th hour showing lower median pain score in paracetamol-tramadol group compared to paracetamol group.

Conclusion: Preemptive combination of paracetamol-tramadol and paracetamol-diclofenac reduce total tramadol consumption and prolongs time to first analgesic request compared to paracetamol alone in patients undergoing laparotomy surgery.

Keywords: Post-operative pain, Multimodal therapy, Preemptive analgesia, Pain management and laparotomy surgery

Background

Pain is defined as "unpleasant emotional and sensory experience due to actual or potential tissue damage", according to international association for study of pain [1]. Studies demonstrates that a significant proportion of patients suffer moderate to severe intensity of pain in the immediate as well as early post-operative period after abdominal surgery [2, 3].

Poorly managed pain after surgery can negatively affect patients wellbeing on multiple levels such as hypertension, myocardial ischemia, arrhythmias, respiratory impairments, poor wound healings, chronic pain, deep vein thrombosis and risk factor for the development of chronic pain syndrome [4–6]. These negative outcomes lead to prolonged hospitalization resulting huge healthcare costs, patient's financial expense as well as involvement of nursing care [7, 8].

Opioids are an alternative to postoperative pain management, although there are considerable side effects and addiction reported. However, in resource limited area, due to cost unaffordability, clinical setup and inaccessibility, managing pain through opioids is too difficult [9–11]. Epidural analgesia and opioid free analgesic techniques are also an alternative techniques but difficult to practice due to lack of resources in a low resources setting like Ethiopia.

Inadequate controlled postoperative pain remains a widespread problem despite the development of specialized acute pain management modalities, especially in developed country [12]. Indeed, current practice guidelines for perioperative pain management recommend the use of multimodal therapy [13, 14].

The adaptation of multimodal analgesic techniques as the standard method for prevention of pain in surgery is one alternative to improve the recovery process [14, 15]. Now a days administering a pain medication before surgery is one of the component in multimodal approach which is called preemptive analgesia. Preemptive analgesia is an antinociceptive treatment to block central nervous system hyperexcitability and leads to a reduced postoperative pain intensity and decrease the risk of postsurgical chronic pain [16, 17].

Despite this evidence-based approach to improve perioperative analgesia, the proportion of patients reporting moderate to severe pain after surgery has remained constant over the past decade [6, 18]. Consequently, for anesthetist in developing countries, providing effective postoperative pain management become practically difficult and open gate for investigating better intervention that are applicable in resource limited setups.Pre-emptive analgesia needs further investigation in order to find out optimal choice of drugs with minimum side effect, which are easy to administer and easily accessible and affordable [19]. Our study assess the combination of drugs which are opioid free analgesic (paracetamol & diclofenac) and the weakest opioid (Tramadol) that are easily available in countries with poor resources to use expensive analgesics. The aim of this study is by taking the pre-emptive analgesia model, to compare effectiveness of paracetamol, paracetamol-tramadol and paracetamol-diclofenac combination as a component of multimodal analgesia on postoperative pain. The study is done on patients undergoing elective abdominal surgery in a resource limited setup.

Methods

A single blind randomized clinical trial was conducted at Hawassa Comprehensive Specialized Teaching Hospital from January 2018 to February 2019. Hawassa Comprehensive Specialized Teaching Hospital is one of the biggest government hospitals in Ethiopia functioning as a teaching and referral hospital since April 2005.

Ethical clearance approval was obtained from Dilla University institutional review board (IRB) with protocol number 007/18–08 on 4th September 2017. In addition, our study was retrospectively registered on July 07, 2019 at Pan African Clinical Trial Registry with the identification number of PACTR201908890749145. The purpose, importance and risk of the study was explained, written informed consent was obtained from each participant. Participants were informed that they can withdraw from the study without any restriction at any time. This study is adhered to CONSORT guidelines.

Patients undergone elective laparotomy surgery at Hawassa Comprehensive Specialized Teaching Hospital in the course of data collection period were included in the study. Patients with age greater than 18 years old and ASA physical status class I–II were included in the study. The exclusion criteria's were concomitant medical or psychiatric problems which prevent completion of the follow-up, acute or chronic pain diagnosis, history of upper gastrointestinal bleeding related to previous NSAI D therapy, comorbidities (Anemia, DM, HTN, Arthritis), moderate or severe renal impairment (serum creatinine > 1.6 mg/dl), known asthmatic patient, history of alcohol, opiate or other drug abuse, use of NSAIDs or Paracetamol within 24 h of surgery and participants with known allergies for the study drugs.

Sample size and sampling procedure

Before this study begun, we conducted a pilot study for estimating a sample size. The Sample size estimation were calculated using a priori power analysis (G Power version 3.1.9.2) based on the pilot study results. The outcomes measure for this study were the mean total analgesic consumption between groups over 24 h, time to first analgesic request and numeric rating scale (NRS) score between groups.

Based on largest sample size, the mean total analgesic (tramadol) consumption was used to estimate the sample size. The observed mean total tramadol consumption from the pilot study was $\mu 1 = 215 \pm 80$ mg $\mu 2 = 170 \pm 60$ mg $\mu 3 = 155 \pm 52$ mg, SDpooled = 51.33. A priori power analysis for a one-way ANOVA with 3 groups was conducted to determine sample size using an alpha = 0.017(Controlling for the probability of a Type I error using a Bonferroni correction). To allow for comparisons of the three groups, a sample of 19 subject per group would have 80% power to detect the difference of the mean total tramadol consumption between groups. The calculated sample size was 57; by adding 10% attrition rate and assuming balanced design the total sample size become 63. The results of that pilot study were not included in the present analysis, and none of the patients from the pilot study were included in the present study.

By reviewing a five-month report, a systemic random sampling method was applied with the probability of 50% to be included in the study (k = ½). Considering the sequential patients scheduled for laparotomy surgery, a random start was used to select every eligible participants. After then, the patients were allocated to one of the three groups randomly with sealed non-transparent envelope containing the name of the group. (Fig. 1).

Data collection procedures

A day prior to the day of surgery, a staff member not involved in data collection performed preoperative assessment and took informed consent. All patients who were scheduled for elective laparotomy, fulfilled the inclusion criteria and volunteer to take part in the study were instructed by data collectors on how to self-report pain using the eleven point Numerical Rating Scale (NRS), a score from 0 to 10. The instruction on how to self-report pain was repeated for study participant on the morning of the surgery.

At midnight, the day before surgery, oral paracetamol (1 g) with sips of water was given for all three groups. At the morning of surgery (60 Minutes before surgery) 1 g of oral (PO) paracetamol (Group P) or 75 mg of Intra muscular (IM) diclofenac (Group- PD) or 100 mg of Intravenous (IV) tramadol (Group- PT) was provided in accordance with the random allocation of the patient to specific group. The time elapsed between the mid night oral paracetamol provided and the morning dose of preemptive analgesia was 8–10 h. The prepared drug was given by the personnel anesthetist assigned to each case who were not involved in the study. Owing to the nature of the study and the study site, blinding was not possible for the patient and anesthetist delivering the interventions.

When the study participant arrived at the waiting room, all participants were premedicated with dexamethasone (8 mg), diazepam (5 mg) and cimetidine (400 mg). Preoperatively, baseline vital sign, the presence and severity of pain (NRS for pain) and demographic data were obtained.

The Numerical Rating Scale (NRS) pain rating system was used for this study. The NRS showed higher compliance rates (across cultures and languages), better responsiveness, easier to use and good applicability than Visual Analogue scale (VAS) in different studies [20–22]. In addition the NRS was the instrument of choice in an age-mixed population making it preferable for this study [21]. (Fig. 2).

The same general anesthesia protocol was applied in all groups without any regional or neuraxial anesthesia. Standard ASA monitors applied to all the patients that include a pulse-oximetry, electrocardiography, noninvasive blood pressure, and a temperature monitor. Induction of general anesthesia were achieved with Propofol at 2.5 mg/kg- ketamine 0.3 mg/kg (analgesia dose),

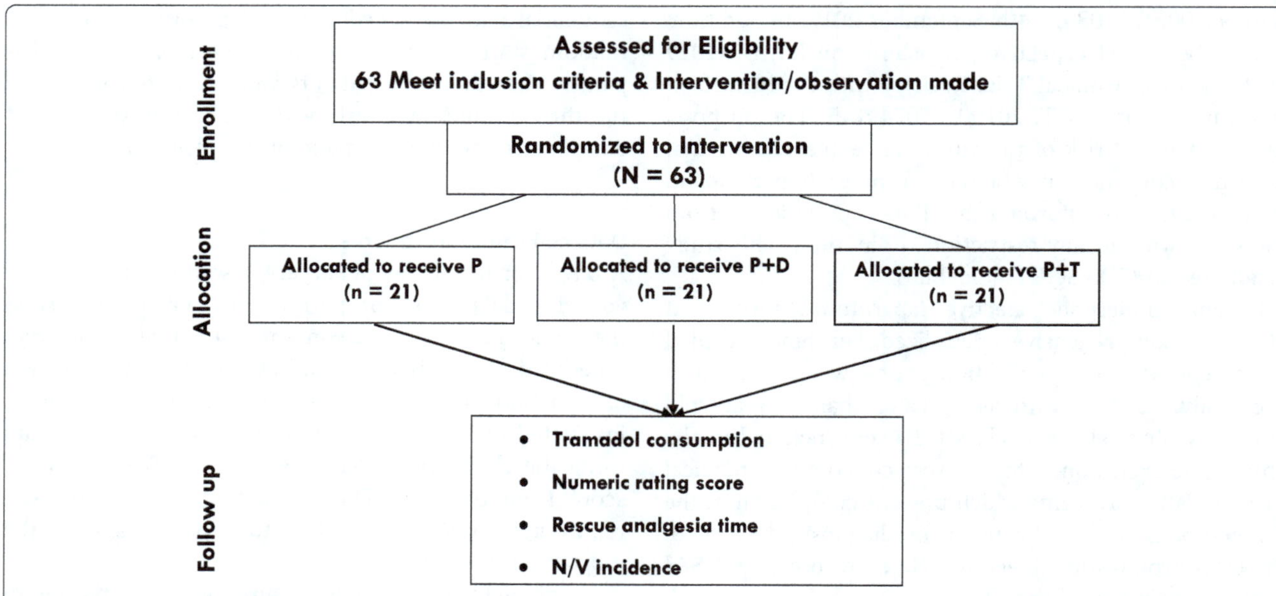

Fig. 1 Enrollment chart for patients scheduled for Laparotomy

fentanyl (50 μg) and tracheal intubation facilitated by succinylcholine (2 mg/kg) after 3 min' of pre-oxygenation.

Anesthesia was maintained by using isoflurane with oxygen (100%) mixture and a low gas flow (3 L/minute) in accordance to clinical needs/assessment of the depth of anesthesia. The patient's mechanical ventilation parameters were adjusted based on the patient's age and weight. Neuromuscular blockage was maintained with Vecuronium. At the end of the surgery, residual neuromuscular block were antagonized with atropine 0.2 mg/kg and neostigmine 0.05 mg/kg. After surgery, participants were transferred to the PACU with adequate emergence from anesthesia.

Outcome data was collected by anesthetists who were blinded to the treatment allocation. Observations begun at post anesthesia care unit. All patients were assessed using systematically structured questionnaire by four trained data collector (BSc Anesthetist with minimum of 3 years' experience). Furthermore, MSc anesthetist was assigned to assist and supervise data collectors. All patient were asked to rate pain intensity on standard numeric rating scale range from 0(no pain) to 10(worst possible pain) at rest (static NRS) and voluntary cough (dynamic NRS).

The pain intensity was rated as mild (NRS: 0–3), moderate (NRS: 4–6), and severe (NRS: 7–10). The NRS score were recorded at recovery after the patient is fully awake from anesthesia, at the 2nd, 4th, 6th, 8th, 12th and 24th hour. Twenty-four-hour postoperative analgesia consumption, time to first analgesia request and incidence of nausea vomiting were recorded. The supervisor checked each questionnaire daily with further cross check by principal investigator for completeness and consistency of data.

In case of nausea or vomiting, intravenous metoclopramide 10 mg and dexamethasone 4 mg was administered. For the first 24 h post-operative analgesic therapy were provided when patients complain of pain (request medication) or a numeric rating scale ≥4 was recorded. The analgesic drug administered were intravenous tramadol (50 mg) according to the hospital protocol. After 24 h post-operative analgesic therapy continue according to the hospital protocol. The post-operative analgesia drug provided to patients were only tramadol since morphine was not available at the study site during the study time.

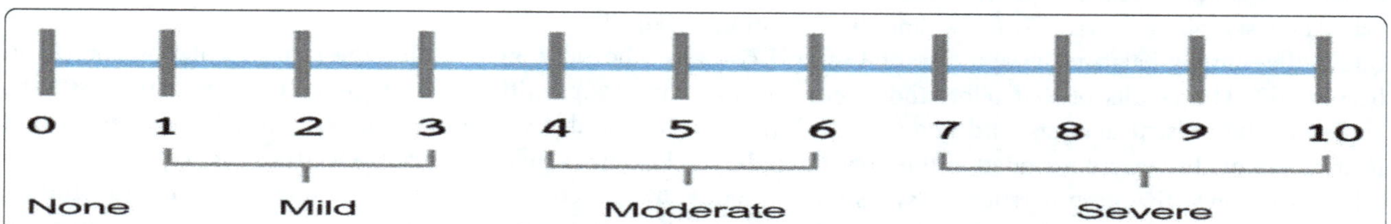

Fig. 2 Numerical pain rating scale (NRS), adopted from the National Initiative on Pain Control™ (NIPC™)

Operational definition

- **Preemptive analgesia** is anti-nociceptive treatment that starts before surgery and prevents the establishment of peripheral and central sensitization [23].
- **Postoperative pain**: the presence of pain in the postoperative period was defined as a pain occurring in a surgical patients following a procedure [24].
- **Numerical pain rating scale (NRS):** is a valid is a method of pain assessment where patients are asked to score their pain ratings on a scale of 0–10, corresponding to current, best, and worst pain experienced over the 24 h. The median value will be used to represent patient's level of pain [25]. (Fig. 2)
- **Total analgesia consumption**: is total amount of analgesic drugs in milligrams used in the first 24 h after the operation.
- **Laparotomy/Abdominal surgery**: any operation that involve opening the abdominal cavity for Diseases affecting the abdominal cavity through the sheath of the rectus abdominis muscles/ midline incision surgery.
- **Time to first analgesic request**: is a time in minutes measured from the end of procedure to time when patient request analgesics.

Data analysis and interpretation

The statistical analyses were performed using SPSS V 23 software. The data was tested for normality using Shapiro–Wilk normality test and homogeneity of variance by Levene's test. Analysis of variance (ANOVA) and Kruskal–Wallis H test were used for normally distributed continuous data and non-normally distributed or non-parametric data respectively. If the ANOVAs or Kruskal–Wallis H test were significant, then Tukey post hoc test was used to compare one group with the others. Categorical data were analyzed using the Pearson Chi-squared test. Data was expressed as a mean and standard deviation (SD) or Median (Q1-Q3). A *P-value* < 0.05 with power of 80% was considered as a statistically significant.

Results

Socio-demographic data

Sixty-three patients participated in this study. There was no significant difference among the three groups with regard to age, gender, weight, operation duration, anesthesia duration, ASA physical status and baseline preoperative pain (p value > 0.05) as depicted in Table 1.

Postoperative numeric rating scale score at rest and during movement

The Kruskal-Wallis test showed that median NRS score were not significant at 2nd, 12th and 24th hours between the three groups ($p > 0.05$). There was statistically significant difference on the NRS score at the 4th, 6th and 8th hour between groups ($p = 0.032$, 0.022 and 0.007 respectively). Post hoc analysis shows a significantly reduced NRS score in the paracetamol-tramadol combination (PT group) than the paracetamol group (P group) at rest with $p = 0.25$, 0.013 and 0.002 respectively. There was no statistically significant difference between the two combination group (PD group & PT group) at all time during 24 h ($p > 0.05$). However, NRS scores of paracetamol-tramadol group were lower than paracetamol-diclofenac at all time. Again there was no statistically significant difference results between paracetamol-diclofenac combination and paracetamol group at all time during 24 h ($p > 0.05$). But, NRS scores of paracetamol-diclofenac group were lower than paracetamol group at all time (Fig. 3).

Table 1 socio demographic characteristics of patients who undergo elective laparotomy surgery at Hawassa compressive specialized hospital

	Group P	Group PD	Group PT	*P*-value
Age (year)[a]	41.67 ± 7.52	45.33 ± 7.72	42.10 ± 9.07	0.286
Gender (M /F)[b]	10/11	12/9	8/13	0.466
Weight (kg)[a]	58.28 ± 3.47	57.52 ± 3.54	59.26 ± 3.67	0.300
ASA I / II[b]	16/5	18/3	17/4	0.734
Operation duration (min)[a]	118.10 ± 23 05	112.38 ± 19.34	114.05 ± 17.51	0.640
Anesthesia duration (min)[a]	134.76 ± 22 28	129.76 ± 19.97	132.14 ± 17.72	0.723
Type of surgery[b]				
Gastrointestinal(n)	13(61.9%)	12 (57.2%)	11 (52.3%)	0.436
Gynecological(n)	8 (38.1%)	9 (42.8%)	10 (47.7%)	
Surgical incision length	15 (14–16)	15 (15–17)	14 (15–17)	0.765

Data are given as mean ± SD or Median (Q1-Q3) or Case number/ proportion (n/%), (ANOVA, Kruskal-Wallis test and Tukey test, Chi-Square Test)
[a]Mean ± SD
[b]Case number (proportion)

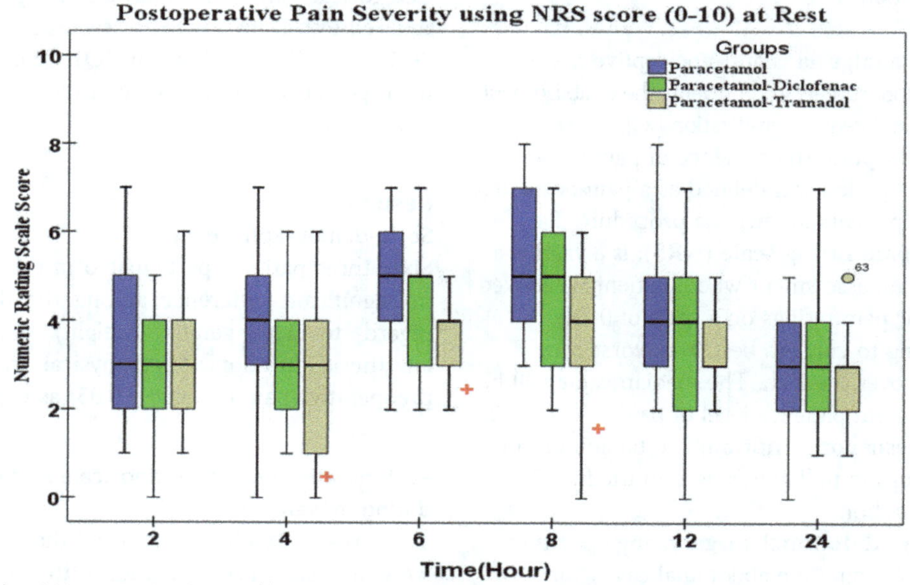

$^{+}p < 0.05$ compared to Group P, $^{++}p < 0.05$ compared to Group PD, $^{+++}p < 0.05$ compared to Group PT (Kruskal-Wallis test and Tukey test), ^{o}= outliers

Fig. 3 Comparison of postoperative pain using 11 point NRS score (0–10) at rest

The Kruskal-Wallis test showed that median NRS score were not significant at 2nd, 12th and 24th hours ($p > 0.05$) between three groups during coughing. There was statistically significant difference results at the 4th, 6th and 8th hour between groups ($p =$ 0.005, 0.008 and 0.007 respectively). Post hoc analysis shows significant reduction in NRS score during coughing in the paracetamol-tramadol combination group when compared to paracetamol alone group with p value ($p =$ 0.003, 0.003 and 0.011 at 4th, 6th and 8th hour respectively). A significant reduction of NRS during coughing was also recorded in the paracetamol-diclofenac combination group compared to paracetamol alone at 4th hour ($p = 0.015$). There was no statistically significant difference results between the two combination group (PD group & PT group) at all time during 24 h ($p > 0.05$). However, NRS scores of paracetamol-tramadol group were lower than paracetamol-diclofenac at all time (Fig. 4).

Time to first analgesia request

The time to first analgesia requirement in the paracetamol group (M ± SD: 87.62 ± 20.95 min) was significantly shorter than in the paracetamol-diclofenac group (103.01 ± 23.53 min, $p = 0.029$) and paracetamol-tramadol groups (144.05 ± 14.72 min, $p < 0.001$). Likewise first analgesia requirement in the paracetamol-diclofenac was significantly shorter than paracetamol-tramadol group ($p < 0.001$) (Table 2).

Total cumulative postoperative analgesia consumption within 24 h

There was statistically significant difference in mean total tramadol consumption within 24 h postoperatively between the groups as shown in Table 2. Post hoc analysis of total tramadol consumed in 24 h showed significantly higher in paracetamol group compared to paracetamol-diclofenac group ($p = 0.008$) and paracetamol-tramadol group ($p = 0.001$). However, no significant difference between paracetamol-diclofenac and paracetamol-tramadol groups (Table 2).

Incidence of nausea and vomiting

The incidence of nausea and vomiting over 24 h was 23.8%. The proportions of patients with nausea and vomiting was lower (19%) in PD group compared to P and PT group ($X^2 = 0.525$) but not significant ($P = 0.769$). No serious complications or life-threatening events occurred in either group.

Discussion

Our study showed that the total tramadol consumption was lower in both paracetamol-diclofenac and paracetamol-tramadol, combination over 24-h compared to paracetamol alone group. The mean total tramadol consumption was 154.76 ± 70.54 mg in paracetamol-tramadol group compared to 173.81 ± 87.49 mg in paracetamol-diclofenac group and 250 ± 79.06 mg in paracetamol group (p = 0.001).

In a study by Samimi et al. the mean total morphine consumption in patients receiving the combination of

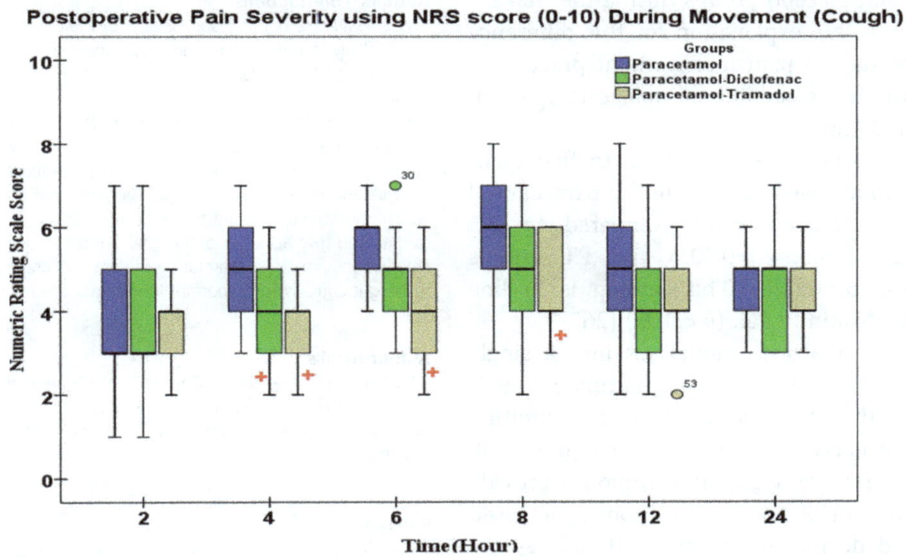

$^{+}p < 0.05$ compared to Group P, $^{++}p < 0.05$ compared to Group PD, $^{+++}p < 0.05$ compared to Group PT (Kruskal-Wallis test and Tukey test), ^{c}= outliers

Fig. 4 Comparison of postoperative pain using 11 point NRS score (0–10) on Movement

paracetamol-diclofenac over the first 24 h was significantly lower (13.9 ± 2.7 mg) compared to diclofenac group (20.1 ± 3.6 mg) with $p < 0.05$. Our study used the weakest opioid (tramadol) for post-operative pain management. To compare our result with the above study by Samimi et al. using opioid conversion factor of tramadol to morphine (0.1), paracetamol-diclofenac group in our study consumed an estimated mean of 17.4 mg morphine [26].

Study done by Montgomery et al, showed total postoperative morphine consumption in paracetamol-diclofenac group (18.5–35.8) (mean, 95% CI) was lower than paracetamol group (36.1–53.6) with $p < 0.01$. Montgomery and colleagues reported that the use of this combination has been shown to reduce the amount of morphine required by about one-third compared with paracetamol alone in women undergoing elective abdominal gynecological procedures [27]. These result was also in line with the study done by Moussa and Riad that assessed total opioid consumption between paracetamol-diclofenac combination and paracetamol alone that found significantly lower total morphine consumption in paracetamol-diclofenac combination: mean (SD) 2.9 (1.5) mg compared to paracetamol alone: 5.5 (1.5) mg with $p < 0.01$ [28].

This study demonstrated a non-significant difference in median (IQR) NRS at 2nd, 12th, and 24th hour between groups. Median (IQR) NRS score significantly lower in paracetamol-tramadol group at 4th, 6th and 8th hours compared to the paracetamol group ($p = 0.032$, $p = 0.022$ and $p = 0.007$ respectively). This result was comparable with the result of a study done by Solmaz and Kovalak which found that significantly lower VAS in acetaminophen- tramadol combination compared to acetaminophen alone at 1st and 2nd hour (2.10 ± 1.48 Vs. 4.75 ± 3.05 $p = 0.030$ and 3.30 ± 1.71 Vs. 6.10 ± 1.86 0.020, respectively). The difference in VAS between the groups disappeared in the second hour (3.45 ± 1.63 Vs. 3.95 ± 1.43 $p = 0.129$) [29].

In contrary to our finding, pain score (VAS) reported by Samimi et al. showed statistically significant difference among paracetamol-diclofenac combination,

Table 2 Time to first analgesic request in minutes and total analgesia consumption over 24 hours

	Group P	Group PD	Group PT	*P*-value
First analgesic requirement time (minutes)[a]	87.62 ± 20.95	103.01 ± 23.53^{+}	144.05 ± 14.72$^{+, ++}$	< 0.001
Total analgesics consumption				
o Tramadol in mg (IV)[a]	250 ± 79.06	173.81 ± 87.49^{+}	154.76 ± 70.54^{+}	0.001

Data are given as mean ± SD (ANOVA and Tukey test)
[a]Mean ± SD
$^{+}p < 0.05$ compared to Group P, $^{++}p < 0.05$ compared to Group PD

diclofenac group and placebo groups during the first 24 h ($p < 0.05$). The possible explanation for this difference in result might be due to pain management practice in study set up or the use of additional analgesic agent in perioperative period [26].

According to our study the mean time to first analgesia request in minutes were shorter in the paracetamol group ($M \pm SD$: 87.62 ± 20.95 min) compared to PD group (103.01 ± 23.53 min, $p = 0.001$) and PT groups (144.05 ± 14.72 min, $p < 0.001$). This finding is in line with study done by Samimi et al. ($p < 0.05$) [26].

Combining several analgesic modalities into a single analgesic regimen often referred to as multimodal analgesia, may hold the greatest promise for limiting sensitization of the nervous systems by noxious stimuli [30]. Effective pre-emptive analgesic techniques provide multi-level interruption of nociceptive inputs, increased pain threshold and decreased activation of nociceptors [23, 31]. Our results showed that combination therapy was superior to paracetamol alone. The low values of the pain scores in combination groups may be explained by decreased excitability in the central nervous system through blockade of nociceptive stimuli at different site before tissue damage.

The current study has certain limitations, including lack of control over the confounding factor like incision size and participation of different anesthetist and surgeon. In addition, one of the potential study design drawbacks is the shorter duration of postoperative follow up. The discussion part is limited by the unavailability of adequate studies to compare with our result.

Conclusion

Analgesic drug combination of paracetamol-tramadol and paracetamol-diclofenac reduce total tramadol consumption and prolongs time to first analgesic request compared to paracetamol before surgical intervention alone in patients undergoing laparotomy surgery. The paracetamol-tramadol combination seems superior to paracetamol-diclofenac combination.

Abbreviations

ASA: American Society of Anesthesiologists; CI: Confidence Interval; GA: General Anesthesia; NRS: Numerical Rating Scale; PACU: Post Anesthesia Care Unit; SPSS: Statistical Package for Social Sciences; VAS: Visual Analogue scale

Acknowledgements

We would like to thank Dilla University, College of Medicine and Health Science for funding this research. Our gratitude goes to supervisors, data collectors and study respondents. Finally, we would like to thank all those, who in one way or another have contributed to this work.

Research registration number

Pan African Clinical Trial Registry with the identification number of PACT R201908890749145.

Authors' contributions

Authors will take public responsibility for the contents, have contributed substantially to the drafting and preparation of the manuscript. All authors have read and approved the final version manuscript. ZA This author helped on substantial intellectual contributions to conception, design, and acquisition of data, analysis, and interpretation of data as well as on preparing the manuscript to this study. FS: have made substantial contributions to conception, design, and acquisition of data, analysis, and interpretation of data as well as on preparing the manuscript to this study. TS: This author contributed to conception, design, analysis and interpretation of data and give approval of the final version to be published. DN: has been involved in analysis, interpretation of data and drafting the manuscript and revising it critically for important intellectual contents.

Author details

[1]Department of Anesthesia, College of Medicine and Health Sciences, Dilla University, Dilla, Ethiopia. [2]Department of Anesthesia, Kotebe Metropolitan University, Menelik II Medical & Health Science College, Addis Ababa, Ethiopia.

References

1. IASP. Pain terminology. International Association for the Study of Pain Committee on Taxonomy. Washington DC: IASP; 2014.
2. Singh PK, Saikia P, Lahakar M. Prevalence of acute post-operative pain in patients in adult age-group undergoing inpatient abdominal surgery and correlation of intensity of pain and satisfaction with analgesic management: a cross-sectional single institute-based study. Ind J Anaesth. 2016;60(10):737.
3. Toro MM, John S, Faruqui AR. Pattern of use of analgesics in post-operative pain management in adults undergoing laparotomy surgery: a prospective observational study. Int Surg J. 2018;5(2):662–7.
4. Gan TJ. Poorly controlled postoperative pain: prevalence, consequences, and prevention. J Pain Res. 2017;10:2287–98 PubMed PMID: PMC5626380.
5. Gerbershagen HJ, Aduckathil S, van Wijck AJ, Peelen LM, Kalkman CJ, Meissner W. Pain intensity on the first day after surgery: a prospective cohort study comparing 179 surgical procedures. Anesthesiology. 2013; 118(4):934–44.
6. Apfelbaum JL, Chen C, Mehta SS, Gan TJ. Postoperative pain experience: results from a national survey suggest postoperative pain continues to be undermanaged. Anesth Analg. 2003;97(2):534–40.
7. Pasero C, Quinlan-Colwell A, Rae D, Broglio K, Drew D. American Society for Pain Management Nursing position statement: prescribing and administering opioid doses based solely on pain intensity. Pain Manag Nurs. 2016;17(3):170–80.
8. Moayedi M, Davis KD. Theories of pain: from specificity to gate control. J Neurophysiol. 2012;109(1):5–12.
9. De Lima L, Pastrana T, Radbruch L, Wenk R. Cross-sectional pilot study to monitor the availability, dispensed prices, and affordability of opioids around the globe. J Pain Symptom Manag. 2014;48(4):649–59.
10. De Lima L, Sweeney C, Palmer JL, Bruera E. Potent analgesics are more expensive for patients in developing countries: a comparative study. J Pain Palliat Care Pharmacother. 2004;18(1):59–70.
11. WHO. Measuring medicine prices, availability, affordability and price components. 2008.
12. Meissner W, Coluzzi F, Fletcher D, Huygen F, Morlion B, Neugebauer E, Pérez AM, Pergolizzi J. Improving the management of post-operative acute pain: priorities for change. Curr Med Res Opin. 2015;31(11):2131–43.
13. Stephens J, Laskin B, Pashos C, Pena B, Wong J. The burden of acute postoperative pain and the potential role of the COX-2-specific inhibitors. Rheumatology. 2003;42(Suppl. 3):iii40–52.
14. Garimella V, Cellini C. Postoperative pain control. Clin Colon Rectal Surg. 2013;26:191–6.
15. Chou R, Gordon DB, de Leon-Casasola OA, Rosenberg JM, Bickler S, Brennan T, et al. Guidelines on the management of postoperative pain management of postoperative pain: a clinical practice guideline from the American Pain Society, the American Society of Regional Anesthesia and Pain Medicine, and the American Society of Anesthesiologists' Committee on regional anesthesia, executive committee, and administrative council. J Pain. 2016; 17(2):131–57.
16. Elia N, Lysakowski C, Martin R. Does multimodal analgesia with acetaminophen, nonsteroidal antiinflammatory drugs, or selective

cyclooxygenase-2 inhibitors and patient-controlled analgesia morphine offer advantages over morphine alone? Meta-analyses of randomized trials. Anesthesiology. 2005;103(6):1296–304.

17. Chou R, Gordon DB, de Leon-Casasola OA, Rosenberg JM, Bickler S, Brennan T, et al. Management of Postoperative Pain: a clinical practice guideline from the American pain society, the American Society of Regional Anesthesia and Pain Medicine, and the American Society of Anesthesiologists' committee on regional anesthesia, executive committee, and administrative council. J Pain. 2016;17(2):131–57.
18. Gan TJ, Habib AS, Miller TE, White W, Apfelbaum JL. Incidence, patient satisfaction, and perceptions of post-surgical pain: results from a US national survey. Curr Med Res Opin. 2014;30(1):149–60.
19. Brennan TJ, Taylor BK. Analgesic treatment before incision compared with treatment after incision provides no improvement in postoperative pain relief. J Pain. 2000;1(2):96–8.
20. Brunelli C, Zecca E, Martini C, Campa T, Fagnoni E, Bagnasco M, Lanata L, Caraceni A. Comparison of numerical and verbal rating scales to measure pain exacerbations in patients with chronic cancer pain. Health Qual Life Outcomes. 2010;8:42.
21. Hjermstad MJ, Fayers P, Haugen DF, Caraceni A, Hanks GW, Loge JH, Fainsinger R, Aass N, Kaasa S. Studies comparing numerical rating scales, verbal rating scales, and visual analogue scales for assessment of pain intensity in adults: a systematic literature review. J Pain Symptom Manag. 2011;41(6):1073–93.
22. van Dijk JFM, van Wijck AJM, Kappen TH, Peelen LM, Kalkmana CJ, Schuurmans MJ. Postoperative pain assessment based on numeric ratings is not the same for patients and professionals: a cross-sectional study. Int J Nurs Stud. 2012;49:65–71.
23. Kissin I. Preemptive analgesia. Anesthesiology. 2000;93:1138–43.
24. American Society of Anesthesiologists Task Force on Acute Pain M. Practice guidelines for acute pain management in the perioperative setting: an updated report by the American Society of Anesthesiologists Task Force on Acute Pain Management. Anesthesiology. 2012;116(2):248–73.
25. McCaffery B. Pain clinical manual for nursing practice. St Louis: Mosby; 1989. p. 14.
26. Samimi SS, Davari TF, Valadan M, Modaressi Z. Comparison between preoperative rectal diclofenac plus paracetamol and diclofenac alone for postoperative pain of hysterectomy. J Family Reprod Health. 2014;8(3):91.
27. Montgomery JE, Sutherland CJ, Kestin IG, Sneyd JR. Morphine consumption in patients receiving rectal paracetamol and diclofenac alone and in combination. Br J Anaesth. 1996;77(4):445–7 PubMed PMID: 894232.
28. Riad W, Moussa A. Pre-operative analgesia with rectal diclofenac and/or paracetamol in children undergoing inguinal hernia repair. Anaesthesia. 2007;62(12):1241–5 PubMed PMID: 17991260.
29. Solmaz FA, Kovalak E. Comparison of tramadol/acetaminophen fixed-dose combination, tramadol, and acetaminophen in patients undergoing ambulatory arthroscopic meniscectomy. Acta Orthop Traumatol Turc. 2018; 52(3):222–5.
30. Kim S-I, Ha K-Y, Oh I-S. Preemptive multimodal analgesia for postoperative pain management after lumbar fusion surgery: a randomized controlled trial. Eur Spine J. 2016;25(5):1614–9.
31. Rosero EB, Joshi GP. Preemptive, preventive, multimodal analgesia: what do they really mean? Plast Reconstr Surg. 2014;134(4 Suppl 2):85S–93S PubMed PMID: 25255012.

22

A prospective observational study testing liquid crystal phase change type thermometer placed on skin against oesophageal/pharyngeal placed thermometers in participants undergoing general anesthesia

G. Simpson[1*] and R. N. Rodseth[1,2]

Abstracts

Background: Patient outcomes are influenced by intraoperative temperature management. Oesophageal/pharyngeal temperature monitoring is the standard of care at our institute but is not well tolerated in awake patients. Many non-invasive temperature monitors have been studied. Only the TraxIt® Wearable Children's Underarm Thermometer which contains liquid crystals that undergo phase changes according to temperature is available at our institution. We tested these non-invasive monitors against our standard of care which is the oesophageal/pharyngeal temperature monitor.

Methods: We conducted a prospective observational study of 100 patients receiving general anaesthesia for elective surgery. Patients were eligible for inclusion if they were ≥ 18 years old, were planned to have a general anaesthetic > 60 min during which no body cavity (chest or abdomen) would be opened. Patient temperature was measured with an oesophageal/pharyngeal thermistor probe and skin surface temperature monitors placed over the forehead, in the axilla, over the sternum, and behind the ear (over major vessels to the brain). Temperatures were recorded and then analysed using Altman-Bland plots. Pre-determined clinically relevant limits of agreement were set at −/+ 0.5 °C.

Results: From the 100 patients we collected 500 data points for each monitor with an average monitoring time of 102 min (30–300 min) across a range of surgical procedures. None of the skin surface temperature monitors achieved the pre-determined limits of agreement and results were impacted by the use of a forced air warmer.

Conclusion: The TraxIt® Wearable Children's Underarm Thermometers are not suitable for temperature monitoring during general anaesthesia.

Keywords: Thermoregulation, Thermometry, Thermometers, Intraoperative monitoring, Observational study

* Correspondence: drgcsimpson@gmail.com
[1]Metropolitan Department of Anaesthetics, Critical Care and Pain Management, University of KwaZulu-Natal, 4 Montrose, Hillcrest, Pietermaritzburg, South Africa

Background

Patient outcome after surgery is strongly influenced by intraoperative temperature management [1–3]. Oesophageal and pharyngeal temperature probes are the standard of care for intraoperative temperature monitoring but are not well tolerated in awake patients [4]. Temperature monitoring in the awake patient is available and range from invasive (e.g. Pulmonary artery catheter thermistor) to semi-invasive (e.g. oral) and non-invasive (e.g. SpotOn Thermometer [5], DoubleSensor thermometer [6] and Temple Touch Pro [7]), however these are not widely endorsed or available for use at our institution.

An alternative temperature monitoring device available at our institution is the Traxit® Wearable Children's Underarm Thermometer. This thermometer utilises liquid crystals that have phase change properties when heated and is read using a dot matrix grid. The purported advantage of such a monitor is that it could be placed on the patient before anaesthesia while in the ward and could serve as the sole temperature monitor throughout the patient's anaesthetic journey from ward to theatre and back again.

We tested the performance of these monitors using an oesophageal/pharyngeal temperature monitor as a reference in a prospective observational study in patients undergoing elective surgery.

Methods

Approval for this study was obtained from the University of KwaZulu-Natal Bio-Ethics Research Committee (BREC BE078/17). Permission was obtained from Grey's Hospital, Pietermaritzburg, KwaZulu-Natal to recruit participants after approval was granted by the Health Research Committee of the KwaZulu-Natal Department of Health (NHRD Ref: KZ_2016RP_297).

We conducted a prospective observational study in 100 adult patients receiving general anaesthesia for elective surgery. Patients were eligible for inclusion if they were ≥ 18 years old, planned to have an anaesthetic for longer than 60 min (to allow sufficient time for monitor warm up and increase the number of data points for analysis) during which no body cavity would be opened, this was to limit possible confounders such as fluid and heat loss from exposed bowel or possible need for rapid or large volume fluid administration that are common in emergency setting and open body cavity procedures. Patient refusal was the only exclusion criteria.

An oesophageal/pharyngeal thermistor temperature probe was placed between 10 and 20 cm from the nares, as insertion to this depth provides temperatures comparable to distal oesophageal temperatures and acted as a reference temperature [5]. This thermistor probe was not calibrated outside of the mandated yearly maintenance. This thermistor probe is the standard of care for temperature monitoring while under general anaesthesia at our institution (i.e. Is routinely inserted to monitor temperature whilst patients are under general anaesthesia). These measurements were then used to test the performance of the study thermometer – a skin temperature monitor that utilises liquid crystal phase change properties and is read using a dot matrix (TraxIt® Wearable Children's Underarm Thermometer, already available and in use at our institution). Study thermometers were placed behind the ear (over major vessels to the brain), in the axillary apex (as recommended by manufacturer), over the sternum (over the precordium/heart), and over the middle of the forehead (may represent temperature of underlying brain) and as directed by previously published studies of temperature monitoring.

Temperatures were recorded at 15-min intervals, time 0 being the time when the probe was first placed. The study thermometers do not require calibration before use and have a manufacture reported accuracy of − 0.1 °C and + 0.2 °C within the range of 35.0 °C to 39.0 °C. Forced air warming devices (FAW) (3 M™ *Bair Hugger*™ System) were used at the discretion of the anaesthesia provider based on the oesophageal/pharyngeal temperature monitor. Upper body FAW were used, these cover the upper chest and both arms when a patient is in a supine position. An upper body FAW does cover the skin temperature monitor placed over the sternum.

Using a standardized data collection tool (Additional file 1) we collected patient demographics (age, gender, weight, height), type of surgery, use of a FAW, and the temperature reading on the monitors at 15-min intervals. In addition, the data collection tool provided a comments section to provide subjective feedback from the anaesthetic provider regarding the use of the monitoring devices.

Eligible study participants were approached and verbally informed about the study. If they were interested in participating, they were provided with written study information in English or isiZulu and written consent was obtained. A written copy of the study information and contact details of the principal investigator were given to the participants. Participants were assigned study numbers and their identifiable details were separated from the study information to ensure anonymity. Data was analysed using Microsoft Excel.

Assuming an effect size difference of 0.5, an α of 0.05, and 80% power we required a sample size of 64 participants. However, as suggested by Professor Martin Bland (https://www-users.york.ac.uk/~mb55/meas/sizemeth.htm) [8], we decided to include 100 participants using pragmatic sequential sampling. We conducted 5 assessments, first a composite comparison and then each monitor site's performance compared to the oesophageal/pharyngeal monitor. We also examined the impact of FAW on the results.

Difference plots, also known as Altman and Bland plots, were used to assess the performance of the skin surface temperature monitor readings as obtained from the four difference sites to the oesophageal/pharyngeal temperature readings. Difference plots aim to compare the test monitoring device to the conventional monitoring device. They plot the difference between the reading of the two monitors against the average of the readings of the two monitors. A bias line is calculated as the average of the difference between the two readings and represents the average discrepancy between the two methods. Upper and lower limits of agreement represent two standard deviations either side of the bias line. However, prior temperature studies have determined that the clinically useful limits of agreement are +/− 0.5 °C [9]. The interpretation of Altman-Bland plots relies on these clinically determined limits of agreement, how wide the limits of agreement are, and whether a trend emerges in the variability of the data points across the plot.

Incomplete and insufficient data points were reported in the results and then excluded from analysis. Participants were examined in the post-anaesthetic care unit to ensure no adverse skin reactions to the skin temperature monitors.

Results

The study recruited 100 participants from October 2017 to January 2018. All potential participants approached consented to be enrolled in the study. The median age of participants was 39.5 years (range 18–73 years), 53% were female and procedures ranged from general surgery with laparoscopic approach (36%) to burns (2%). Other procedures included orthopaedic upper and lower limb surgery, laparoscopic gynaecological procedures and cystoscopic urological procedures. Participants were under anaesthesia for a median time of 90 min with 60 min being the most frequent duration of anaesthesia (range 30 to 300 min). FAW devices were used for 75% of the participants. Fifty-five of the 400 monitors tested failed to heat up during the recording period: 23% of the forehead monitors, 10% of sternal, 9% of temperature monitor placed behind the ear (over major vessels to the brain), and 13% of axillary monitors. There were 8 incomplete data sheets and 4 participants were not monitored for the correct length of time - these incomplete data points were not included in the analysis.

Interpretation of the Altman Bland plots are included below each plot. The aim of this study was to determine the agreement between the two monitors. If the monitors perfectly agreed all data points would fall on the zero-line indicating no difference in readings. The bias line (i.e. the extent to which one method varies with respect to another when the two methods are compared is plotted as a red solid line) shows the mean difference or average discrepancy between the two monitors. Two standard deviations above and below the bias line represent the upper and lower limits of agreement (yellow broken lines). In this study we also included predetermined limits of agreement of +/− 0.5 °C to indicate clinically utility (green broken lines).

Figure 1, a composite average of all readings at specific time intervals, does not accurately represent the usefulness of the skin temperature monitors but merely offers a visual representation of the trends of the monitors studied. The oesophageal monitor started at a higher base line temperature when compared to the skin temperature monitors and approximated core temperature within 15 min, this is a function of the relatively rapidly responding oesophageal monitor when compared to the skin monitors. Only the axillary skin temperature appeared to visually approach the trend of the oesophageal temperature monitor. The sternally placed probe overshot the oesophageal temperature readings, while the forehead monitor appeared to initially approximate the trend of the

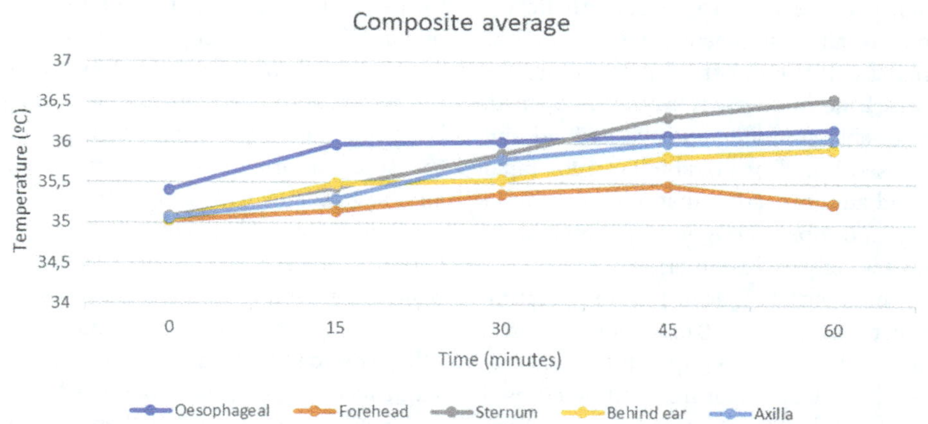

Fig. 1 Composite averages of temperature monitors placed on the forehead, sternum, behind the ear, in the axilla and compared to an oesophageal monitor

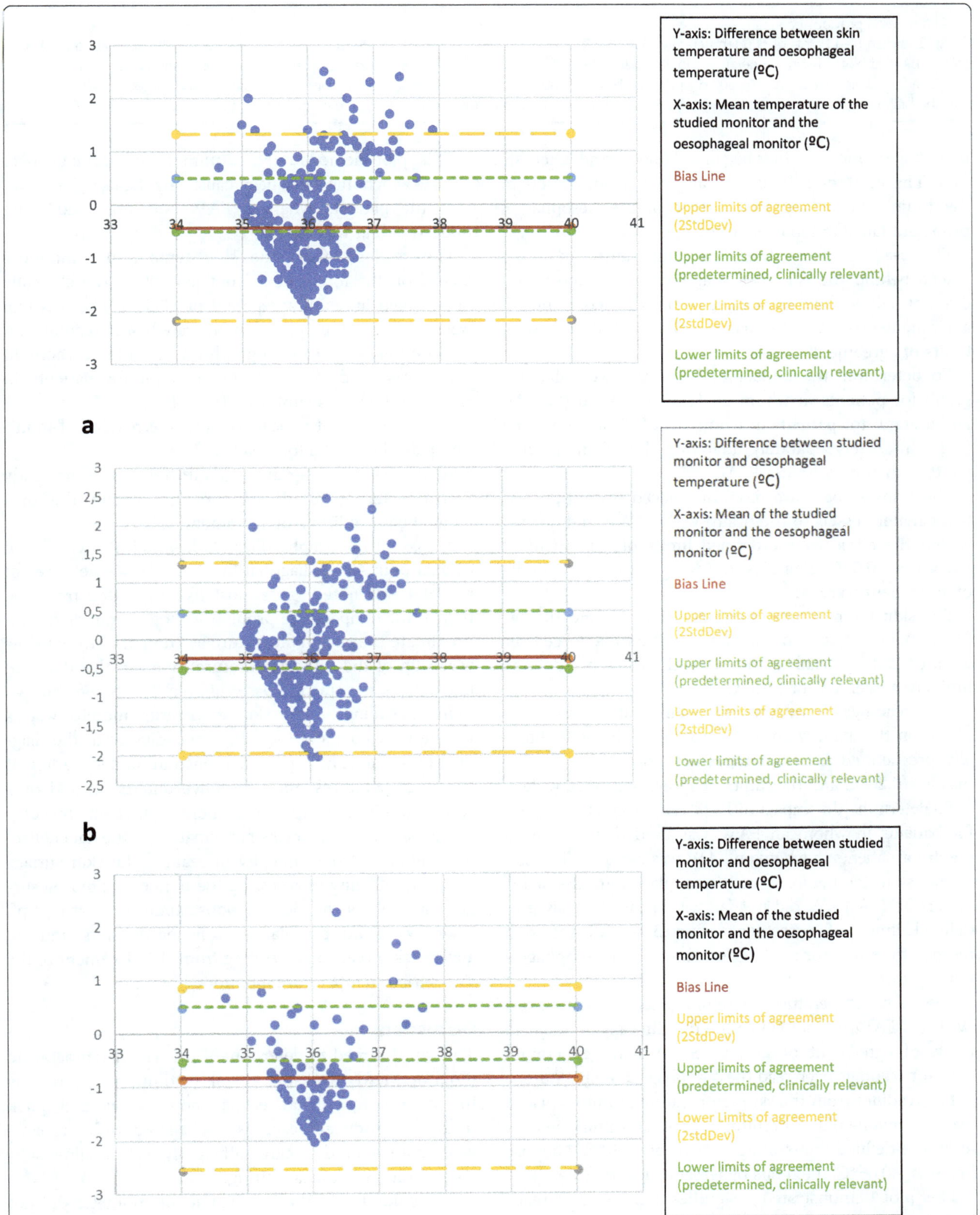

Fig. 2 (See legend on next page.)

(See figure on previous page.)
Fig. 2 Altman-Bland plots of skin temperature monitor placed behind ear as compared to oesophageal temperature. (n = 92; 368 data points). **a** Altman-Bland plots of skin temperature monitor placed behind the ear (over major vessels to the brain) compared to oesophageal temperature WITH a forced air warmer (n = 75; 300 data points). **b** Altman-Bland plots of skin temperature monitor placed behind the ear (over major vessels to the brain) compared to oesophageal temperature WITHOUT a forced air warmer (n = 17; 68 data points)

oesophageal monitor but began to under read after 45 min. The monitor behind the ear (over major vessels to the brain) slowly approached that of the oesophageal probe but failed to follow its trend.

The readings from the skin temperature monitors placed behind the ear (over major vessels to the brain) did not fall within the clinically pre-defined limits of agreement (±0.5 °C), the bias is – 0.43 °C but with wide limits of agreement.

To determine the impact of FAW use we created a graph for patients in whom an FAW was used (Fig. 2a) and a graph for patients in whom an FAW was not used (Fig. 2b). After separately analysing data from participants with and without a FAW.

The skin temperature monitors placed behind the ear (over major vessels to the brain) with a FAW did not fall within the clinically pre-defined limits of agreement of – 0.5 and + 0.5 °C. The bias line was – 0.31 °C, the limits of agreement were wide.

The skin temperature monitors placed behind the ear (over major vessels to the brain) without a forced air warmer did not fall within the clinically pre-defined limits of agreement of ±0.5 °C.

The readings from the skin temperature monitors placed in the axillary apex did not fall within the clinically pre-defined limits of agreement of ± – 0.5 °C. The bias is – 0.26 °C and the limits of agreement were wide.

To determine the impact of FAW use we created a graph for patients in whom an FAW was used (Fig. 3a) and a graph for patients in whom an FAW was not used (Fig. 3b).

The skin temperature monitors placed in the axilla WITHOUT A FAW did not fall within the clinically pre-defined limits of agreement of ±0.5 °C. All the skin temperature monitor readings under-read the oesophageal temperature.

The skin temperature monitors placed in the axilla WITH A FAW did not fall within the clinically pre-defined limits of agreement of ±0.5 °C. Some skin temperature monitor readings over-read the oesophageal temperature.

The readings from the skin temperature monitors placed over the middle of the sternum did not fall within the clinically pre-defined limits of agreement of ±0.5 °C. The bias line was – 0.66 °C, the limits of agreement were wide.

This plot demonstrated a significant number of readings over 37.5 °C which may have been caused using an FAW. To explore this, we created a graph for patients in whom an FAW was used (Fig. 4a) and a graph for patients in whom an FAW was not used (Fig. 4b).

This plot demonstrated a number of readings over 37.5 °C which may have been caused by the use of a FAW.

In the patients where a FAW was not used more under-reading was noted.

The readings from the skin temperature monitors placed on the forehead did not fall within the clinically pre-defined limits of agreement of ±0.5 °C. The bias line was – 0.66 °C. This plot demonstrated over-reading. To explore this, we created a graph for patients in whom an FAW was used (Fig. 5a) and a graph for patients in whom an FAW was not used (Fig. 5b).

A FAW does not appear to affect the reading of monitors placed over the forehead.

Surface skin temperature monitoring using the study thermometers (TraxIt®) did not fall within the pre-defined clinical limits of agreement.

Across all the graphs (Figs. 2, 3, 4 and 5) a clustering of data points in a diagonal line in the lower left area of the plot was noted. This most likely resulted from the thermistor temperature probe warming up rapidly to approximate the core temperature as compared to the slow warm up of the skin temperature monitor; this diagonal line acts as the starting/base difference between the two monitor readings. As the skin temperature monitor warms up the data points are spread perpendicular to the diagonal base line. These plots demonstrate under reading at lower temperatures (more negative difference) and over reading at higher temperature (more positive difference).

Feedback from clinicians participating in the data collection bemoaned the difficulty of reading the skin surface monitor; difficulty in accessing these monitors during surgery; as well as the slow response time in "heating up". There were no complaints from participants and no adverse skin reactions resulting from the placement of the skin surface temperature monitors.

Discussion

This study aimed to determine if the Traxit temperature monitor (newly available at our institution, cheap, easy to use in many clinical settings, non-invasive and quick to apply) produced readings that agreed with the conventional standard of care sufficiently well to allow substitution in our clinical setting.

This study found that the Traxit thermometer did not perform adequately enough to be used during general anaesthesia. None of the sites tested achieved the clinically relevant predetermined limits of agreement (+/– 0.5 °C).

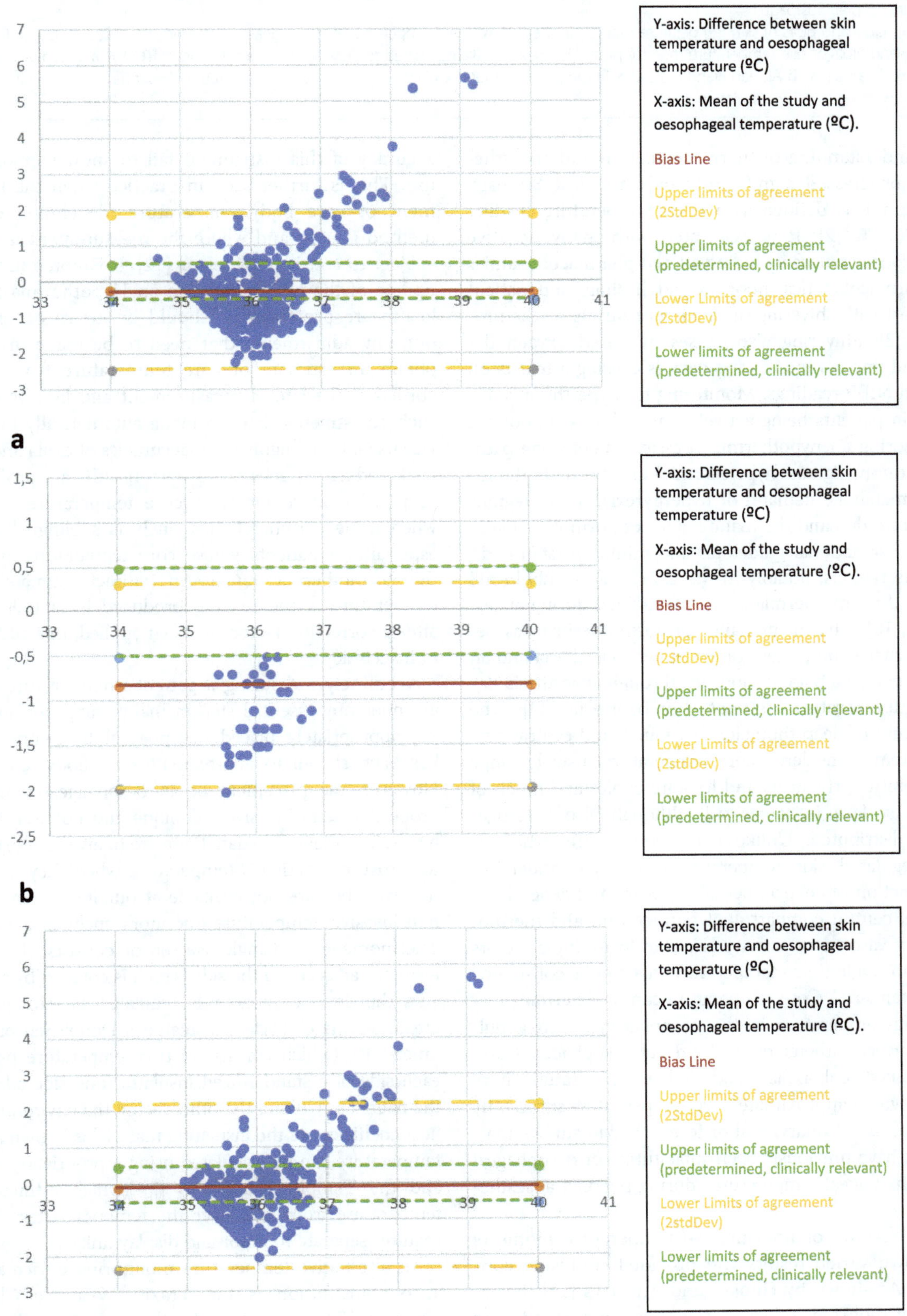

Fig. 3 (See legend on next page.)

(See figure on previous page.)

Fig. 3 Altman-Bland plots of skin temperature monitor in the axillary apex compared to oesophageal temperature. ($n = 92$; 368 data points). **a** Altman Bland Plots of skin temperature monitor placed in apex of axilla compared to Oesophageal temperature WITHOUT a forced air warmer ($N = 17$; 68data points). **b** Altman Bland Plots of Skin temperature monitor placed in apex of axilla compared to Oesophageal temperature WITH a forced air warmer. ($N = 75$; 300 data points)

Our understanding of thermoregulation and anaesthesia has progressed significantly over the last 30 years. Hypothermia is defined as a body temperature reading below 36.0 °C [2]. It is associated with many negative clinical consequences including altered pharmacodynamics and pharmacokinetics, poor wound healing, and patient discomfort with shivering on waking or during awake procedures [2]. Shivering also causes increased oxygen demand and impairs monitoring devices causing artefacts on ECG and NIBP readings. Monitoring for hyperthermia, especially in patients being actively warmed, is as important as monitoring for hypothermia. It assists in detecting pathologies (e.g. malignant hyperthermia) and prevents the increased metabolic demand of hyperpyrexia. Many regions in the world demand the maintenance of normothermia as part of their national guidelines and minimum standards, and some regions, notably in the USA, may withhold full payment if normothermia is not maintained during anaesthesia [9, 10]. The maintenance of normothermia has become a crucial component of providing anaesthesia and an essential part of a patient's journey through anaesthesia [9].

Body temperature is not homogeneous [2]: the temperature of deep thoracic, abdominal, and central nervous system (considered core temperature) usually range in temperature, the arms and legs are cooler and much of the skin surface is cooler still although also heterogeneously distributed. Unlike core temperature, which is tightly regulated, skin temperature can vary considerably. It is a function of environmental exposure and depends on exposure, central compartment temperature and thermoregulatory vasomotor activity [1]. Due to multiple factors there is no single tissue temperature that can be considered a "gold standard". Core temperature can be determined by measuring temperature in the nasopharynx, with a pulmonary artery catheter or in the distal oesophagus. Carefully obtained oral, axillary and bladder temperatures have been shown to approximate core temperatures sufficiently for clinical use. Axillary, oral or forehead skin surface temperatures have previously been substituted for oesophageal or nasopharyngeal temperatures during regional anaesthesia [11].

Earlier reviews of non-invasive temperature monitors have shown varied results and provided confusing conclusions. As shown by Hooper and Andrews [11] the results they reported indicated that tympanic monitoring is commonly used but high-quality evidence supporting the accuracy of tympanic thermometry is lacking, and in fact, the most recent high-quality studies evaluating the accuracy of this instrument fail to show support for its use. This is further seen in practice when the measurement of core body temperature, depending on what method is used and where the measurement is made, is subject to considerable error [12]. It is noted in the 2018 update of the NICE guidance on Hypothermia [13] that healthcare professionals should be aware of, and carry out, any adjustments that need to be made in order to obtain an estimate of core temperature from that recorded at the site of measurement and be aware of any such adjustments that are made automatically by the device used. It highlights the inaccuracies of axilla and sublingual readings. It goes on to warn health care professionals of possible inaccuracies in core temperature estimation when using peripheral sites, such as sublingual or axilla, especially in patients whose core temperature is outside the normothermic range. An indirect estimate of core temperature is the reading produced by a thermometer after a correction factor has been applied, this adds a layer of inaccuracy.

Accurately measuring a patient's temperature remains an inherently essential step in maintaining normothermia. An appropriately placed oesophageal temperature probe has been shown to approximate core body temperature. However, the placement of an oesophageal temperature probe is a semi-invasive technique and not well tolerated by awake patients. To date there are many suitable methods to measure a patient's temperature when they are awake, however they are not available at our institution. Semi or non-invasive temperature monitors include the SpotOn Thermometer [5] (single-use sensor consists of a thermal insulator adjacent to the skin which is covered by a flex circuit, the flex circuit actively regulates its temperature to create a zone of perfect insulation), DoubleSensor thermometer [6] (which consists of two temperature probes on each side of a standardized insulator, one side adjacent to the patient's skin and the other facing the environment, the heat coefficient of the insulating material is known and core temperature can be calculated using a proprietary formula) and the Temple Touch Pro [7] (which estimates core temperature from skin over the temporal artery but also requires separate monitor and display unit).

An alternative temperature monitoring device available at our institution is the Traxit® Wearable Children's Underarm Thermometer. This thermometer utilises liquid crystals that have phase change properties when heated and is read using a dot matrix grid. The purported advantage of such a monitor is that it could be placed on the

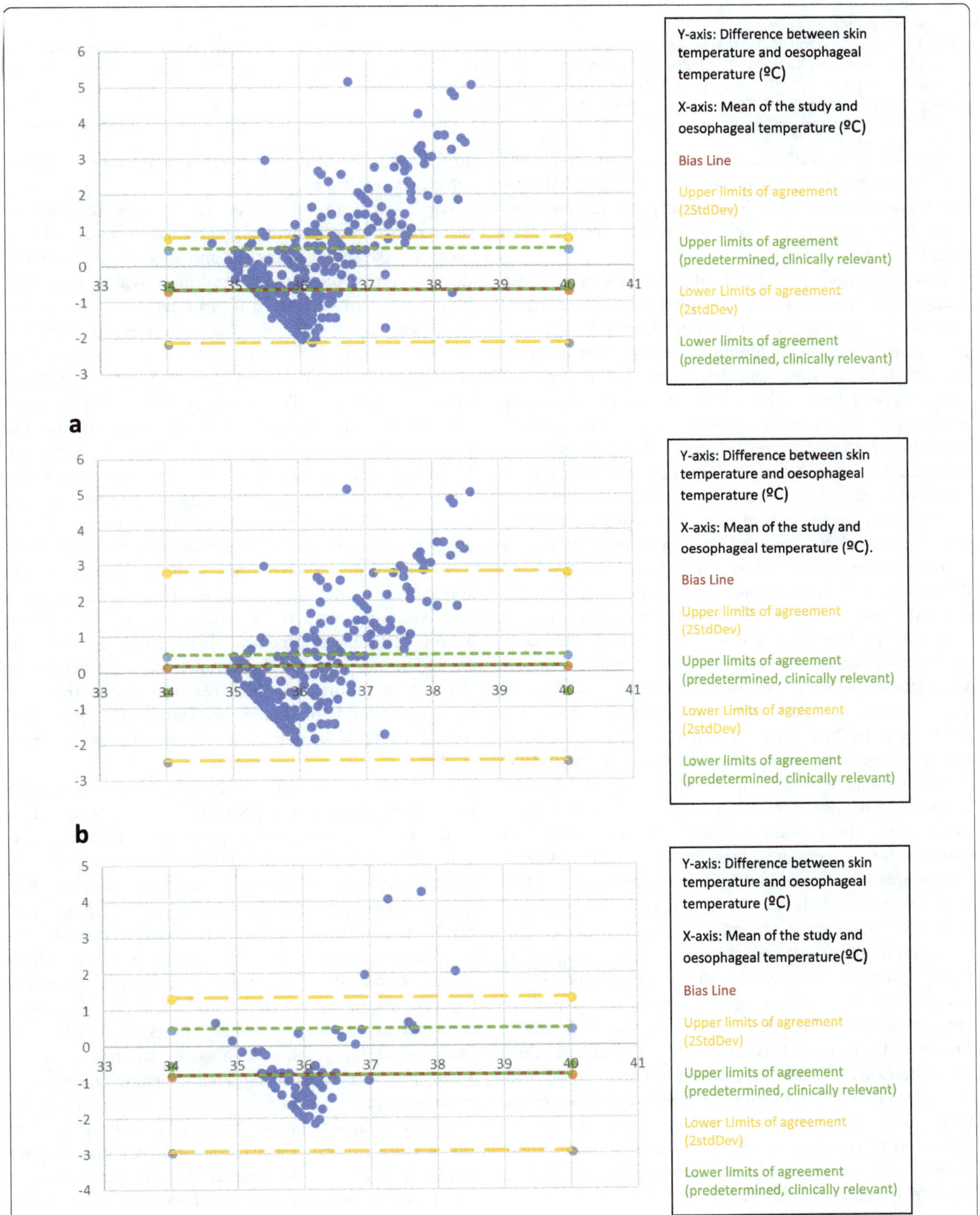

Fig. 4 (See legend on next page.)

(See figure on previous page.)
Fig. 4 Altman-Bland plots of skin temperature monitor on the middle of the sternum as compared to oesophageal temperature. (n = 92; 368 data points). **a** Altman-Bland Plots of skin temperature monitor on the middle of the sternum compared to oesophageal temperature WITH a forced air warmer (N = 75 [300 data points]). **b** Altman-Bland Plots of skin temperature monitor on the middle of the sternum compared to oesophageal temperature WITHOUT a forced air warmer (N = 17; 68 data points)

patient before anaesthesia while in the ward and could serve as the sole temperature monitor throughout the patient's anaesthetic journey from ward to theatre and back again. Unfortunately, they were shown not to be of clinical value.

This study used Altman-bland plots to compare two methods of measurement, the pharyngeal/oesophageal thermistor (the standard of care at our institution) and the Traxit® Wearable Children's Underarm Thermometer. Altman-bland plots are considered superior to simple regression/correlation analysis. Previous studies comparing non-invasive temperature monitors used similar methods to analysis performance of monitors. Kimberger et al. [6] collected data from 56 patients (general anaesthesia and regional anaesthesia) and found the average bias to be − 0.13 °C with narrow limits of agreement (− 0.65 to 0.40 °C). The Spoton deep forehead non-invasive temperature monitor was evaluated by Kato [5] in 2015. Kato examined 20 patients following cardiac surgery and compared the Spoton thermometer to the pulmonary artery catheter thermometer, they were able to collect and analyse over 16,000 data points. Altman-Bland plots were again used and clinical limits of agreement were agreed to be +/− 0.5 °C. A bias of − 0.28 °C with narrow limits of agreement were found. In 2017 Evron and colleges [7] examined the Temple Touch Pro device, they also used Altman-bland plots to compare the Temple Touch Pro to reference temperature measured in the naso-pharynx or oesophagus. Evron tested the hypothesis that the Temple touch pro non-invasive temperature measurement system estimates core temperature to within 0.5 °C of reference values. They were able to conclude cutaneous temporal TTP temperatures were sufficiently accurate for routine clinical use, with 94% of all measurements across a range of ages and types of surgery being within ±0.5 °C of reference distal oesophageal or naso-pharyngeal reference core temperatures. This study clearly shows that the Traxit® Wearable Children's Underarm Thermometer is not of clinical value. Traxit® Wearable Children's Underarm Thermometer had bias values of − 0.43 °C (behind the ear (over major vessels to the brain)), − 0.26 °C (in the axilla), − 0.66 °C (sternum) and − 0.66 °C (forehead) with wide limits of agreement. None of the results fell within the pre-defined clinical limits of agreement of +/− 0.5 °C.

Importantly, 55 of the 400 (14%) monitors failed to give a reading above 35 °C, the minimum displayed temperature of the Traxit® Wearable Children's Underarm Thermometer. This was a notable finding when compared to the reliability of the oesophageal temperature monitor which never failed to heat up.

Forced air warming devices (FAW) were placed at the discretion of the individual anaesthetic providers based on their assessment of patient and surgical factors. FAW devices consist of a heat generating device and a fan or blowing system connected to a perforated 'blanket' that is placed over the patient. Many devices are available, the Bair Hugger 3 M is available in the intuition that conducted this study. It has three temperature settings and two fan modes. They work by radiant shielding and convection. They provide a buffer of warm air over the patient's skin so heat loss via radiation is minimised. FAW devices heat the patient's skin by convection/facilitated conduction by inducing a flow of warm air over the patient's skin. Ambient temperature should not affect the monitor as they are insulated but the mechanism of FAW devices may impact on the accuracy of the surface skin temperature monitors. This was investigated by separating out the study participants into those where a FAW device was used and those where one was not used. The use of a FAW did not impact the results, in that no monitors provided reading within the pre-determined limits of agreement. The use of a FAW impacted readings by falsely increasing the temperature readings.

A theoretical limitation of skin temperature monitoring is the establishment of a peripheral to core temperature gradient. This gradient develops as the patient vasoconstricts in the presence of hypothermia to preserve heat and maintain core temperature. Skin temperature is often quoted as being up to 2 °C cooler than core temperature. However, the thermoregulatory response to hypothermia is reduced when under general anaesthesia. The threshold for skin vasoconstriction is reduced, and only becomes active at core temperatures less than 34.5 °C [9, 10]. This, in combination with the vasodilatory effects of general anaesthetic agents (propofol, volatile agents and regional techniques), makes interpreting and assigning a definitive number to skin temperatures in relation to core temperatures under anaesthesia difficult. It is also noted that temperature of vital organs is not homogenous, for example the brain may be warmer than the kidneys. Also, skin temperature has a wide variation determined by exposure and proximity to the central components. Big toe temperatures are different to axillary temperatures which in turn are different to forehead temperatures. This study aimed to find a suitable device that could substitute the

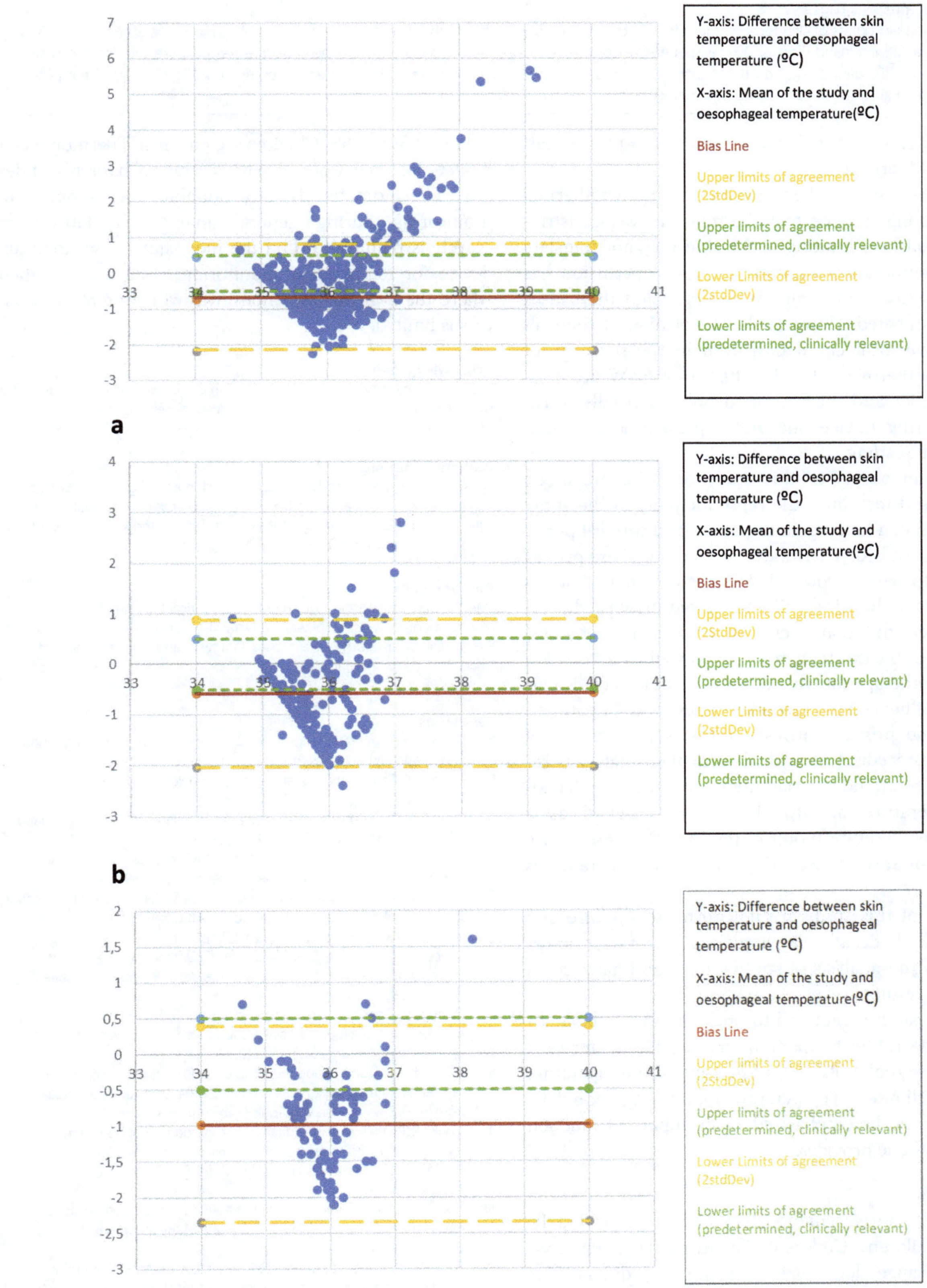

Fig. 5 (See legend on next page.)

(See figure on previous page.)
Fig. 5 Altman-Bland plots of skin temperature monitor over the middle of the forehead as compared to oesophageal temperature. (n = 92; 368 data points). **a** Altman-Bland Plots of skin temperature monitor over the forehead as compared to oesophageal temperature WITH a forced air warmer. (N = 75; 300 data points). **b** Altman-Bland Plots of skin temperature monitor over the forehead as compared to oesophageal temperature without a forced air warmer. (N = 17; 68 data points)

standard of care in our facility which is the pharyngeal/oesophageal thermistor.

FAW devices may be better at preventing hypothermia than correcting it once hypothermia and vasoconstriction is established. Heating of the skin may not translate into core temperature warming until skin perfusion has improved, vasoconstriction has reversed and the causes of heat loss abated. However, local warming of the skin may improve local circulation even in the presence of central hypothermia [14]. The effect of a FAW are difficult to predict and may serve to only externally warm the monitoring device and not represent a true skin temperature reading.

Further limitations to this study are, the pragmatic sampling used may limit the reproducibility of the study as it resulted in a heterogenous patient and surgical population being studied. Thermodynamics of an obese patient presenting for laparoscopic cholecystectomy may differ as compared to a chronically ill and wasted orthopaedic patient. Further limitations include non-uniformity of ambient operating theatre temperatures, as well as a variation in pharmacotherapy for which data was not collected. This may have influenced the vasodilatory response of patients. Although the principal investigator was present at the start of the procedure, individual participants data was recorded by the attending anaesthetic provider. The Traxit Skin temperature monitor has been designed as a paediatric temperature monitor, the impact of probe size and foot print area on measuring an adult's temperature is unknown.

Strengths of this study are its prospective nature and pragmatic study design. The large number of data points has allowed sub-analysis of study groups and has yielded meaningful results.

Future research is required to find the most suitable location and device for temperature monitoring in an awake patient where the availability of non-invasive temperature monitors is limited. Temperature monitoring should be compulsory and be emphasized as an important function of the anaesthetic provider.

Conclusion

Temperature measurements recorded with a TraxIt® Wearable Children's Underarm Thermometer (liquid crystal phase change dot matrix thermometer) did not fall within the clinically applicable predefined limits of agreement. They also demonstrated a high failure rate and were found to be poorly responsive. They proved to be unreliable, unresponsive and inaccurate. The practicality of using a TraxIt® Wearable Children's Underarm Thermometer is limited. Placement of a TraxIt® Wearable Children's Underarm Thermometer is not suitable for temperature monitoring during general anaesthesia. Future research is required to find the most suitable location and device for temperature monitoring in an awake patient where the availability of non-invasive temperature monitors is limited.

Acknowledgements
The authors have no conflict of interest. Financial assistance was provided by UKZN Department of anaesthesia Grey's Hospital Research Fund in purchasing the study probes.

Authors' contributions
GS and RNR conceived the study and shared in its design. GS undertook data collection, data capturing and handling. GS coordinated data analysis with assistance and review by RNR. GS and RNR drafted the manuscript. Both GS and RNR read and approved the final manuscript.

Author details
[1]Metropolitan Department of Anaesthetics, Critical Care and Pain Management, University of KwaZulu-Natal, 4 Montrose, Hillcrest, Pietermaritzburg, South Africa. [2]Jones, Bhagwan and Partners, Specialist Anaesthetists, Pietermaritzburg, South Africa.

References

1. Sessler DI. Temperature monitoring and perioperative thermoregulation. Anesthesiology. 2008;109(2):318–38.
2. Sessler DI. Complications and treatment of mild hypothermia. Anesthesiology. 2001;95(2):531–43.
3. Hopf HW. Perioperative temperature management: time for a new standard of care? Anesthesiology. 2015;122(2):229–30.
4. Frank SM, Nguyen JM, Garcia CM, Barnes RA. Temperature monitoring practices during regional anesthesia. Anesth Analg. 1999;88(2):373–7.
5. Kato H, Kawashima S, Mimuro S, Obata Y, Doi M, Nakajima Y. An evaluation of deep-forehead temperature (spoton®) in ICU patients after cardiac surgery. Intensive Care Med Exp. 2015;3(1):A111.
6. Kimberger O, Saager L, Egan C, Sanchez IP, Dizili S, Koch J, et al. The accuracy of a disposable noninvasive core thermometer. Can J Anaesth. 2013;60(12):1190–6.
7. Evron S, Weissman A, Toivis V, Shahaf DB, You J, Sessler DI, et al. Evaluation of the temple touch pro, a novel noninvasive core-temperature monitoring system. Anesth Analg. 2017;125(1):103–9.
8. Bland M. How can I decide the sample size for a study of agreement between two methods of measurement? 2004. Updated 2004. Available from: https://www-users.york.ac.uk/~mb55/meas/sizemeth.htm.
9. Matika R, Ibrahim M, Patwardhan A. The importance of body temperature: an anesthesiologist's perspective. Temperature (Austin). 2016;4(1):9–12.
10. Sessler DI. Mild perioperative hypothermia. N Engl J Med. 1997; 336(24):1730–7.
11. Hooper VD, Andrews JO. Accuracy of noninvasive core temperature measurement in acutely ill adults: the state of the science. Biol Res Nurs. 2006;8(1):24–34.
12. Torossian A, Bräuer A, Höcker J, Bein B, Wulf H, Horn E-P. Preventing inadvertent perioperative hypothermia. Dtsch Arztebl Int. 2015;112(10):166–72.
13. excellence NNifhac. Hypothermia: prevention and management in adults having surgery. NICE clinical guidline. 2008;23 April 2008.
14. Sheffield CW, Sessler DI, Hopf HW, Schroeder M, Moayeri A, Hunt TK, et al. Centrally and locally mediated thermoregulatory responses alter subcutaneous oxygen tension. Wound Repair Regen. 1996;4(3):339–45.

23

Monitoring of anesthetic depth and EEG band power using phase lag entropy during propofol anesthesia

Hye Won Shin[1*], Hyun Jung Kim[2], Yoo Kyung Jang[1], Hae Sun You[1], Hyub Huh[1], Yoon Ji Choi[3], Seung Uk Choi[1] and Ji Su Hong[1]

Abstract

Background: Phase lag entropy (PLE) is a novel anesthetic depth indicator that uses four-channel electroencephalography (EEG) to measure the temporal pattern diversity in the phase relationship of frequency signals in the brain. The purpose of the study was to evaluate the anesthetic depth monitoring using PLE and to evaluate the correlation between PLE and bispectral index (BIS) values during propofol anesthesia.

Methods: In thirty-five adult patients undergoing elective surgery, anesthesia was induced with propofol using target-controlled infusion (the Schneider model). We recorded the PLE value, raw EEG, BIS value, and hemodynamic data when the target effect-site concentration (Ce) of propofol reached 2, 3, 4, 5, and 6 μg/ml before intubation and 6, 5, 4, 3, 2 μg/ml after intubation and injection of muscle relaxant. We analyzed whether PLE and raw EEG data from the PLE monitor reflected the anesthetic depth as the Ce of propofol changed, and whether PLE values were comparable to BIS values.

Results: PLE values were inversely correlated to changes in propofol Ce (propofol Ce from 0 to 6.0 μg/ml, $r^2 = -0.83$; propofol Ce from 6.0 to 2.0 μg/ml, $r^2 = -0.46$). In the spectral analysis of EEG acquired from the PLE monitor, the persistence spectrogram revealed a wide distribution of power at loss of consciousness (LOC) and recovery of consciousness (ROC), with a narrow distribution during unconsciousness. The power spectrogram showed the typical pattern seen in propofol anesthesia with slow alpha frequency band oscillation. The PLE value demonstrated a strong correlation with the BIS value during the change in propofol Ce from 0 to 6.0 μg/ml ($r^2 = 0.84$). PLE and BIS values were similar at LOC (62.3 vs. 61.8) ($P > 0.05$), but PLE values were smaller than BIS values at ROC (64.4 vs 75.7) ($P < 0.05$).

Conclusions: The PLE value is a useful anesthetic depth indicator, similar to the BIS value, during propofol anesthesia. Spectral analysis of EEG acquired from the PLE monitor demonstrated the typical patterns seen in propofol anesthesia.

Keywords: Anesthetic depth monitoring, Bispectral index, Phase lag entropy, Propofol

Background

Level of consciousness is related to the complexity and variability of communication between the brain regions [1]. The diverse functional connectivity of the brain in awake state is diminished during anesthesia [2]. There are increases in the phase synchronization or shifts between electroencephalography (EEG) signals of the frontal brain during anesthesia, indicating a reduction in communication diversity [3]. The state of consciousness is more closely related to the temporal dynamics of the functional network configuration than to the strength of static connectivity [4, 5]. The processed EEG signal is an integral part of the brain function monitors used to measure the level of consciousness during anesthesia [6].

Unconsciousness is a fundamental component of general anesthesia; however, anesthesiologists have no reliable way of confirming that a patient is unconscious.

* Correspondence: drhwshin@naver.com
[1]Department of Anesthesiology and Pain Medicine, Korea University Anam Hospital, College of Medicine, Korea University, Goryodae-ro 73, Seongbuk-gu, 02841 Seoul, Republic of Korea

Generally, loss of consciousness (LOC) is marked by an increase in low-frequency (< 1 Hz) EEG power, the loss of spatially coherent occipital alpha (8–12 Hz) oscillations, and the appearance of spatially coherent frontal alpha oscillations [7]; these dynamics are then reversed during recovery of consciousness (ROC) [8]. There have been reports of changes in functional connectivity and disruptions of frontal EEG communication in the brain during anesthesia with propofol [4, 9, 10], sevoflurane [10–12], and ketamine [10].

The Bispectral Index™ (BIS™, Aspect Medical Systems, USA), the most widely used monitor in clinical practice, is based on spectral analysis of frequency powers from one-channel EEG [4, 13, 14]. BIS™ is useful for titration of anesthetics and postoperative recovery [15, 16]. However, BIS monitors cannot provide information regarding functional connectivity in the brain. Previous studies have reported a poor correlation between BIS and depth of anesthesia or sedation [6, 13, 17].

Phase lag entropy (PLE) is an EEG-based anesthetic depth indicator that calculates diversity in temporal patterns of the phase relationship in the brain [4, 10]. The recently developed PLE monitor (PLEM™, Inbody Co., Ltd., Republic of Korea), which measures the PLE value, is a four-channel EEG anesthetic depth monitoring device [4, 18–20].

The purpose of this study was to evaluate the clinical performance of the PLEM™ to monitor anesthetic depth and to evaluate the correlation between PLE and BIS values during propofol anesthesia.

Methods

The study was approved by an institutional review board (Korea University Anam Hospital, Institutional Review Board) (IRB No. 2017AN0268), and was prospectively registered, prior to patient enrollment, at ClinicalTrials.gov (NCT03299621, date of registration: October 2017). We also obtained written informed consent from all patients participating in the trial. This study used a prospective, observational, one-group design. The primary end-point of this study was to evaluate the clinical performance of the PLEM™ to monitor anesthetic depth during propofol anesthesia. The secondary end-point was to evaluate the correlation between the PLE and BIS values during propofol anesthesia.

Anesthesia and monitoring

Thirty-five adult patients undergoing elective surgery under general anesthesia were enrolled for the study. Patients were aged 20–60 years with an American Society of Anesthesiologists (ASA) physical status I or II. Exclusion criteria were presence of cardiovascular disorders, cerebrovascular disorders, respiratory disorder, and an anticipated difficult airway. Table 1 summarizes the patient characteristics. All patients were premedicated with glycopyrrolate 0.2 mg intramuscularly 1 h before induction of anesthesia. In the operating room, routine standard monitoring was followed, including electrocardiogram, non-invasive blood pressure monitoring, pulse oximetry, capnography, and temperature monitoring. General anesthesia was induced using a propofol target-controlled infusion (TCI, Orchestra®, Fresenius Kabi, France), and intravenous (iv) rocuronium 0.9 mg/kg was administered for tracheal intubation. To maintain propofol TCI, we used a "staircase" TCI that automatically reached the target effect-site concentrations (Ce) after the propofol Ce was set. After endotracheal intubation, we maintained controlled ventilation with a tidal volume of 6–10 ml/kg, respiration rate of 10–12/min, and inspired oxygen concentration of 0.5. Anesthesia was maintained with remifentanil Ce 0–10 ng/ml (Minto model) and propofol Ce 0–6 μg/ml (Schneider model). Hemodynamics were maintained within a 20% range of baseline value using fluids, phenylephrine 100–200 μg iv (< 20% from baseline blood pressure), or hydralazine 5–10 mg iv (> 20% from baseline blood pressure).

Table 1 Characteristics of included patients

Patient characteristics (n = 35)	
Age (years)	38.3 ± 12.2
Male/Female (number)	21/14
Weight (kg)	69.9 ± 12.5
Height (cm)	168.7 ± 9.6
ASA I/ASA II (number)	23/12
Duration of anesthesia (min)	66.1 ± 47.5
Type of surgery	
Orthopedic surgery	24
Genitourinary surgery	5
Breast surgery	2
Gynecologic surgery	4

Data are mean ± standard deviation or number of patients. American Society of Anesthesiologists (ASA) physical status I; A normal healthy patient, ASA physical status II; A patient with mild systemic disease

Preparation of the PLEM™ and BIS™ sensor

The PLEM™ and BIS™ were placed on the left temporal-frontal area, with the BIS™ sensor above the PLEM™ sensor as recommended by the manufacturer (Fig. 1). Both monitors displayed PLE and BIS values and trends, as well as electromyography (EMG) recordings of the forehead muscle, signal quality index (SQI), and real-time EEG waveforms. The anesthesiologist maintained an SQI > 70 for both devices to ensure accuracy of PLE and BIS values. Both PLEM™ and BIS™ monitors provide a calculated numeric PLE or BIS value between 0 (isoelectric EEG) and 100 (patient fully awake). The smoothing rates of the PLEM™ and was BIS™ were 4 s and 10 s, respectively.

Data collection and EEG acquisition

Frontal raw EEG signals were recorded using the PLEM™ sensor. EEG data were recorded with a preamplifier bandwidth of 0.5–45 Hz and sampling rate of 128 Hz. In order to minimize noise in the EEG signal, we analyzed the data after filtering it through baseline correction and reducing non-specific artifacts. The PLEM™ electrode array was configured with electrodes positioned approximately at FP1 (L_1), FP2 (R_1), AF5 (L_2), and AF6 (R_2). The ground electrode was at Fpz, and the reference electrode was at position T3 on the temporal area of the face (T) (Fig. 1). Electrode impedance was less than 7 kΩ in each channel.

Data measurement at time points

We collected data regarding patient demographics and anesthetic management. We acquired the data for PLE value, EEG band power, and BIS value using a USB memory card on PLEM™ and BIS™ devices at the following points in time: (1) prior to intubation as propofol Ce increased from 0 μg/ml to 2, 3, 4, 5, and 6 μg/ml, and after intubation as propofol Ce decreased from 6 μg/ml to 5, 4, 3, and 2 μg/ml; (2) two min after muscle relaxant injection and tracheal intubation; (3) at LOC, defined as when a patient no longer responds to the verbal command "open your eyes" (modified Observer's Assessment Alertness/Sedation [OAA/S] scale = 2) repeated every 10 s during induction; and (4) at ROC, defined as when a patient once again obeys the verbal command "open your eyes" (modified OAA/S scale = 3) repeated every 10 s during emergence from anesthesia.

Calculation of PLE

The PLE value was calculated following the approach used in Lee et al.'s study [4]. The degree of communication between different areas of the brain is correlated with the phase relationship among multi-channel EEG signals [8, 15]. In order to calculate the PLE value, the data from the frontal and prefrontal lobes were recorded using PLEM™ sensor electrodes arranged at FP1, FP2, AF5, and AF6 (Fig. 1). EEG signals were segmented into 4-s time series with 50% overlapping epochs. All filters used a zero-phase finite impulse response to prevent changes in phase. In addition, the correction algorithm employing nonlinear signal decomposition was used to correct the amplitude and base line of the signals. Calculations were performed after removal of signals outside the range of biological noise and EEG signals. Because the amplitude of noise is also physiologically significant, we used correction methods to limit the elimination of noise. However, the calculation was not performed if the

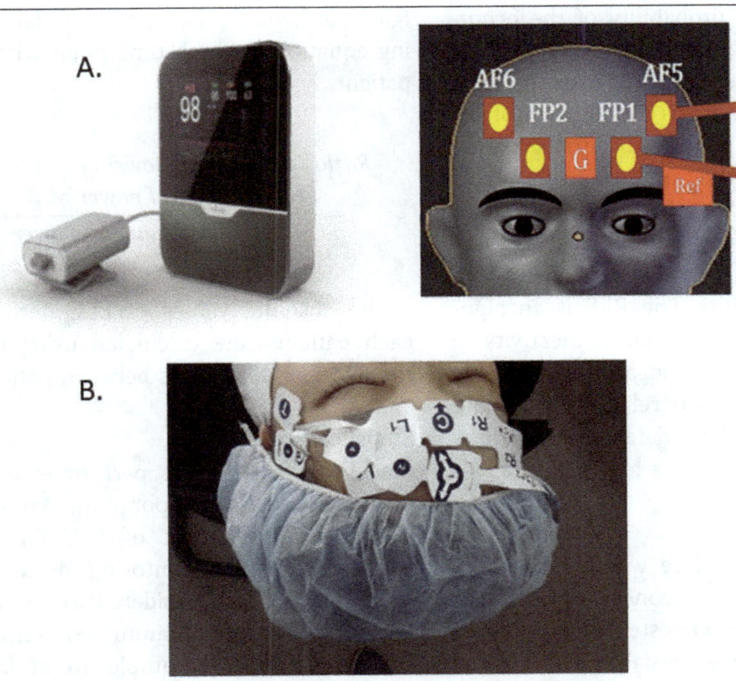

Fig. 1 Illustration of electroencephalogram (EEG) channels and phase difference sign measurement. **a** PLEM™ measures the phase lag entropy (PLE) value. The PLE electrode array consists of electrodes positioned approximately at FP1 (L_1), FP2 (R_1), AF5 (L_2), and AF6 (R_2). The ground electrode is at F_{PZ} (G), and the reference electrode is at T3 of the temporal area of the face (T). **b** Both sensors are placed on the left temporal-frontal area with the bispectral index (BIS) sensor placed above the PLE sensor.

data exceeded 50% of the epoch. PLEM™ operates by extracting and combining EEG signals from the frontal and prefrontal regions. The instantaneous phase was extracted via Hilbert transform using the signal processing toolbox in MATLAB (version 2017b, Mathworks Inc., Co., Ltd., USA). The PLE value was quantified using the entropy of regularity or irregularity in the temporal variation of phase difference between two EEG signals. In order to calculate the PLE value, the instantaneous phase signal was extracted from two signals and the difference value of the instantaneous phase was encoded. $S_t = 1$ if $\Delta\phi_t > 0$ (i.e., first signal is phase leading the second signal), and $S_t = 0$ if $\Delta\phi_t < 0$ (i.e., first signal is phase lagging the second signal). Thus, the vector S_t, representing the temporal pattern of the phase relationship is given by

$$S_t = \{\ s_t, s_{t+\tau}, \ldots s_{t+(m-1)\tau}\ \}t = 1, 2, \ldots, N-(m-1)\tau \quad (1)$$

where, m and s represent pattern size (word length) and time lag, respectively. For example, with $m = 3$, eight patterns ("000," "001," "010," "100," "011," "101," "110," and "111") can be generated. Finally, the PLE value was calculated by applying the standard Shannon entropy formula for the distribution of the phase patterns:

$$\text{PLE} = -\frac{\sum p_j\ log p_j}{log(2^m)} \quad (2)$$

In Eq. (2), p_j represents the probability of the occurrence of the jth pattern in a given input signal, and m represents the size of one pattern. Eq. (2) is in the form of a fraction, where the numerator is the entropy of the probability of different phase patterns occurring in the signal, and the denominator is the number of all possible patterns. The normalization term in the denominator scale of the PLE value is the range [0 1]. PLEM™ displays the index value on the screen in a linear scale (× 100) with a value between 0 and 100. The PLE is an algorithm designed to reflect the functional connectivity of the frontal area in the brain. In the awake state, the histogram distribution of patterns is relatively even and thus has a high PLE value. In the sedated state, the distribution of patterns is biased toward a low PLE value.

Spectral analysis

We used spectral analysis to analyze whether the EEG signal acquired from PLEM™ was consistent with the typical known patterns in the persistence and power spectrograms during propofol anesthesia [7, 12].

The persistence spectrogram was analyzed using MATLAB. We divided the EEG signal into segments with a uniform epoch length (4 s), then overlapped the spectrogram (2 s) such that the frequency power at each frequency (0.125 Hz) represented a high percentage of the spectrogram. EEG signals were divided into three states during propofol anesthesia: awake state (A-state), unconscious state (UC-state), and recovery of consciousness state (ROC-state). The frequency and frequency power were plotted on the x-axis and y-axis, respectively. The distribution of power was shown using color to visually represent a decibel ratio (%) [21].

For the power spectrogram, we estimated the standard Multitaper Power Spectral Density (MPSD) using MATLAB [22]. For computing the power spectrogram, we obtained individual four-channel EEG signals acquired from PLEM™. We computed four-channel median spectrograms by taking the median across all time epochs. The time was plotted on the x-axis and frequency on the y-axis; the signal frequency power was expressed in scale color. The power spectrogram quantifies the frequency distribution of energy or power within the EEG signal over time. We calculated the MPSD using 8-s EEG segments (4 s before to 4 s after each EEG measurement point) to quantify the frequency power ratio for a given propofol Ce. We set the following parameters: window length (2 s), overlap (1 s), time-half bandwidth product (3 Hz), and spectral resolution (0.25 Hz). We calculated the average of the listed four-channel MPSD values for all band power values.

Calculation of EEG band power

We also computed the ratio of EEG band powers (gamma, beta, alpha, theta, and delta) using the following equation for each time point with propofol Ce in all patients:

$$\textit{Ratio of EEG band power}\,(\gamma,\beta,\alpha,\theta,\delta) = \frac{\textit{Frequency band power}(\gamma,\beta,\alpha,\theta,\delta)}{\textit{Total frequency power}}$$

The absolute values of EEG-derived band power in each patient were calculated using the ratio to reduce the effect of differences between patients.

Statistical analysis

Statistical analysis was performed using SPSS software version 20 (IBM Corporation, Armonk, NY, USA). A correlation coefficient of 0.7, for the index of the anesthetic depth monitoring device according to the propofol Ce, was considered to be clinically significant. We calculated a minimum requirement of 29 patients. We also calculated a sample size of 32 based on previous observational studies correlating EEG-based anesthetic depth monitoring (a difference of 10 between BIS and entropy based on pilot study, a power of 90% with an α value of 0.05) [23]. Considering possible data loss, we decided to study 35 patients.

The data are presented as mean ± SD or median for continuous variables, and number of patients for categorical variables. Spearman correlation analysis was performed between the PLE value and propofol Ce and displayed using box and whiskers plots. Repeated measures analysis of variance (ANOVA) was performed for changes in PLE value before and after muscle relaxant injection, and for the change in EEG-band power during propofol anesthesia, displayed using box and whiskers plots. Post-hoc multiple comparisons were then performed using the Tukey test. A comparison between the PLE value and BIS value at the same points in time was performed using the *t*-test with the Bland-Altman graph. *P*-values < 0.05 were considered statistically significant.

Results

Of the 35 patients, one was excluded because of a technical error during recording with the sensor electrode. Therefore, 34 patients were included in the statistical analysis. The demographic data of these patients are shown in Table 1.

Correlation between PLE value and changes in propofol Ce

The PLE values were inversely correlated to changes in propofol Ce (propofol Ce from 0 to 6.0 μg/ml, Spearman correlation coefficient $r^2 = -0.835$; propofol Ce from 6.0 to 2.0 μg/ml, $r^2 = -0.467$) (Fig. 2a). The PLE value at LOC was 62.3 ± 10.9 with propofol Ce 4.4 ± 0.8 μg/ml, whereas the PLE value at ROC was 64.4 ± 9.6 with propofol Ce 1.0 ± 0.2 μg/ml.

Spectral analysis of EEG acquired from PLEM™

The persistence spectrogram showed a wide distribution of power for a given frequency in the LOC-state and ROC-state compared to the dense distribution of power for a given frequency in the UC-state (Fig. 3a). The power spectrogram showed a typical pattern of propofol-induced sedation with slow alpha (8–12 Hz) band oscillations (Fig. 3b) [7]. PLE and BIS values were inversely proportional to propofol Ce (Fig. 3c). For each EEG band power, as propofol Ce increased, the alpha-, beta-, and theta-band powers showed a tendency to increase, and the gamma-band power showed a tendency to decrease. There was no significant change in the delta-band power. However, the changes in EEG band power were not statistically significant because of the wide range of SD and some outliers (Fig. 4).

A comparison of PLE and BIS

The PLE value demonstrated a strong correlation with the BIS value during the change in propofol Ce from 0 to 6.0 μg/ml ($r^2 = 0.84$) (Fig. 5). The PLE was significantly higher than the BIS at all propofol Ce values prior to intubation ($P < 0.05$), and lower than the BIS at all propofol Ce values after intubation ($P < 0.05$) (Table 2) (Fig. 5). The PLE values were similar to the BIS at LOC (PLE: 62.3 ± 10.9, BIS: 61.8 ± 10.5), but lower at ROC (PLE: 64.4 ± 9.6, BIS: 75.7 ± 6.4) ($P < 0.05$).

Effect of muscle relaxants

Both PLE and BIS values significantly decreased after injection of the muscle relaxant (PLE: 43.8 ± 11.6 vs 38.3 ± 4.2, BIS: 49.7 ± 14.5 vs 36.5 ± 9.7) ($P < 0.05$).

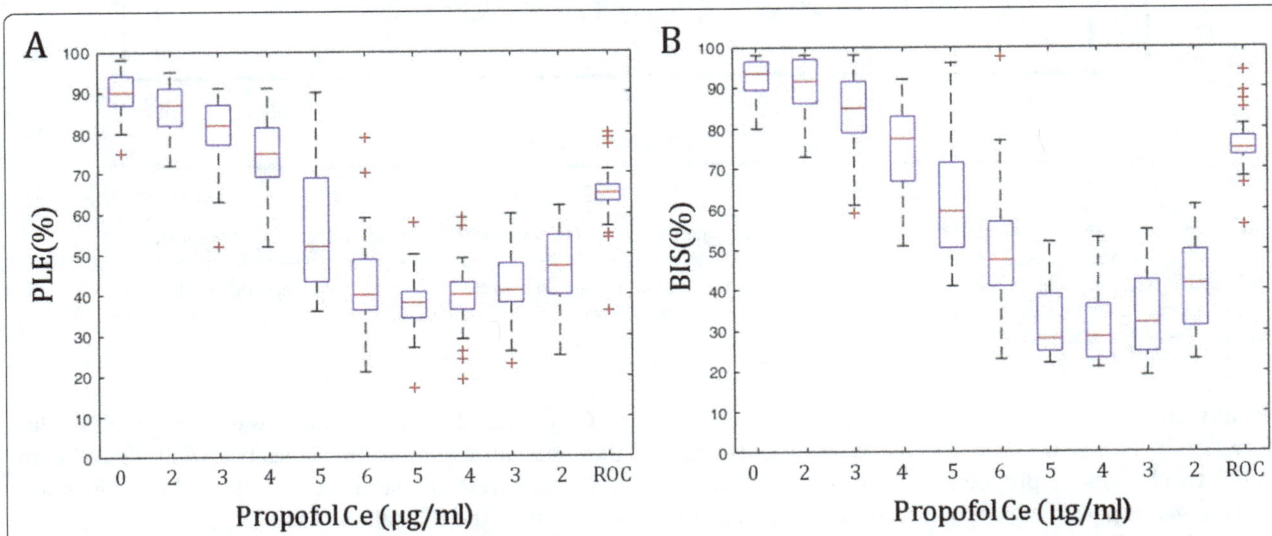

Fig. 2 The change in PLE and BIS values during propofol anesthesia. The box and whiskers plots show PLE and BIS values at the time when a given propofol target effect concentration (propofol Ce) was reached. **a** For PLE, Spearman correlation coefficient = 0.835 (from propofol Ce 0 to propofol Ce 6.0 μg/ml). **b** For BIS, Spearman correlation coefficient = 0.781 (from propofol Ce 0 to propofol Ce 6.0 μg/ml). Abbreviations: PLE, phase lag entropy; BIS, bispectral index; LOC, loss of consciousness; ROC, recovery of consciousness. The boxes depict the median values and the 25th and the 75th percentiles (lower whisker = − 1.5 × IQR, upper whisker = + 1.5 × IQR, IQR; inter-quartile range, +; outlier)

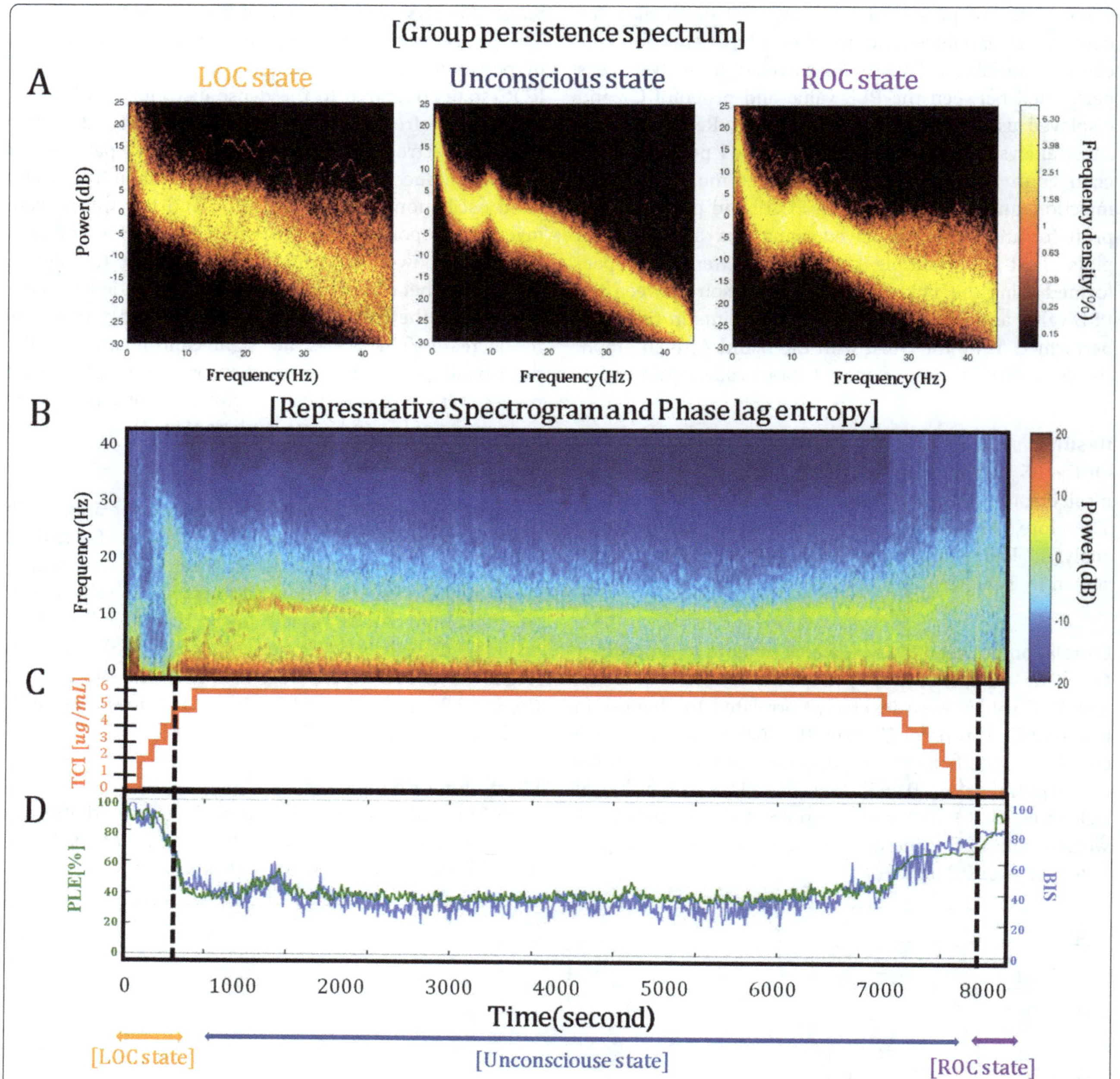

Fig. 3 The spectrograms obtained from PLEM™ during propofol anesthesia. **a** Group-level persistence spectrogram for different states of consciousness (LOC-state, UC-state, and ROC-state). **b** Representative power spectrogram showing the power of the slow and delta (0.1 to 4 Hz) and alpha (8 to 13 Hz) band oscillations, and **c** the time domain phase lag entropy (PLE) obtained from PLEM™ during propofol anesthesia. Abbreviations: TCI, target-controlled infusion; LOC, loss of consciousness; UC, unconsciousness; ROC, recovery of consciousness. The black dashed line indicates when LOC and ROC occurred

Discussion

In this study, PLE values from PLEM™ were inversely correlated to changes in propofol Ce during the induction and emergence period of propofol anesthesia. The persistence spectrogram and power spectrogram using EEG signals acquired from the PLEM™ were consistent with the typical known patterns seen in propofol anesthesia. The PLEM™ was similarly comparable for anesthetic depth monitoring with BIS™ during the change of propofol Ce 0 to Ce 6.0 μg/ml. The PLE value was lower at BIS values above 40, but higher at BIS values below 40. The PLE and BIS values were similar at LOC, but the PLE values were smaller than the BIS values at ROC.

To date, there have been many studies for developing a method of assessing anesthetic depth using processed EEG data [8]. The most widely used processed EEG-based anesthetic depth monitor, BIS™, quantifies the consistency of phase-coupling and frequency of single-

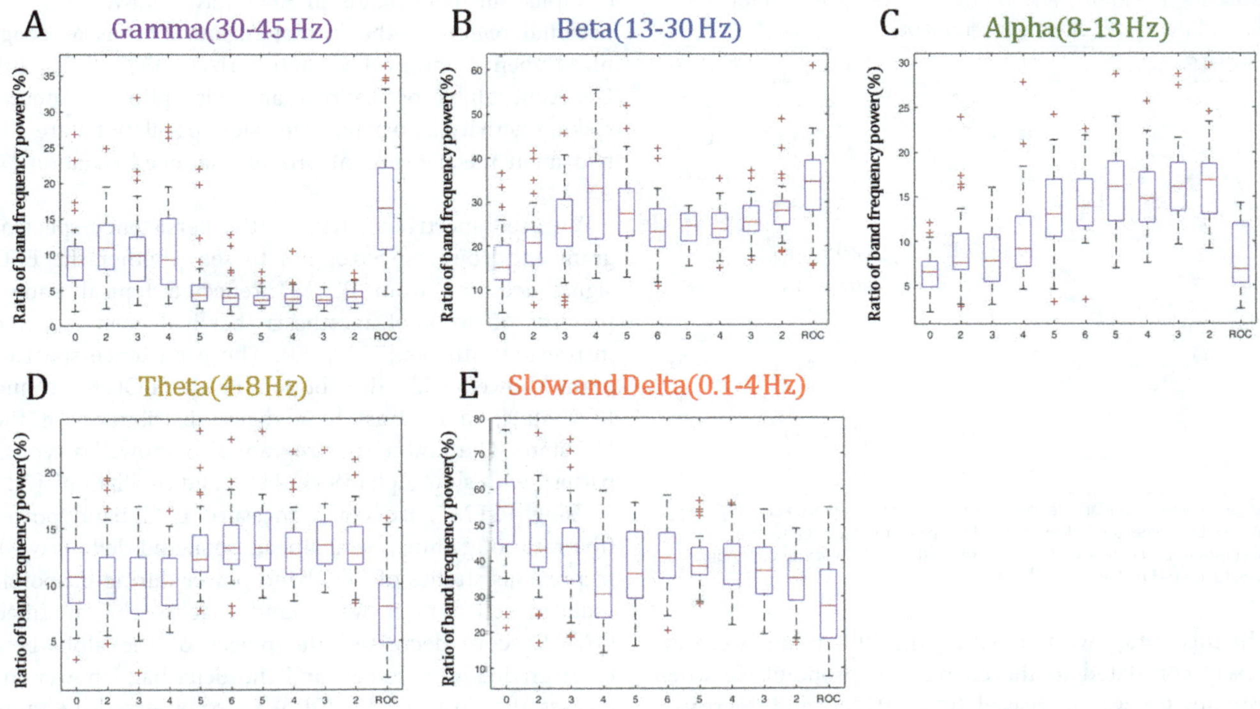

Fig. 4 The change in the ratio of electroencephalogram (EEG) band power during propofol anesthesia. The box and whiskers plots show the ratio of EEG band power (gamma, beta, alpha, theta, and delta) at the time when a given propofol target effect concentration (propofol Ce) was reached. The boxes depict the median values and the 25th and the 75th percentiles (lower whisker = − 1.5 × IQR, upper whisker = + 1.5 × IQR, IQR; inter-quartile range, +; outlier)

channel EEG in the brain, whereas PLEM™ quantifies the entropy based on the spatial or connectivity information of four-channel EEG signals by measuring the regularity of variations in the temporal phase difference between two separate areas of the brain [4, 8].

PLEM™ is a recently developed anesthetic depth monitoring device that uses four-channel EEG [4]. The PLE value in PLEM™ is composed of three sub-parameters, PLE1 (8–32 Hz), PLE2 (0.1–1 and 32–45 Hz), and BSR (2–32 Hz). PLE1 (light hypnotic state) is calculated from the alpha (8–13 Hz) and beta (13–30 Hz) bands, whereas PLE2 (deep hypnotic state) is calculated from the slow-frequency (0.1–1 Hz) and gamma (30–45 Hz) bands. BSR is composed of two types of burst-suppression detection, such as the portions of the isoelectric EEG and/or a very low power frequency. The PLE value (scale 0–100) is calculated by combining PLE1, PLE2, and BSR with appropriate weights.

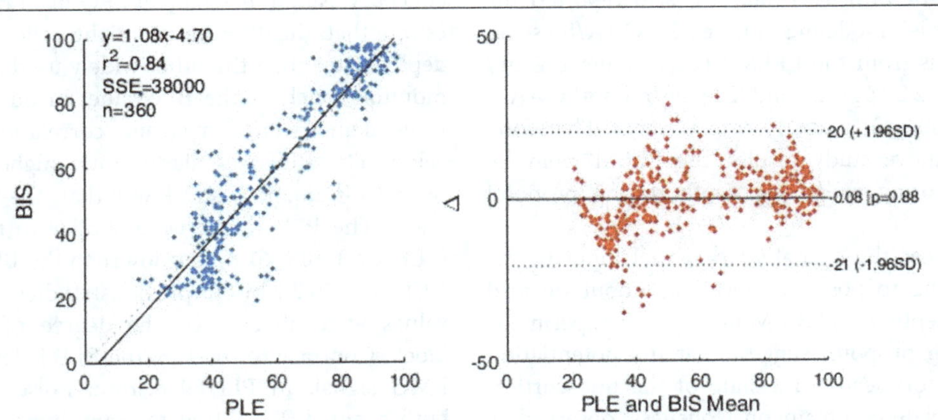

Fig. 5 A comparison of PLE and BIS using the Spearman correlation graph and Bland-Altman graph. Abbreviations: PLE, phase lag entropy; BIS, bispectral index; SD, standard deviation

Table 2 PLE and BIS values at the time point when propofol reached the target effect concentration

Propofol Ce (μg/ml)	PLE	BIS	*P*-value
0	89.1 ± 8.5*	91.6 ± 5.7	0.042
2	83.9 ± 12.7*	90.7 ± 6.4	0.002
3	79.0 ± 10.7*	83.5 ± 10.7	0.000
4	74.5 ± 9.2	74.9 ± 11.1	0.798
5	56.8 ± 14.8*	62.0 ± 14.8	0.001
6	43.7 ± 11.4*	49.7 ± 14.5	0.002
Intubation			
5	37.3 ± 7.1*	31.6 ± 8.2	0.005
4	39.3 ± 7.8*	30.8 ± 8.8	0.000
3	41.7 ± 9.1*	34.5 ± 10.7	0.000
2	47.2 ± 9.1*	41.1 ± 11.6	0.000

Data are mean ± standard deviation or values. Abbreviations: PLE, phase lag entropy; BIS, bispectral index; propofol Ce, propofol target effect-site concentration. * *P*-value < 0.05 compared with BIS at the same time points for propofol Ce 0–6 μg/ml

In this study, we found that the PLE values were inversely correlated to the changes in propofol Ce when propofol Ce was increased ($r^2 = -0.835$) and decreased ($r^2 = -0.467$). The PLE values at LOC and ROC were similar (62.3 and 64.4, respectively). Koo et al.'s study [24] results of propofol Ce at LOC and ROC (4.4 ± 1.1 μg/ml, 1.1 ± 0.3 μg/ml) are similar to that in our study. In Lee et al.'s study [4] that compared recently used anesthetic depth monitors, the PLE value exhibited the highest agreement with the level of consciousness (using the modified OAA/S score) relative to other monitors such as the BIS, relative beta ratio (RBR), approximate entropy (ApEn), and permutation entropy (PeEn) values. Recently, clinical studies have been reported for PLEM™ during propofol-induced sedation [18–20]. Jung et al. [20] reported that PLEM™ was comparable with BIS™ in correlational studies using the OAA/S score during propofol-induced sedation (Spearman's Rho: 0.755 for PLE, 0.788 for BIS). Ki et al. [18] also reported the pharmacodynamic modeling for each OAA/S score using PLE values from the PLEM™ (Ce_{50} value: 1.67 μg/ml, 1.96 μg/ml, 2.22 μg/ml, and 2.69 μg/ml for OAA/S scores of ≤4, ≤3, ≤2, and ≤ 1, respectively). Therefore, based on the above study results, the PLEM™ may be used for monitoring anesthetic depth during propofol anesthesia.

Propofol reduces the excitation potential input to the cortex by binding to post-synaptic γ-aminobutyric acid A ($GABA_A$) receptors [8, 25]. Modeling and experimental studies using propofol suggest that the potentiation of GABA receptors leads to a state of thalamo-cortical synchrony associated with unconsciousness, observed as frontal slowing and alpha band oscillations [8]. In the states bordering consciousness, such as LOC, the power of alpha and beta bands in EEG waves move from the occipital region to the frontal region. This is a recognized phenomenon called "anteriorization" [7, 8, 15, 26]. Coherent alpha oscillations and disruption of neural spiking activity associated with slow oscillations are the two main mechanisms of propofol-induced sedation [7, 27, 28].

We used spectral analysis of the persistence spectrogram and power spectrogram to see whether the EEG signal acquired from PLEM™ reflected typical known patterns of propofol anesthesia that had been reported in previous studies [7, 12, 29]. The persistence spectrogram showed wide distribution in the LOC-state and ROC-state, in contrast to a dense distribution in the UC-state. The power spectrogram also showed a typical pattern with slow alpha (8–12 Hz) band oscillations [7].

Using PLEM™, we could measure EEG band power (the ratio of gamma, beta, alpha, theta, and delta waves). In previous studies of EEG band power during propofol-induced sedation, it was found that as the modified OAA/S score decreases, the power of the alpha-beta band gradually increases, and the delta-band power increases after LOC [7, 12, 30]. We also observed the same results in our study; as propofol Ce increased, alpha-, beta-, and theta- band powers showed the tendency to increase, and gamma-band power showed the tendency to decrease. However, these changes were not statistically significant because of the wide SD and some outliers. Generally, as the anesthetic depth increases, the frequency of the EEG band power shifts toward the lower frequencies (beta to alpha to theta to delta). If the propofol Ce was increased any further in our study, burst suppression activity would ensue [7]. In our study, the gamma-band power increased during the start of propofol TCI and then decreased at propofol Ce 4–5 μg /ml; this might be because of noise interference with the EEG [25].

Before the start of our study, by prioritizing spatial concepts using four-channel EEG in PLEM™, we hypothesized that the PLE value might reflect the anesthetic depth better than the other widely used anesthetic depth monitors, such as the BIS value. In our study, the PLE value demonstrated a strong correlation with the BIS value. The PLE was significantly higher than the BIS prior to intubation, and lower than the BIS after intubation. The PLE values were similar to the BIS at LOC (PLE: 62.3, BIS: 61.8), but lower to the BIS at ROC (PLE: 64.4, BIS: 75.7). In the previous studies [31–33], the BIS values were affected by the degree of neuromuscular block. Contrary to the BIS, the PLE is less influenced by EMG signal. In PLE algorithm, noise introduced into both channel (R1, R2) at the same time is removed during the binarization process ("000," "001," "010," "100," "011," "101," "110," and "111") of phase difference by phase extraction. The EMG activity in our result was higher in ROC compared to LOC (27.9 ± 41.7% vs. 67.4 ± 22.5%). We suspect the observed differences between the BIS and PLE, especially during ROC phase, may be due to the difference in the EMG-EEG interferences of both devices. However, in the results, both PLE and BIS values significantly decreased after injection of the muscle relaxant. Further studies are suggested for the effect of EMG signals on the PLE and the BIS.

The limitations of our study are as follows. First, BIS sensor (circle 3) was slightly mal-positioned (the commercially recommended location of the BIS sensor is as follows: circle 1 at the center of the forehead, approximately 4 cm above the nose, circle 2 at 2.8 cm lateral right to circle 1, and circle 3 on the temple area between the corner of the eye and the hairline). Second, the disagreement between the PLE value and the BIS value at each time point showed large standard deviation. Third, the PLE and BIS values were not measured at the same point in time because of the different smoothing rates of the devices. The smoothing rates for PLE and BIS were 4 s and 10 s, respectively. Fourth, PLE and BIS values changed continuously after reaching propofol Ce. The inter-trial variability of these values was related to time. Fifth, we only investigated the performance of PLEM™ in young adults during propofol anesthesia [7]. Further studies are needed to validate the PLE value from PLEM™ for pediatric or geriatric patients and with other drugs such as other GABAnergic anesthetic drugs and non-GABAnergic drugs such as ketamine, dexmedetomidine, and N_2O.

Conclusion

The PLE value obtained using PLEM™ is a useful anesthetic depth indicator, similar to the BIS value, in patients subjected to propofol anesthesia. Spectral analysis of the raw EEG signals acquired from the PLEM™ demonstrated the typical patterns of propofol anesthesia.

Abbreviations

ANOVA: Analysis of variance; ApEn: Approximate entropy; ASA: American Society of Anesthesiologists; A-state: Awake state; BIS: Bispectral index; Ce: Target effect-site concentration; EEG: Electroencephalography; EMG: Electromyography; GABA: γ-aminobutyric acid; LOC: Loss of consciousness; MPSD: Multitaper power spectral density; OAA/S: Observer's Assessment Alertness/Sedation; PeEn: Permutation entropy; PLE: Phase lag entropy; RBR: Relative beta ratio; ROC: Recovery of consciousness; ROC-state: Recovery of consciousness state; SQI: Signal quality index; TCI: Target-controlled infusion; UC-state: Unconscious state

Acknowledgments

We thank Kyoung Soo Kim (Neuroscience researcher, InBody, Seoul, Korea) for the support in the data analysis. We would like to thank Editage (www.editage.co.kr) for English language editing.

Authors' contributions

Study conception and design: HW Shin, HJ Kim. Experiment performed by: HW Shin, HJ Kim, YK Jang, HS You. Data acquisition: HJ Kim, YK Jang, YJ Choi, H Huh, JS Hong. Data analysis: YK Jang, HW Shin, SU Choi. Data processing and data interpretation: HW Shin, SU Choi, H Huh. Statistical analysis: HW Shin, JS Hong, HS You. Manuscript drafted by: HW Shin, YJ Choi, JS Hong. Draft revised critically for important intellectual content by: HW Shin. All authors read and approved the final manuscript.

Author details

[1]Department of Anesthesiology and Pain Medicine, Korea University Anam Hospital, College of Medicine, Korea University, Goryodae-ro 73, Seongbuk-gu, 02841 Seoul, Republic of Korea. [2]Department of Anesthesiology and Pain Medicine, Ewha University Magok Hospital, College of Medicine, Ewha University, Seoul, Republic of Korea. [3]Department of Anesthesiology and Pain Medicine, Korea University Ansan Hospital, College of Medicine, Korea University, Gyeonggi-do, Republic of Korea.

References

1. Dehaene S, Changeux JP. Experimental and theoretical approaches to conscious processing. Neuron. 2011;70:200–27.
2. Alkire MT, Hudetz AG, Tononi G. Consciousness and anesthesia. Science. 2008;322:876–80.
3. Lee U, Kim S, Noh GJ, Choi BM, Hwang E, Mashour GA. The directionality and functional organization of frontoparietal connectivity during consciousness and anesthesia in humans. Conscious Cogn. 2009;18:1069–78.
4. Lee H, Noh GJ, Joo P, Choi BM, Silverstein BH, Kim M, et al. Diversity of functional connectivity patterns is reduced in propofol-induced unconsciousness. Hum Brain Mapp. 2017;38:4980–95.
5. Barttfeld P, Uhrig L, Sitt JD, Sigman M, Jarraya B, Dehaene S. Signature of consciousness in the dynamics of resting-state brain activity. Proc Natl Acad Sci. 2015;112:887–92.
6. Fahy BG, Chau DF. The Technology of Processed Electroencephalogram Monitoring Devices for assessment of depth of anesthesia. Anesth Analg. 2018;126:111–7.
7. Purdon PL, Sampson A, Pavone KJ, Brown EN. Clinical electroencephalography for anesthesiologists. Anesthesiology. 2015;123: 937–60.
8. Purdon PL, Pierce ET, Mukamel EA, Prerau MJ, Walsh JL, Wong KFK, et al. Electroencephalogram signatures of loss and recovery of consciousness from propofol. Proc Natl Acad Sci. 2013;110:E1142–51.
9. Hudetz AG, Liu X, Pillay S. Dynamic repertoire of intrinsic brain states is reduced in Propofol-induced unconsciousness. Brain Connect. 2015;5:10–22.
10. Lee U, Ku S, Noh G, Baek S, Choi B, Mashour GA. Disruption of frontal–parietal communication by ketamine, Propofol, and Sevoflurane. Anesthesiology. 2013;118:1264–75.
11. Ward LM, Ku S-W, Lee U, Noh G-J, Jun I-G, Mashour GA. Preferential inhibition of frontal-to-parietal feedback connectivity is a neurophysiologic correlate of general anesthesia in surgical patients. PLoS One. 2011;6: e25155.
12. Akeju O, Westover MB, Pavone KJ, Sampson AL, Hartnack KE, Brown EN, et al. Effects of Sevoflurane and Propofol on frontal electroencephalogram power and coherence. Anesthesiology. 2014;121:990–8.
13. Hajat Z, Ahmad N, Andrzejowski J. The role and limitations of EEG-based depth of anaesthesia monitoring in theatres and intensive care. Anaesthesia. 2017;72:38–47.
14. Johansen JW. Update on bispectral index monitoring. Best Pract Res Clin Anaesthesiol. 2006;20:81–99.
15. Cimenser A, Purdon PL, Pierce ET, Walsh JL, Salazar-Gomez AF, Harrell PG, et al. Tracking brain states under general anesthesia by using global coherence analysis. Proc Natl Acad Sci. 2011;108:8832–7.
16. Punjasawadwong Y, Phongchiewboon A, Bunchungmongkol N. Bispectral index for improving anaesthetic delivery and postoperative recovery. Cochrane Database Syst Rev. 2014;17:CD003843.
17. Nasraway SA, Wu EC, Kelleher RM, Yasuda CM, Donnelly AM. How reliable is the Bispectral index in critically ill patients? A prospective, comparative, single-blinded observer study. Crit Care Med. 2002;30:1483–7.
18. Ki S, Kim KM, Lee YH, Bang JY, Choi BM, Noh GJ. Phase lag entropy as a hypnotic depth indicator during propofol sedation. Anaesthesia. 2019;74: 1033–40.
19. Seo KH, Kim KM, Lee SK, John H, Lee J. Comparative analysis of phase lag entropy and Bispectral index as anesthetic depth indicators in patients undergoing thyroid surgery with nerve integrity monitoring. J Korean Med Sci. 2019;34:e151.

20. Jun MR, Yoo JH, Park SY, Na S, Kwon H, Nho J-H, et al. Assessment of phase-lag entropy, a new measure of electroencephalographic signals, for propofol-induced sedation. Korean J Anesthesiol. 2019;72:351.
21. Fulop SA, Fitz K. Algorithms for computing the time-corrected instantaneous frequency (reassigned) spectrogram, with applications. J Acoust Soc Am. 2006;119:360–71.
22. Babadi B, Brown EN. A review of multitaper spectral analysis. IEEE Trans Biomed Eng. 2014;61:1555–64.
23. Musialowicz T, Lahtinen P, Pitkänen O, Kurola J, Parviainen I. Comparison of spectral entropy and BIS VISTA™ monitor during general anesthesia for cardiac surgery. J Clin Monit Comput. 2011;25:95–103.
24. Koo BN, Lee JR, Noh GJ, Lee JH, Kang YR, Han DW. A pharmacodynamic analysis of factors affecting recovery from anesthesia with propofol-remifentanil target controlled infusion. Acta Pharmacol Sin. 2012;33:1080–4.
25. Hemmings HC Jr, Akabas MH, Goldstein PA, Trudell JR, Orser BA, Harrison NL. Emerging molecular mechanisms of general anesthetic action. Trends Pharmacol Sci. 2005;26:503–10.
26. Tinker JH, Sharbrough FW, Michenfelder JD. Anterior shift of the dominant EEG rhytham during anesthesia in the Java monkey: correlation with anesthetic potency. Anesthesiology. 1977;46(4):252–9.
27. Lewis LD, Weiner VS, Mukamel EA, Donoghue JA, Eskandar EN, Madsen JR, et al. Rapid fragmentation of neuronal networks at the onset of propofol-induced unconsciousness. Proc Natl Acad Sci. 2012;109:E3377–86.
28. Devor M, Zalkind V. Reversible analgesia, atonia, and loss of consciousness on bilateral intracerebral microinjection of pentobarbital. Pain. 2001;94:101–12.
29. Lee JM, Akeju O, Terzakis K, Pavone KJ, Deng H, Houle TT, et al. A prospective study of age-dependent changes in Propofol-induced electroencephalogram oscillations in children. Anesthesiology. 2017;127:293–306.
30. Choi B-M. Characteristics of electroencephalogram signatures in sedated patients induced by various anesthetic agents. J Dent Anesth Pain Med. 2017;17:241–51.
31. Messner M, Beese U, Romstöck J, Dinkel M, Tschaikowsky K. The bispectral index declines during neuromuscular block in fully awake persons. Anesth Analg. 2003;97:488–91.
32. Shin YC, Kim SI, Ok SY, Kim SC. The influence of a muscle relaxant on bispectral index during the propofol induction of anesthesia. Korean J Anesthesiol. 2008;54:373–7.
33. Bruhn J, Bouillon TW, Shafer SL. Electromyographic activity falsely elevates the bispectral index. Anesthesiology. 2000;92:1485–7.

24

Early versus delayed postoperative oral hydration in children following general anesthesia

Xiaorong Yin[1], Xiaoqi Zeng[1], Ting Wang[1], Binbin Dong[1], Menghang Wu[1], Anna Jia[1] and Ling Ye[2*]

Abstract

Background: Oral hydration has typically not been administered for between 4 and 6 h postoperative for children's safety in China. But children are more likely to suffer from apnea, crying and agitation, wound bleeding, and other complications during the post-anesthesia recovery period because of thirsty and fear. This Prospective, randomized study sought to assess the compare the early and late oral hydration (EOH and DOH, respectively) in children following general anesthesia, with the goal of assessing relative safety and tolerability and thereby improving patient comfort.

Methods: A total of 2000 children corresponding to the American Society of Anesthesiology (ASA) I-III were randomized into an EOH group ($n = 1000$) and a DOH group (n = 1000). For the former group, children were administered a small amount of drinking water following recovery of the swallowing reflex, and children's vital signs were monitored for 20 min in a postanesthesia care unit (PACU). DOH group patients received water at 4 h following general anesthesia). All patients underwent monitoring to assess their thirst, satisfaction, oropharyngeal discomfort, nausea, and vomiting.

Results: Complete data were collected from a total of 1770 patients (EOH = 832, DOH = 938) and was compared via chi-squared and t-tests as appropriate. There was no hypoxemia in either group, nor did the incidence of nausea and vomiting differ between the two groups ($P > 0.05$). The thirst score of the EOH group was significantly decreased relative to the DOH group in the children over 5 years old after drinking for 10 to 20 min ($P < 0.05$).

Conclusions: For children undergoing general anesthesia, a small amount of drinking water in the early stages of recovery will not increase the incidence of nausea, vomiting, or hypoxemia, but will decrease thirst and improve satisfaction. It is important, however, that medical staff carefully monitor the swallowing reflex and vital signs of all children.

Keywords: General anesthesia, Oral intake, Postoperative nausea, Vomitting

* Correspondence: zerodq_hx@163.com
[2]Department of Pain Management, West China Hospital, Sichuan University, Chengdu, Sichuan Province 610041, People's Republic of China

Background

Compared with adult patients, children are more likely to suffer from apnea, crying and agitation, wound bleeding, and other complications during the post-anesthesia recovery period because of their own physiological and psychological characteristics [1–3]. Crying and agitation during the recovery period may cause airway spasms, severe hypoxemia leading to respiratory depression or apnea, postoperative bleeding, accidental falls, and other adverse events. It therefore represents a safety concern during anesthesia recovery period, and remains a difficult problem for nursing care [4]. Through several years of clinical observation, we found that hunger and thirst were the primary causes of agitation in children.

In order to ensure postoperative safety and prevent coughing, vomiting, and aspiration caused by drinking water following general anesthesia for non-gastrointestinal operations, postoperative oral hydration has typically not been administered for between 4 and 6 h in China [2, 3]. However, many researchers have found more rapid administration of oral hydration to be beneficial and safe [5–10]. The optimal timing for such administration of fluids, however, has remained unclear in China. For example, certain researchers have suggested that in children undergoing relatively minor operations water could safely be provided 1 h after anesthesia [8, 9]. This study sought to compare early and delayed oral hydration (EOH and DOH, respectively) after general anesthesia in order to assess the relative safety of these approaches, and to gauge their ability to decrease thirst and improve satisfaction and high-quality nursing service. Thirst, oropharyngeal discomfort, satisfaction, and incidence of nausea/vomiting, as well as the time from PACU arrival to first oral fluid intake, served as the primary outcome measurements for this study. Data was additionally collected regarding nausea and vomiting after returning to the ward, the incidence of postoperative complications, and the PACU observation time and hospitalization time.

Materials and methods

Sample

This prospective, randomized, controlled trial received approval from the Clinical trial and Biomedical Ethics Committee, West China Hospital, Sichuan University, Chengdu, China. This study was registered on the Chinese Clinical Trial Registry (ChiCTR-IOR-16008197) (http://www.chictr.org.cn/index.aspx. On April 2, 2016 the first patients was enrolled and on March 31, 2016 the trial was registered). From April 2016 – March 2018, a computer-generated list of random numbers served to mediate prospective randomization of a total of 2000 children corresponding to the American Society of Anesthesiology (ASA) I-III status who were in a post-anesthesia care unit (PACU) after general anesthesia. Exclusion criteria included: preoperative colds, respiratory infections, facial, oropharyngeal, thoracic, gastrointestinal, neuro-, or laryngeal surgery, altered mental state, or dysphagia.

On the basis of pilot study, a sample size of 628 allowed a 20% difference between the two groups, with an α of 0.05 (two-tailed) and a $\beta$of 0.20, power of 0.8. to account for attrition, a sample size of 785 was selected for each group.

Study design

For all study participants, a complete medical history was taken, and patients and their parents were then informed of the study protocols (including the hydration regimens, follow-up plans, and thirst/satisfaction scoring systems). We additionally informed both groups of possible complications associated with the EOH treatment, such as nausea or vomiting. We then obtained written informed consent from the parents of all participating children. After surgical treatment was complete, patients were transferred to the PACU where they were monitored via pulse oximetry, electrocardiography, and noninvasive blood pressure monitoring. Patients were also provided with fluid intravenously. Thirst was rated verbally using a scale of 0–100, with the former representing no thirst and the latter representing the most significant possible thirst. Oropharyngeal discomfort similarly used a 0–100 scale, with 0 representing comfort and 100 representing the most worst discomfort ever suffered. One day postoperatively, patient satisfaction regarding their assigned treatment regimen was also assessed on a 0–100 scale from not satisfied to most satisfied.

A total of 2000 patients were randomized into the EOH and DOH groups ($n = 1000$/group). For the EOH group, medical professionals in the PACU monitored patient recovery until patients exhibited a normal mental status, degree V muscle recovery, stable vitals, and a normal swallowing reflex, at which time children were asked to consume water (< 5 ml/kg, 5% GS). The water was administered by a trained doctor or nurse by first aspirating the appropriate amount of water in an empty needle according to the child's weight, tilting the child's head to one side, and then slowly administering the water in the corner of the mouth. Patients in the DOH group were given oral water 4 h following anesthesia according to standard protocols. Immediately following recovery from anesthetization, patients were assessed for thirst and discomfort.

Measures

Primary outcome and secondary outcome were recorded. Children over 5 years of age used self-reporting scales for thirst and hunger, with both scales extending from 0 to 100 (0: not hungry/thirsty; 100: very hungry/thirsty).

Statistical analysis

SPSS v18.0 (SPSS Inc., Chicago, IL) was used for all analyses. Data are given as means ± SD. Continuous values were compared via Student's t-tests and ANOVAs, while categorical variables were compared via chi-squared tests with Fisher's test. $P < 0.05$ was the significance threshold.

Results

A total of 2000 children were enrolled in this study, with complete data being available for 1770 of these study participants. Of the remaining patients, 88 were excluded due to a failure to drink following anesthesia, while 142 were excluded due to their unavailability for follow-up (Fig. 1). Table 1 summarizes the demographics of the patients included in the final study dataset, with no significant differences in age, gender, weight, surgical operation, or ASA status between groups.

Rates of nausea and vomiting were comparable between the DOH and EOH groups ($P > 0.05$) (Table 2). A similar finding was observed with respect to oropharyngeal discomfort scales ($p < 0.0001$). EOH group patients exhibited higher postoperative satisfaction scores ($P < 0.001$) (Table 3). With respect to the thirst and hunger scores of children over 5 years of age, compared with the DOH group, the scores of thirst and hunger in the EOH group at 10 and 20 min after general anesthesia were significantly lower ($P < 0.05$). After the patients were sent back to the ward, the thirst and hunger in the EOH group were significantly lower than those in the DOH group ($P < 0.05$) (Table 3).

Discussion

The results of this randomized study indicate that EOH is safe in children immediately after general anesthesia associated with non-gastrointestinal surgery, significantly reducing thirst and discomfort while increasing satisfaction.

Postoperative hunger and thirst in children primarily occur due to prolonged preoperative fasting. In order to prevent reflux and aspiration during the operation, fasting for 2 h before anesthesia is necessary [9].

In this study, after recovery from general anesthesia, a small amount of water was given to children, and it did not increase the incidence of postoperative nausea or vomiting. This EOH treatment effectively lowered the thirst and hunger of children in the PACU, improving their comfort. Xiaoping Chen et al. found that the postoperative fasting time for patients undergoing non-

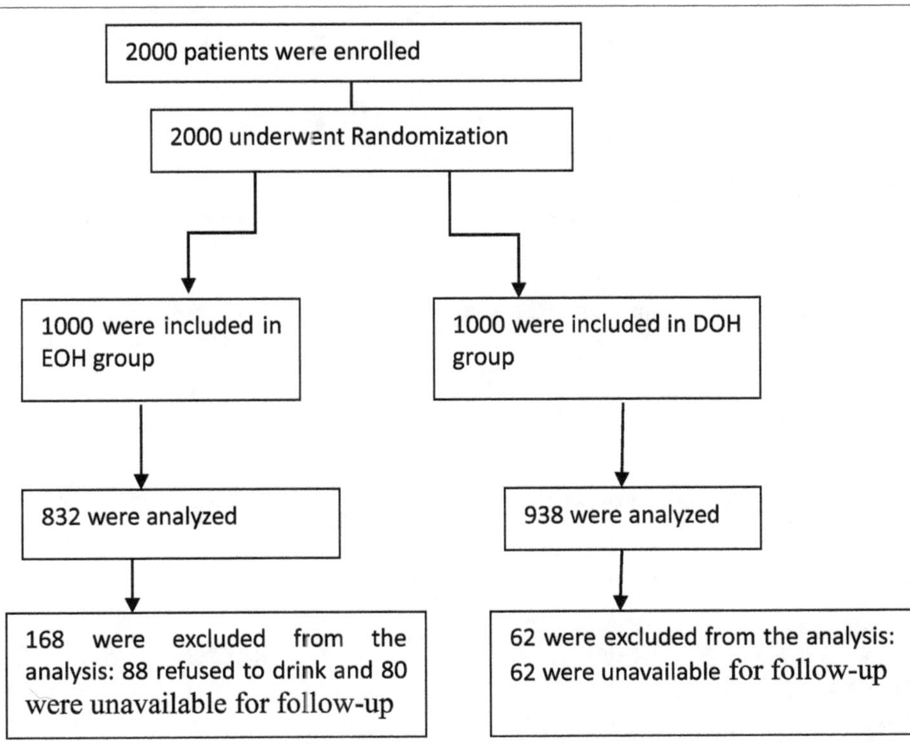

Fig. 1 Randomization, treatment, and inclusion in Analysis. EOH group: early oral hydration group; DOH group: delayed oral hydration group

Table 1 Characteristics of the patient population and the surgical procedures performed

Characteristic and surgical procedure	Early oral hydration group ($n = 832$)	Delayed oral hydration group 4 h after operation group ($n = 938$)	P
Age (y)	5.59 ± 3.25	5.55 ± 3.21	0.79
Sex (%)			0.44
Male	483 (58.1)	562 (59.9)	
Female	349 (41.9)	376 (40.1)	
Weight (Kg)	21.51 ± 9.87	21.59 ± 10.20	0.87
Anesthesia time (min)	80.99 ± 51.45	78.53 ± 48.13	0.30
ASA (%)			0.88
I	179 (21.5)	194 (20.7)	
II	645 (77.5)	736 (78.5)	
III	8 (1.0)	8 (0.9)	
Type of peration			0.55
Polydactyly surgery	13 (1.6)	26 (2.8)	
Burn and plastic surgery	149 (17.9)	145 (15.5)	
orthopedic surgery	239 (28.7)	256 (27.3)	
Hemangioma surgery	22 (2.6)	29 (3.1)	
Ear surgery	43 (5.2)	49 (5.2)	
Ophthalmologic surgery	271 (32.6)	332 (35.4)	
Clubfeet surgery	6 (0.7)	11 (1.2)	
Ambulatory Stitches remove	12 (1.4)	11 (1.2)	
Hypospadias surgery	75 (9.0)	76 (8.1)	
Double J stent remove	2 (0.2)	3 (0.3)	0.75

ASA American Society of Anesthesiologists

Table 2 Drugs used during general anesthesia

Drugs	Early oral hydration group ($n = 832$)	Delayed oral hydration group ($n = 938$)	P
Propofol (%)	742 (89.2)	823 (87.7)	0.37
Fentanyl (%)	707 (85.0)	796 (84.9)	1.00
Midazolam (%)	717 (86.2)	790 (84.2)	0.26
Sevoflurane (%)	832 (100)	938 (100)	1.00
Sulfentanyl (%)	64 (7.7)	77 (8.2)	0.73
Remifentanil (%)	163 (19.6)	174 (18.6)	0.59
Cisatracurium Besilate (%)	534 (64.2)	600 (64.0)	0.96
Succinylcholine chloride (%)	5 (0.6)	6 (0.6)	1.00
Vecuronium bromide (%)	1 (0.1)	5 (0.5)	0.22
ketamine (%)	1 (0.1)	3(0.3)	0.63
Ropivacaine (%)	122 (14.7)	168 (17.9)	0.07
Ondansetron Hydrochloride (%)	656 (78.8)	748 (79.7)	0.68
Tropisetron Hydrochloride (%)	4 (0.5)	3 (0.3)	0.71
Neostigmine (%)	259 (31.1)	330 (35.2)	0.08

Table 3 Incidence of the postoperative nausea and vomiting in PACU and ward

	Early oral hydration group ($n = 332$)	Delayed oral hydration group ($n = 938$)	P
PACU nausea after 20 min (%)	1 (0.1)	5 (0.5)	0.22
PACU: vomiting after 20 min (%)	1 (0.1)	2 (0.2)	1.00
Ward: nausea after 4 h (%)	6 (0.7)	11 (1.2)	0.47
Ward: vomiting after 4 h (%)	5 (0.6)	7 (0.7)	0.78

abdominal surgery should be determined according to operation size, anesthesia method, and patient's reactions following general anesthesia, with patients eating following recovery and elimination of nausea/vomiting symptoms [10]. Another study by Ding Chuanzhong et al. [11], included a control group given a gradually increasing fluid diet 6 h after operation, as well as a control group in which children without nausea and vomiting were evaluated and given warm water after they had recovered from general anesthesia. These children were first given 15–30 ml water, and, if they did not experience discomfort, some milk 15–30 min later, followed by glutinous rice porridge or noodles. In this study, the incidence of postoperative hyperpyrexia, thirst, hunger, crying, agitation, and family anxiety in the experimental group was significantly lower than that in the control group. We previously found it to be feasible for children to drink a small amount of GS after general anesthesia [12]. This work suggested that it was feasible and safe to drink a small amount of water after the recovery from general anesthesia once the cough and swallowing reflex had recovered.

Some researchers [13] have found that complete recovery of the swallowing reflex occurs within 24 min after anesthetization with propofol. Kerz et al. [14] concluded that it was safe to eat via the oral route at early time points after anesthetization when propofol is the only anesthetic used. Children have stomachs that empty rapidly, and preoperative fasting leads to hunger, crying, and significant swallowing of air, thereby leading to increased pressure in the stomach, abdominal distension, prolonged recovery of gastrointestinal peristalsis, and delayed recovery [15].

It is important that water intake in children be carefully monitored following general anesthesia. Children must be completely awake, with a recovered cough and swallowing reflex, as well as muscle strength that has recovered to grade V. When drinking water, children's heads should be tilted to one side, and children should be monitored for cough, nausea, and hypoxemia. There were no instances of hypoxemia during this study. Doctors or nurses must carefully conduct this water administration, monitoring patient vital signs at all times. A small amount of water intake after recovery from general anesthesia can improve the comfort of children, improve their perioperative metabolic state, reduce thirst and hunger, reduce crying, and thereby help facilitate an earlier recovery.

Limitations

Children did not drink or eat from 4 h after returning to the ward, based on standard protocols. There were no statistical differences in thirst or hunger scores from 2 to 4 h after returning to the ward. Further assessment of oral hydration should be continued after returning to the ward.

Conclusions

Postoperative oral intake of fluids is very important for children following general anesthesia. This prospective randomized trial provided evidence that administering oral hydration at early post-anesthesia time points was safe in those children, improving satisfaction and decreasing thirst. Perioperative oral intake of fluids is very important for children following general anesthesia.

Abbreviations

DOH: Late oral hydration; EOH: Early oral hydration; ASA: American Society of Anesthesiology; PACU: Postanesthesia care unit; ChiCTR: Chinese Clinical Trial Registry

Acknowledgments

The authors would like to thank Department of Anesthesiology and Department of Pain Management of West China Hospital.

Authors' contributions

LY contributed to the conception and design of the study, manuscript writing and final approval of the manuscript. XYR contributed to the design of the study, with emphasis on the statistical analysis and sample size analyses, and final approval of the study. XQZ, TW, BBD, MHW and ANJ contributed to the design of the study, statistics analysis and manuscript writing. All authors have read and approved the final manuscript.

Author details

[1]Department of Anesthesiology, West China Hospital, Sichuan University/ West China School of Nursing, Sichuan University, Chengdu, Sichuan Province 610041, People's Republic of China. [2]Department of Pain Management, West China Hospital, Sichuan University, Chengdu, Sichuan Province 610041, People's Republic of China.

References

1. Ting L. Analysis and prevention of concerns in nursing care of patients in anaesthesia recovery room. J Aerospace Med. 2014;25(6):889–90.
2. Xiaoqing L. Perianaesthesia management of agitation during general anesthesia recovery period in children. Chin Modern Med. 2010;17(19):94.
3. Yuanfang C. Nursing care of children during anaesthesia recovery period after operation. Chin Foreign Med Res. 2012;10(21):78.
4. Hao L, Li X, Zhao Z. Study on risk factors and prevention and treatment of emergence agitation. Modern Med J China. 2014;16(10):106–8.
5. Mendelson CL. The aspiration of stomach contents into the lungs during obstetric anesthesia. Am J Obstet Gynecol. 1946;52:191–205.
6. Exarhos ND. The importance of pH and volume in tracheobronchial aspiration. Dis Chest. 1965;47(2):167–9.
7. James CF. Pulmonary aspiration effects of volume and pH in the rat. Anesth Analg. 1984;63(7):665–8.
8. Xi S. Eye, ear, nose, throat and oral nursing. Beijing: People's Medical Publishing House; 2006. p. 147–50.
9. Weixin C. Surgical nursing. 3rd ed. Beijing: People's Medical Publishing House; 2006. p. 18–46.
10. Xiaoping C. Surgery, vol. 57. Beijing: People's Medical Publishing House; 2006.
11. Chuanzhong D, Ailian W, Zhuo L. Application of early food intake in children after general anesthesia undergoing non-gastrointestinal operation. Modern Clin Nurs. 2011;10(6):9.
12. Xiaorong Y, Ling T, Liao YA. Feasibility of a small mount of water intake at early stage after general anesthesia in children. Chin J Anesthesiol. 2012; 32(3):282–3.
13. Xiaojing H, Nanhai P, Jiwei J. Prolonged fasting before surgery should be abolished in patients undergoing elective surgery. J Clin Med Pract. 2007; 11(5):21–2.
14. Kerz T, Wahlen BM. How long should patients refrain from oral food and fluid intake after general anaesthesia?An assessment of the swallowing reflex of postoperative neurosurgical patients. Minim Invasive Neurosurg. 2004;47(6):378–81.
15. Lu G. Evaluation of the effect of individualized health education on fasting before operation in children. Guangxi Med J. 2008;30(7):1053–4.

Prevalence and multivariable factors associated with inadvertent intraoperative hypothermia in video-assisted thoracoscopic surgery

Yinan Li, Hansheng Liang and Yi Feng*

Abstract

Background: Inadvertent intraoperative hypothermia increases the risk of adverse events, but its related risk factors have not defined in video-assisted thoracoscopic surgery (VATS). This study aimed at analyzing the prevalence and factors related to inadvertent intraoperative hypothermia in adults undergoing elective VATS under general anesthesia.

Methods: This was a retrospective study using data from the Peking University People's Hospital from January through December, 2018. Data were collected on age, sex, height, weight, American Society of Anesthesiologists physical status, the duration of preparation and surgery, timing of surgery, surgery types, anesthesia types, intraoperative core temperature and the length of stay (LOS) in the hospital from the electronic database in our center. Patients were covered with a cotton blanket preoperatively and the surgical draping during the operation. A circulation-water warming mattress set to 38 °C were placed under the body of the patients. Inadvertent intraoperative hypothermia was identified as a core temperature monitored in nasopharynx < 36 °C. Multivariate logistic regression analysis was used to identify independent risk factors of hypothermia.

Results: We found that 72.7% (95% CI 70.5 to 75.0%) of 1467 adult patients who underwent VATS suffered hypothermia during surgery. The factors associated with inadvertent intraoperative hypothermia included age (OR = 1.23, 95% CI 1.11 to 1.36, $p < 0.001$), BMI (OR = 1.83, 95% CI 1.43 to 2.35, $p < 0.001$), the duration of preparation (OR = 1.01, 95% CI 1.00 to 1.02, $p = 0.014$), the duration of surgery (OR = 2.10, 95% CI 1.63 to 2.70, $p < 0.001$), timing of surgery (OR = 1.64, 95% CI 1.28 to 2.12, $p < 0.001$), ambient temperature in the operating room (OR = 0.67, 95% CI 0.53 to 0.85, $p = 0.001$) and general anesthesia combined with paravertebral block after induction of anesthesia (OR = 2.30, 95% CI 1.31 to 4.03, $p = 0.004$). The average LOS in the hospital in the hypothermia group and the normothemic group was 9 days and 8 days, respectively ($p < 0.001$).

Conclusions: We highlight the high prevalence of inadvertent intraoperative hypothermia during elective VATS and identify key risk factors including age, duration of surgery more than 2 h, surgery in the morning and general anesthesia combined with paravertebral block (PVB) after intubation. We also find that hypothermia did prolong the LOS in the hospital.

Keywords: Hypothermia, Video-assisted thoracoscopic surgery (VATS), Incidence, Risk factors, Paravertebral block (PVB)

* Correspondence: doctor_yifeng@sina.com
Department of Anesthesia, Peking University People's Hospital, Beijing 100044, China

Background

Hypothermia can be divided into therapeutic hypothermia and inadvertent hypothermia. Inadvertent intraoperative hypothermia, a recognized common perioperative complication, is defined as a core temperature (Tc) < 36 °C with an incidence as high as 70% in adults undergoing elective and emergency surgery [1]. Meanwhile, hypothermia might be associated with increased risk of several different kinds of adverse events. For instance, morbid cardiac events and ventricular tachycardia, blood loss, wound infections, delayed post-anesthetic recovery time and hospitalization, and postoperative cognitive dysfunction [2–6].

Compared to open thoracic surgery, video-assisted thoracoscopic surgery (VATS) is minimally invasive and lowers the exposure of the thoracic viscera to the environment; however, VATS is still vulnerable to perioperative hypothermia [7]. Accordingly, we performed a retrospective study to determine the incidence and factors associated with inadvertent intraoperative hypothermia in adult patients during elective VATS under general anesthesia combined with paravertebral block (PVB) or not.

Methods

This single-center retrospective study was approved by the Ethical Review Committee of Peking University People's Hospital (Beijing, China) and informed consent was waived (No.2019PHB135–01). We retrieved electronic medical information from databases in our center and reviewed data from adult patients who underwent elective VATS under general anesthesia or combined with PVB in the Peking University People's Hospital from January through December, 2018. Patients < 18 years were excluded. Patients who underwent thoracotomy, laparotomy, hyperthermia intrapleural chemotherapy, emergency surgery, non-surgical or cardiac procedures, or under local anesthesia were excluded. Those lacking ambient temperature records or temperature monitoring were also excluded.

We recorded information in an electronic anesthetic documentation system certified by the Healthcare Information and Management Systems Society and rated to Electronic Medical Records Adoption Model stage 7 (HIMSS EMRAM7) in our center in 2014. Our data were all obtained from the electronic database on the server. We collected demographic data including age, sex, height and weight (used to calculate the body mass index, BMI and body surface area, BSA) and American Society of Anesthesiologists physical status (ASA). Clinical data including duration of preparation and surgery, time of surgery (morning or afternoon), types of surgery (wedge resection, lobectomy, mediastinoscopy and others), modes of anesthesia (general anesthesia or general anesthesia combined with PVB) and intraoperative core temperature were collected from the anesthetic documentation. The total time in the operating room (OR) including the preparation time from patients arriving in the OR to the start of surgery, the duration of surgery from surgical incision to the last suture, and the interval from the end of surgery to patients leaving the OR were recorded. The length of stay (LOS) in the hospital was also collected. The ambient temperature and relative humidity in the OR were obtained from the records of the hospital's control center. Patients received routine nasopharyngeal temperature monitoring as intraoperative core temperature in our study. All patients were covered with an unheated cotton blanket preoperatively and the surgical draping during operation for thermal insulation. A circulation-water warming mattress under the body of the patients was set to 38 °C intraoperatively. We didn't use fluid warming or forced air warming device until the core temperature dropped to 35.5 °C. Inadvertent intraoperative hypothermia was defined as a core temperature (Tc) below 36 °C during the intraoperative phase while normothemic referred to a temperature of Tc ≥36 °C throughout the operation. Although Our monitoring system automatically recorded the temperature data every 10s, we collected nasopharyngeal temperature data at intervals of 5 min, and determine the occurrence of hypothermia with all records less than 36 °C within 5 min after the start of the 5 min-data less than 36 °C in order to exclude "false" hypothermia due to factors such as equipment problems or accidental probe displacement.

Continuous variables are shown as the mean (standard deviation) in the normal distribution or the median [interquartile range] where abnormally distributed data were encountered. Frequency (percentages) distributions are shown in categorical variables. Univariate logistic regression analyses were used to explore the influencing factors for inadvertent intraoperative hypothermia, and brought variables with *p*-value less than 0.1 into multivariate logistic regression analyses with backward stepwise regression. The results were expressed as odds ratios with a 95% confidence interval. All statistical analyses were carried out by IBM SPSS, version 22.0. A *p*-value less than 0.05 was considered statistically significant.

Results

After retrieving data from 1720 patients, 1467 were finally analyzed. The flow diagram is shown in Fig. 1 (page 17). Patients ranged 51–66 years of age (58 yrs. [51-66 yrs]), and 50.4% were overweight (BMI ≥ 24 kg/m^2, $n = 740$). Most patients underwent lobectomy ($n = 856$, 58.4%) and were ASA II class ($n = 1113$, 75.9%). The mean ambient temperature and humidity was 22.6 °C (standard deviation 0.5 °C) and 41% (standard deviation 9%), respectively. PVB was widely applied in our study, with 73.6% patients ($n =$ 1079) were applied either before or after induction of anesthesia. More than half of the patients ($n = 778$, 53%) had surgery in the morning (from 8 am to 2 pm) with the

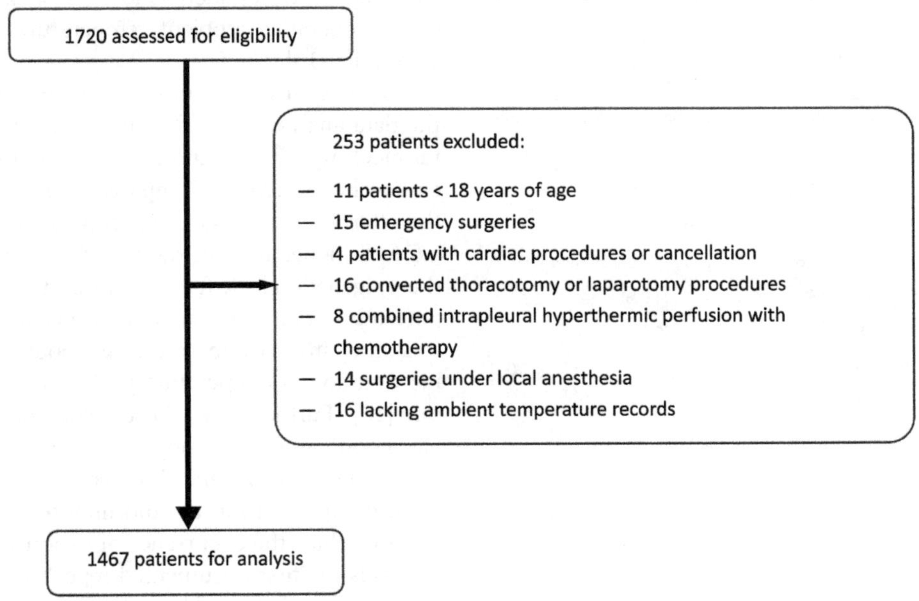

Fig. 1 Study Flow

remainder having surgery in the afternoon (from 2 pm to 8 pm). Statistical differences were observed for all variables excluding sex ($p = 0.057$) and ASA ($p = 0.516$) between the two groups. And the average LOS in the hospital in the hypothermia group and the normothemic group was 9 days and 8 days, respectively ($p < 0.001$) (Table 1, page 13 to 14). Of the 1467 cases, only one in the hypothermia group died before discharge due to post-operative myocardial infarction.

Among the total population, 1067 (72.7, 95% CI 70.5 to 75.0%) patients suffered from intraoperative hypothermia. According to the univariate logistic regression (Table 2, page 15), p-values ≤0.1 were analyzed by multivariate logistic regression, and ultimately, there were seven variables independently related to inadvertent intraoperative hypothermia (Table 3, page 16). High ambient temperature (OR = 0.67, 95% CI 0.53 to 0.85, $p = 0.001$) in the OR was protective against hypothermia; and age (OR = 1.23, 95% CI 1.11 to 1.36, $p < 0.001$), BMI < 24 kg/m^2 (OR = 1.83, 95% CI 1.43 to 2.35, $p < 0.001$), duration of preparation (OR = 1.01, 95% CI 1.00 to 1.02, $p = 0.014$), duration of surgery more than 2 h (OR = 2.10, 95% CI 1.63 to 2.70, $p < 0.001$), undergoing surgery in the morning (OR = 1.64, 95% CI 1.28 to 2.12, $p <$ 0.001) and general anesthesia combined with PVB after intubation (OR = 2.30, 95% CI 1.31 to 4.03, $p = 0.004$) were independent risk factors for hypothermia.

Discussion

In the current study, the prevalence of inadvertent intraoperative hypothermia in VATS was 72.7%, with related risk factors including older age, longer preparation and surgery time, lower ambient temperature, receiving surgery in the morning and general anesthesia combined with PVB after intubation. Being overweight was a protective factor.

In a previous report, the overall incidence of hypothermia was 64.3% during thoracic surgery. We included a more strict definition of hypothermia ≤36 °C and our study cohort had a lower mean BMI than previous studies, explaining such discrepancies [8]. Being overweight is protective owing to the body fat maintaining heat balance through triggering vasoconstriction early when core temperatures decreased in obese patients [9]. Other studies divided patients into hypothermic groups at the end of surgery, which of lower incidence due to the active warming measures performed intraoperatively [10].

It was not surprised that intraoperative hypothermia is more likely to occur at an advanced age, at low room temperature, or during prolonged surgery. This was consistent with patients receiving abdominal surgery under general anesthesia [11]. Previous studies demonstrated that thermoregulatory vasoconstriction threshold is reduced in elderly patients under general anesthesia [12]. The duration of surgery was related to the decline of Tc, in agreement with the results of Suneerat et al. [13]. A longer duration of surgery results in a longer intrathoracic organ exposure time and a longer duration of anesthesia. Both general and neuraxial anesthesia could impair thermoregulatory control [14]. In this study, ambient temperatures were positively associated with core temperatures. This was in accordance with a previous study which demonstrated a higher temperature in the operating room being a strong protective factor against hypothermia [13]. However, if patients used active

Table 1 Demographic and clinical characteristics of the patients ($n = 1467$)

Variable	Hypothermia ($n = 1067$)	Normothermia ($n = 400$)	P value
Age (yr)	60 [53–67]	56 [48–64]	< 0.001*
Sex			0.057
female	577 (54.1%)	194 (48.5%)	
male	490 (45.9%)	206 (51.5%)	
BMI (kg/m^2)	23.81 [21.80–25.80]	24.75 [22.68–26.89]	< 0.001*
< 24	563 (52.8%)	164 (41.0%)	
≥ 24	504 (47.2%)	236 (59.0%)	
BSA (m^2)	1.80 [1.69–1.92]	1.86 [1.73–2.01]	< 0.001*
≤ 1.83	626 (58.7%)	186 (46.5%)	
> 1.83	441 (41.3%)	214 (53.5%)	
ASA			0.516
I	175 (16.4%)	73 (18.3%)	
II	811 (76.0%)	302 (75.5%)	
III	81 (7.6%)	25 (6.3%)	
Duration of Preparation (min)	60 [49–72]	54 [46–66]	< 0.001*
≤ 1 h	551 (51.6%)	263 (65.8%)	
> 1 h	516 (48.4%)	137 (34.3%)	
Time of Surgery			< 0.001*
Morning	616 (57.7%)	162 (40.5%)	
Afternoon	451 (42.3%)	238 (59.5%)	
Duration of Surgery (min)	122 [94–156]	100.5 [74–130]	< 0.001*
≤ 2 h	511 (47.9%)	267 (66.8%)	
> 2 h	556 (52.1%)	133 (33.3%)	
Time in OR (min)	201 [168–237]	174 [140.5–210]	< 0.001*
≤ 3 h	378 (35.4%)	227 (56.8%)	
> 3 h	689 (64.6%)	173 (43.3%)	
OR temperature (°C)	22.6 [22.3–23.0]	22.7 [22.4–23.1]	< 0.001*
OR humidity (%)	40 [36–51]	39 [36–48]	< 0.001*
Type of Surgery			< 0.001*
wedge resection	281 (26.3%)	153 (38.3%)	
lobectomy	667 (62.5%)	189 (47.3%)	
mediastinum	98 (9.2%)	46 (11.5%)	
others	21 (2.0%)	12 (3.0%)	
Type of Anesthesia			< 0.001*
general anesthesia alone	289 (27.1%)	99 (24.8%)	
PVB before intubation	632 (59.2%)	283 (70.8%)	
PVB after intubation	146 (13.7%)	18 (4.5%)	
LOS in the hospital (day)	9 [7–11]	8 [7–10]	< 0.001*

Values are shown as the median [interquartile range] or number (%), analyzed using a Mann-Whitney U test or chi-square test
OR operating room, *BMI* body mass index, *BSA* body surface area, BSA = 0.0061*height (cm) + 0.0124*weight (kg)-0.0099; *ASA* American Society of Anesthesiologists physical status, *PVB* paravertebral block, *LOS* length of stay
Duration of preparation refers to the interval from arrival in the OR to incision
Time in the OR refers to minutes from arrival in the OR to leaving the OR

warming strategies such as forced-air blankets, the effects of intraoperative ambient temperatures on hypothermia were mild [15].

A significant finding of this retrospective study was that the data analysis showed timing of surgery or paravertebral block were also important factors influencing intraoperative hypothermia. Compared to surgery performed in the afternoon, the risk of intraoperative hypothermia was 1.6 fold higher than in the morning. This may be due to the epigenetic clock function in body temperature as reported in different seasons in a previous study. According to a study investigating individual body temperature, diurnal variation in temperature peak at 4 pm compared to 12 pm [16]. Furthermore, those undergoing surgery in the afternoon provide perioperative myocardial protection [17]. Hence, it is beneficial to perform surgery in the afternoon compared to in the morning to regarding in reduction of reduce the occurrence of hypothermia.

This is the first documented report to establish relationships between PVB and hypothermia. There were no statistical differences between general anesthesia with PVB and general anesthesia alone related to hypothermia in univariate logistic regression. According to the blocking time, ultrasound-guided PVB was further divided into the pre-induction PVB group and the post-induction PVB group. Patients who received ultrasound-guided PVB first and then underwent general anesthesia were referred to as pre-induction PVB, while patients who received ultrasound-guided PVB after general anesthesia were referred to as post-induction PVB. After regrouping PVB according to blocking time, compared with general anesthesia alone, the risk of intraoperative hypothermia was 2.3 fold higher in patients undergoing general anesthesia combined with post-induction PVB by multivariate logistic regression analysis. Compared to the epidural anesthesia (EA), PVB blocks ipsilateral sympathetic nerves and is associated with a reduction in hypotension [18]. As known, EA leads to hypothermia through its ability to redistribute heat [19]. PVB may therefore promote hypothermia through the same mechanism. However, it may have a "hypothermic preconditioning" function which differs from EA due to its unilateral sympathetic block. PVB may neutralize variations in Tc by enhancing thermogenesis before general anesthesia impairing thermoregulatory control. Further randomized controlled studies are required to establish the relationship between PVB and hypothermia.

There were some limitations in this study. First, only the relationship between hypothermia and variations were analyzed but the etiology associated was not discussed. Then, the core temperature data of PACU cannot be obtained retrospectively, so we did not analyze the correlation between intraoperative core temperature and PACU temperature. And a further limitation was the study being single-centered, limiting its external validity.

Table 2 Univariate logistic regression for inadvertent intraoperative hypothermia rates

	β	Wald	Odds ratio	95% confidence interval		*P* value
Age (per decade)	.256	27.188	1.292	1.173	1.423	.000*
Female	.223	3.623	1.250	.993	1.574	.057
BMI (kg/m^2)	−.100	26.662	.905	.871	.940	.000*
< 24	.475	15.985	1.607	1.274	2.029	.000*
BSA (m^2)	−2.101	36.946	.122	.062	.241	.000*
≤ 1.83	.491	17.293	1.633	1.296	2.058	.000*
ASA						
I	/	1.319	/	/	/	.517
II	.114	.538	1.120	.827	1.517	.463
III	.301	1.265	1.352	.799	2.285	.261
Duration of Preparation (min)	.019	23.995	1.019	1.012	1.027	.000*
> 1 h	.587	23.160	1.798	1.416	2.283	.000*
Surgery in the morning	.696	34.122	2.007	1.588	2.535	.000*
Duration of Surgery (min)	.009	45.492	1.009	1.007	1.012	.000*
> 2 h	.781	40.642	2.184	1.718	2.777	.000*
Time in OR (min)	.008	46.178	1.008	1.006	1.010	.000*
> 3 h	.872	53.239	2.392	1.892	3.023	.000*
OR temperature (°C)	−.388	11.685	.678	.543	.847	.001*
OR humidity (%)	.026	11.132	1.026	1.011	1.042	.001*
Type of Surgery						
lobectomy	/	28.149	/	/	/	.000
wedge resection	−.653	25.264	.520	.403	.671	.000*
mediastinum	−.505	6.577	.604	.410	.888	.010*
others	−.701	3.572	.496	.240	1.026	.590
Type of Anesthesia						
general anesthesia alone	/	26.221	/	/	/	.000
PVB before intubation	−.268	3.842	.765	.585	1.000	.050*
PVB after intubation	1.022	13.747	2.779	1.619	4.769	.000*

BMI body mass index, *BSA* body surface area, BSA = 0.0061*height (cm) + 0.0124*weight (kg)-0.0099; *ASA* American Society of Anesthesiologists physical status, *OR* operating room, *PVB* paravertebral block
Time in OR refers to minutes from arrival in OR to leaving OR

Table 3 Multivariate logistic regression for inadvertent intraoperative hypothermia rates

	β	Wald	Adjusted odds ratio	95% confidence interval		*P* value
Age (per decade)	.206	15.898	1.229	1.111	1.360	.000*
BMI < 24 kg/m^2	.606	23.351	1.833	1.434	2.345	.000*
Surgery in the morning	.497	14.915	1.644	1.278	2.117	.000*
Duration of Preparation (min)	.010	5.995	1.011	1.002	1.019	.014*
Duration of Surgery> 2 h	.742	33.426	2.099	1.633	2.699	.000*
OR temperature (°C)	−.401	11.243	.670	.530	.847	.001*
Type of Anesthesia						
general anesthesia alone	/	10.797	/	/	/	.005
PVB before intubation	−.084	.309	.920	.685	1.235	.579
PVB after intubation	.832	8.441	2.298	1.311	4.029	.004*

Method = Backward Stepwise (Likelihood Ratio)
BMI body mass index, *OR* operating room, *PVB* paravertebral block
**p*-value less than 0.05 was considered statistically significant

Conclusions

The prevalence of inadvertent intraoperative hypothermia in adult patients during elective VATS under general anesthesia is high. And we find that hypothermia did prolong the length of stay. Being overweight prevented patients from hypothermia, while independent risk factors associated with hypothermia were old age, a duration of surgery more than 2 h, morning surgery and general anesthesia combined with PVB after intubation. Advanced prospective studies are now required evaluate the relationship between PVB and inadvertent intraoperative hypothermia.

Abbreviations

ASA: American Society of Anesthesiologists physical status; BMI: Body mass index; EA: Epidural anesthesia; HIMSS EMRAM7: the Healthcare Information and Management Systems Society and rated to Electronic Medical Records Adoption Model stage 7; OR: Operating room; PVB: Paravertebral block; Tc: Core temperature; VATS: Video-assisted thoracoscopic surgery

Acknowledgements

We thank Xu Guo for his designing of data retrieval program, Huixin Liu and Xiaohua Zhou for their statistical consultation, and Kehong Zhang for his scientific writing instruction, sincerely.

Authors' contributions

All authors designed the study and revised the manuscript. YL conducted the study, collected and analyzed the data, and drafted the manuscript. HL and YF made contributions to the conception of the work and substantively revised the manuscript. All authors read and approved the final manuscript.

References

1. NICE: The Management of Inadvertent Perioperative Hypothermia in Adults Vol. NICE Clinical Guideline 65. 2008.
2. Frank SM. Perioperative maintenance of normothermia reduces the incidence of morbid cardiac events. JAMA. 1997;277(14):1127.
3. Schmied H, Reiter A, Kurz A, Sessler DI, Kozek S. Mild hypothermia increases blood loss and transfusion requirements during total hip arthroplasty. Lancet. 1996;347(8997):289–92.
4. Lenhardt R, Marker E, Goll V, Tschernich H, Kurz A, Sessler DI, Narzt E, Lackner F. Mild intraoperative hypothermia prolongs Postanesthetic recovery. Anesthesiology. 1997;87(6):1318–23.
5. Kurz A, Sessler DI, Lenhardt R. Perioperative Normothermia to reduce the incidence of surgical-wound infection and shorten hospitalization. N Engl J Med. 1996;334(19):1209–16.
6. Ma H, Lai B, Dong S, Li X, Cui Y, Sun Q, Liu W, Jiang W, Xu F, Lv H, et al. Warming infusion improves perioperative outcomes of elderly patients who underwent bilateral hip replacement. Medicine. 2017;96(13):e6490.
7. Franke R, Brandes I, Hinterthaner M, Danner B, Bauer M, Bräuer A, Emmert A. Comparison of conductive and convective warming in patients undergoing video-assisted thoracic surgery: a prospective randomized clinical trial. Thorac Cardiovasc Surg. 2016;65(05):362–6.
8. Emmert A, Gries G, Wand S, Buentzel J, Bräuer A, Quintel M, Brandes IF. Association between perioperative hypothermia and patient outcomes after thoracic surgery. Medicine. 2018;97(17):e0528.
9. Kasai T, Hirose M, Matsukawa T, Takamata A, Tanaka Y. The vasoconstriction threshold is increased in obese patients during general anaesthesia. Acta Anaesthesiol Scand. 2003;47(5):588–92.
10. Sumida H, Sugino S, Kuratani N, Konno D, J-i H, Yamauchi M. Effect of forced-air warming by an underbody blanket on end-of-surgery hypothermia: a propensity score-matched analysis of 5063 patients. BMC Anesthesiol. 2019;19(1):50.
11. Kim EJ, Yoon H. Preoperative factors affecting the intraoperative Core body temperature in abdominal surgery under general anesthesia. Clin Nurse Spec. 2014;28(5):268–76.
12. Ozaki M, Sessler DI, Matsukawa T, Ozaki K, Atarashi K, Negishi C, Suzuki H. The threshold for thermoregulatory vasoconstriction during nitrous oxide/sevoflurane anesthesia is reduced in the elderly. Anesth Analg. 1997;84(5):1029–33.
13. Kongsayreepong S, Chaibundit C, Chadpaibool J, Komoltri C, Suraseranivongse S, Suwannanonda P, Raksamanee E-o, Noocharoen P, Silapadech A, Parakkamodom S, et al. Predictor of Core hypothermia and the surgical intensive care unit. Anesth Analg. 2003;93:826–33.
14. Sessler DI. Perioperative thermoregulation and heat balance. Lancet. 2016; 387(10038):2655–64.
15. Pei L, Huang Y, Xu Y, Zheng Y, Sang X, Zhou X, Li S, Mao G, Mascha EJ, Sessler DI. Effects of ambient temperature and forced-air warming on intraoperative core temperature. Anesthesiology. 2018;128(5):903–11.
16. Obermeyer Z, Samra JK, Mullainathan S. Individual differences in normal body temperature: longitudinal big data analysis of patient records. BMJ. 2017;359:j5468.
17. Montaigne D, Marechal X, Modine T, Coisne A, Mouton S, Fayad G, Ninni S, Klein C, Ortmans S, Seunes C, et al. Daytime variation of perioperative myocardial injury in cardiac surgery and its prevention by rev-Erbα antagonism: a single-Centre propensity-matched cohort study and a randomised study. Lancet. 2018;391(10115):59–69.
18. Davies RG, Myles PS, Graham JM. A comparison of the analgesic efficacy and side-effects of paravertebral vs epidural blockade for thoracotomy—a systematic review and meta-analysis of randomized trials. Br J Anaesth. 2006;96(4):418–26.
19. Glosten B, Hynson J, Sessler DI, McGuire J. Preanesthetic skin-surface warming reduces redistribution hypothermia caused by epidural block. Anesth Analg. 1993;77(3):488–93.

The effect of brief pre-anesthetic exercise therapy of jaw and neck joints on mouth opening, neck extension and intubation conditions during induction of general anesthesia

Sue Young Lee[1†], Sung Il Bae[2†], Sang-Hwan Do[3,4], Ju-Tae Sohn[2,5] and Jin-Woo Park[3*]

Abstract

Background: The effort to improve tracheal intubation process is clinically valuable. We hypothesized that a preoperative brief exercise therapy would increase mouth opening and neck extension, enhancing intubation conditions during general anesthesia.

Methods: Patients undergoing general anesthesia were randomized into two groups. The exercise group performed the exercise regimen including masseter muscle massage and stretching of jaw and neck joints before anesthetic induction, while the control did not. Before (baseline) and after the intervention, we evaluated Mallampati score, mouth aperture size, and sternomental distance. After tracheal intubation, intubation difficulty scale with direct laryngoscope and oropharyngeal soft tissue injury were also evaluated.

Results: A total of 138 patients completed the analysis (control = 68, exercise = 70). Baseline characteristics did not differ between groups. At anesthetic induction, there was a significant difference in Mallampati score between the two groups ($P = 0.039$) and the incidence of Mallampati scores of 1 was higher in the exercise group (odds ratio [95% CI]: 2.1 [1.0–4.3], $P = 0.043$). Mouth opening after the intervention was greater in the exercise group than in the control group (estimated difference [95% CI]: – 2.4 [– 4.8 – -0.1], $P = 0.042$) and sternomental distance was similar between the two groups (estimated difference [95% CI]: – 3.7 [– 9.0–1.7, $P = 0.175$). The exercise group showed less soft tissue injuries (odds ratio [95% CI]: 0.2 [0.1–0.8], $P = 0.009$), however, intubation difficulty scale did not differ between the study groups ($P = 0.112$).

Conclusions: The brief pre-anesthetic exercise improved intubation conditions and enabled faster tracheal intubation with less injury to oropharyngeal soft tissue.

Keywords: Anesthesia, general, Exercise, Intubation, Mouth opening, Neck extension

* Correspondence: jinul8282@gmail.com
†Sue Young Lee and Sung Il Bae contributed equally to this work.
[3]Department of Anesthesiology and Pain Medicine, Seoul National University Bundang Hospital, 82 Gumi-ro, 173 Beon-gil, Bundang-gu, Seongnam, Gyeonggi-do 13620, Republic of Korea

Background

Limited neck movement and a short inter-incisor gap may interfere with exposure of the larynx during direct laryngoscopy and are significant risk factors for difficult tracheal intubation [1–5]. When glottic exposure is inadequate with a direct laryngoscope, other instruments such as intubation stylet, video laryngoscope, or fiberoptic bronchoscope can be utilized to access the larynx [6, 7]. However, difficult intubation cannot be exactly predicted in advance [3, 5, 8]. Complications such as soft tissue injuries and dental trauma may also occur during successful intubation [9, 10]. Without a doubt, improvement of intubation conditions is of clinical significance for patients undergoing general anesthesia.

Various exercise regimens based on stretching and muscle massage have been proposed to treat patients with temporomandibular joint disorders and impaired mouth opening [11]. Furthermore, previous studies demonstrated that brief stretching or massage of joint muscles could increase range of motion and decrease muscle stiffness in healthy volunteers as well as subjects with musculoskeletal abnormalities [12–18]. Therefore, we hypothesized that pre-anesthetic exercise therapy of jaw (temporomandibular) and neck (cervical vertebral) joints could enhance mouth opening and neck mobility during anesthetic induction and facilitate the process of orotracheal intubation.

We performed a randomized controlled trial to evaluate the effects of a single brief pre-anesthetic exercise therapy session on mouth opening, neck extension, intubation difficulty, and soft tissue injuries to the oropharyngeal area in patients undergoing general anesthesia.

Methods

Study

The protocol for this prospective multicenter trial was approved by the Institutional Review Boards of Seoul National University Bundang Hospital (study number: B-1709-423-307) and Jinju Gyeongsang National University Hospital (study number: GNUH 2018–05–019-001). It was registered at the Clinical Research Information Service (https://cris.nih.go.kr; registration number: KCT0002618; date of registration: December 28, 2017). Written informed consent was obtained from all patients before surgery. Patients were enrolled from January to October 2018 at both institutions. This study adhered to CONSORT guidelines.

Patients

Adult patients with American Society of Anesthesiologists physical status I–II, aged 20–70 years, who were scheduled to undergo elective surgery under general anesthesia were enrolled in this study. We excluded patients who were likely to encounter difficulties or pain when actively performing the jaw and neck exercises: Patients with cognitive disorders, temporomandibular joint disorders, or cervical spine diseases. For safety reasons, we excluded patients under consideration for awake intubation using a fiber-optic bronchoscope, such as those with craniofacial anomaly or mechanical airway obstruction. Patients with tracheostomy or who were to receive oropharyngeal surgery during this protocol were also excluded. Enrolled patients were randomly allocated to either the exercise or the control group, using a computer-generated randomization code (Random Allocation Software Version 1.0; University of Medical Sciences, Isfahan, Iran). The allocation ratio was 1:1. Randomization was performed by an independent anesthesiologist in each hospital. These individuals were only involved in patient allocation and coaching of the exercise, and not in any aspects of anesthesia, data analysis or interpretation.

Intervention, anesthesia, and study outcomes

At the reception area, each patient's basal characteristics related to tracheal intubation difficulty were assessed [2–5]. These included mouth aperture size defined as the maximum interincisal distance, Mallampati score, sternomental distance (SMD) as an indicator of neck mobility, thyromental distance, and the presence of buck teeth, were assessed by an anesthesiology resident in each hospital who only participated in these examinations and did not know the patient group. We used a single assessor in each hospital, to minimize inter-rater bias. In this protocol, Mallampati scoring was performed in sitting position, with the tongue fully protruded, and without phonation [19]. During the measurements, the sitting patients were encouraged to open their mouths as wide as possible and to fully extend their head on the neck. After the baseline examination, patients in the exercise group were guided to perform exercise therapy for 5 min at the reception area, before transferral to the operating room. This brief exercise regimen comprises masseter muscle massage and active/passive stretching of the jaw and neck joints (Fig. 1). Stretching was performed to the maximum range of motion within the level not causing pain. The patients in the control group waited at the reception area, without any exercise, before transfer to the operating room. No pre-medication was given to patients in either group. Patients were instructed not to reveal their group information to anyone after the intervention. The importance of blindness was emphasized repeatedly to all patients throughout the protocol.

After transport to the operating room, standard non-invasive monitoring of vital signs was started.

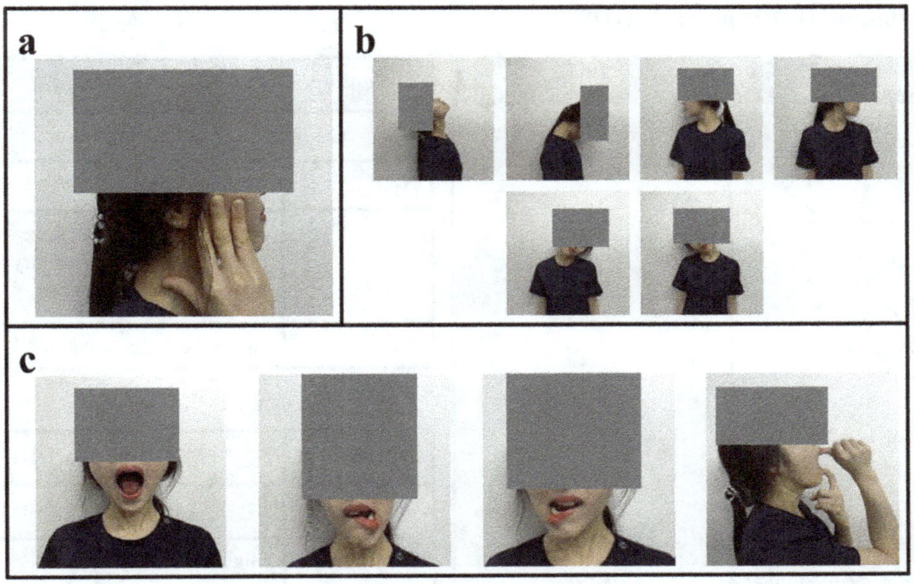

Fig. 1 The exercise regimen on jaw and neck joints (Exercise sequence: a – b – c – a). **a** Manual massage of masseter muscle (30 s); **b** Extension, flexion, rotation, and lateral flexion of neck (2 min); **c** Active and passive maximum mandibular opening and lateral deviation of temoporomandibular joint (2 min)

Mouth aperture, Mallampati score, and SMD were measured again, just before anesthetic induction. In each hospital, the induction of general anesthesia and intubation were performed by a blinded anesthesiologist (clinical professor) who was unaware of patient allocation, and had more than 7 years of experience with anesthesia. After denitrogenation with 100% oxygen, propofol 1.5–2 mg/kg was intravenously administered, and target-controlled infusion of remifentanil with 4 ng/ml effect site concentration was started to inhibit hemodynamic responses to tracheal intubation. After patient consciousness and eyelash reflex were lost, rocuronium 0.6 mg/kg was administered, and facial mask ventilation was performed. Muscle relaxation was assessed using train-of-four stimuli every 10 s. Following the disappearance of T1 of train-of-four stimuli, orotracheal intubation was performed using a direct laryngoscope with Macintosh blade. During intubation, the anesthesiologist placed the laryngoscope into the mouth and raised the blade up and away from the patient to obtain a clear view of the glottis. The subjective necessity of increased lifting force compared to routine practice, and the Cormack-Lehane grade, were checked. To facilitate intubation, laryngeal compression (backward, upward, and rightward pressure) was sometimes applied by an assistant [20]. If we could not obtain an adequate view, orotracheal intubation was attempted with alternative techniques including intubation stylet, video laryngoscope, and/or fiber-optic bronchoscope. If the first anesthesiologist failed to intubate within 3 attempts, the fourth trial was performed by another senior anesthesiologist [21]. The requirements for laryngeal compression or alternative techniques, the number of intubation attempts and additional anesthesiologists, and the intubation time from the end of mask ventilation to the passage of an orotracheal tube through the vocal cords, were recorded by an independent and blinded anesthetic nurse in each hospital. Intubation difficulty scale (IDS) was calculated based on these values (Fig. 2) [2, 22, 23].

After anesthetic induction, anesthetic depth was maintained using 1–1.5 minimum alveolar concentration inhalation (sevoflurane or desfluane), or target-controlled infusion of propofol at a 40–60 bispectral index, with remifentanil target-controlled infusion adjusted to maintain hemodynamic stability. At the end of the operation, neostigmine 0.03 mg/kg and glycopyrrolate 0.01 mg/kg were administered to reverse residual neuromuscular block. When the train-of-four ratio increased over 90% and sufficient spontaneous breathing was confirmed, oropharyngeal secretions were gently cleared by suction, and the endotracheal tube removed.

At the post anesthesia care unit of each hospital, 15 min after the extubation, injuries of oropharyngeal soft tissue including lip, gum, tongue, buccal mucosa, palate, and pharynx were examined using a penlight by a single blinded anesthesiologist who participated only in this measurement and had no other involvement in the study. Except in nasal surgery cases, the appearance of bloody secretions in the oropharyngeal suction before extubation was also interpreted as incidence of oropharyngeal injury.

Intubation Difficulty Scale (IDS)

Parameter	Score
Number of Attempts > 1	N_1
Number of Operators > 1	N_2
Number of Alternative techniques	N_3
Cormack and Lehane Grade - 1	N_4
Lifting Force Required Normal Increased	 $N_5=0$ $N_5=1$
Cricoid Compression Not applied Applied	 $N_6=0$ $N_6=1$
Vocal cord Mobility Abduction Adduction	 $N_7=0$ $N_7=1$
TOTAL: IDS = SUM OF SCORES	N_1 - N_7

Score	Rule
N_1	Every additional attempt adds 1 pt.
N_2	Each additional operator adds 1 pt.
N_3	Each alternative technique adds 1 point: intubation stylet, video laryngoscope, and/or fiber-optic bronchoscope.
N_4	Apply Cormack grade for 1st oral attempt.

IDS Score	Degree of Difficulty
0	Easy
$0 < IDS \leq 5$	Slight Difficulty
$5 < IDS$	Moderate to Major Difficulty

Fig. 2 Intubation difficulty scale

Statistical analysis

Continuous variables are expressed as mean (SD). Categorical variables are shown as number or percentage (%). The primary outcome was the Mallampati score before and after exercise. Secondary outcomes were as follows: mouth aperture size, SMD, Cormack-Lehane grade, intubation time, numbers of intubation attempts, number of anesthesiologists who attempted orotracheal intubation, number of alternative techniques required, increased lifting pressure or laryngeal compression, soft tissue injuries after using direct laryngoscope, and IDS. To compare continuous variables between control and exercise groups, we used the independent Student's t-test. Differences between categorical variables were assessed using the chi-square or Fisher's exact test between the two groups. For grading characteristic of Mallampati score and Cormack-Lehane grade, linear-by-linear association was performed to compare the trend between groups. To analyze within-group change between before and after the exercise therapy, a paired t-test was used. SPSS version 19.0 software (SPSS Inc., IBM, Chicago, IL, USA) was used for the statistical analysis. All reported *P*-values are two-sided, and a *P*-value < 0.05 was considered statistically significant.

Sample size

In a pilot study of 20 patients (10 patients in each group), the effect size for Mallampati score was used to calculate the required sample size (number of patients). The Mallampati score indicates mouth aperture size relative to tongue size, and therefore reflects the adequacy of mouth opening during displacement of the tongue by the laryngoscope [3, 19, 24]. Mallampati score is one of the well-recognized predictive factors for the condition of orotracheal intubation, and a Mallampati score other than 1 was reported as one of the criteria for predicting the condition [3, 5]. The incidence of Mallampati scores of 1 after the exercise regimen were 15% for the control group, and 35% for the exercise group. Based on the results of the pilot study, a power analysis was performed with G*Power 3.1.2 (Heinrich-Heine University, Düsseldorf, Germany). This suggested that in each group, 70 patients were required for a power of 80%, a risk of 0.05 for a type-I error in two-tailed statistical analysis, and a dropout rate of 7.5%.

Results

Of the 151 eligible patients, 11 were excluded because 8 declined to participate, and 3 met the exclusion criteria for cervical pain. The remaining 140 patients were randomly allocated to one of the two study groups, with 70 patients per group. Two patients in the control group withdrew after the training intervention. Thus, 138 patients completed the study (number of patients in the control and exercise groups, 44 and 47 respectively in Seoul National University Bundang Hospital, and 24 and 23 in Jinju Gyeongsang National University Hospital; Fig. 3).

Patients' baseline characteristics did not differ between groups, including mouth aperture size, SMD, pre-intervention Mallampati score, anesthesia, and surgery data affecting the intubation difficulty or the postoperative soft tissue assessment between the study groups (Tables 1 and 2).

At anesthetic induction, there was a significant difference in Mallampati score between the two groups (P = 0.039) and the incidence of Mallampati scores of 1 was higher in the exercise than in the control group (2.1 (1.0–4.3), odds ratio (95% CI); $P = 0.043$; Table 2). Mouth opening was after the intervention greater in the exercise group than in the control group ($P = 0.042$), however, SMD was indistinguishable between the control and exercise groups ($P = 0.175$; Table 2). Analysis of pre- to post-exercise therapy changes within the exercise group showed that the exercise intervention increased mouth aperture size and SMD ($P < 0.001$; Table 2).

The incidences of increased lifting force and laryngeal compression required to obtain the intubation pathway were lower in the exercise than in the control group ($P = 0.034$ and 0.027, respectively; Table 3). All other variables of IDS, the IDS score itself, and IDS difficulty group did not differ significantly between the two groups (Table 3). In both groups, there was no case in which an additional anesthesiologist was requested to attempt tracheal intubation (Table 3). Compared to the control group, the exercise group showed shorter intubation time and fewer soft tissue injuries ($P = 0.032$ and 0.009, respectively; Table 3). There were 58 patients with a baseline Mallampati score III or IV, who were deemed to show smaller mouth opening during tracheal intubation. In the subgroup analysis performed for those patients, there was a significant difference in the IDS grade between the control and exercise groups ($P = 0.029$; Table 4). The Cormack-Lehane grade did not significantly differ between the groups in the subgroup comparison (Table 4).

Discussion

The beneficial effects of stretching or massage on different joints have been studied for various therapeutic applications [12–18]. A variety of exercise-treatments have been demonstrated to relieve clinical symptoms and restore range of motion in joint disorders, including

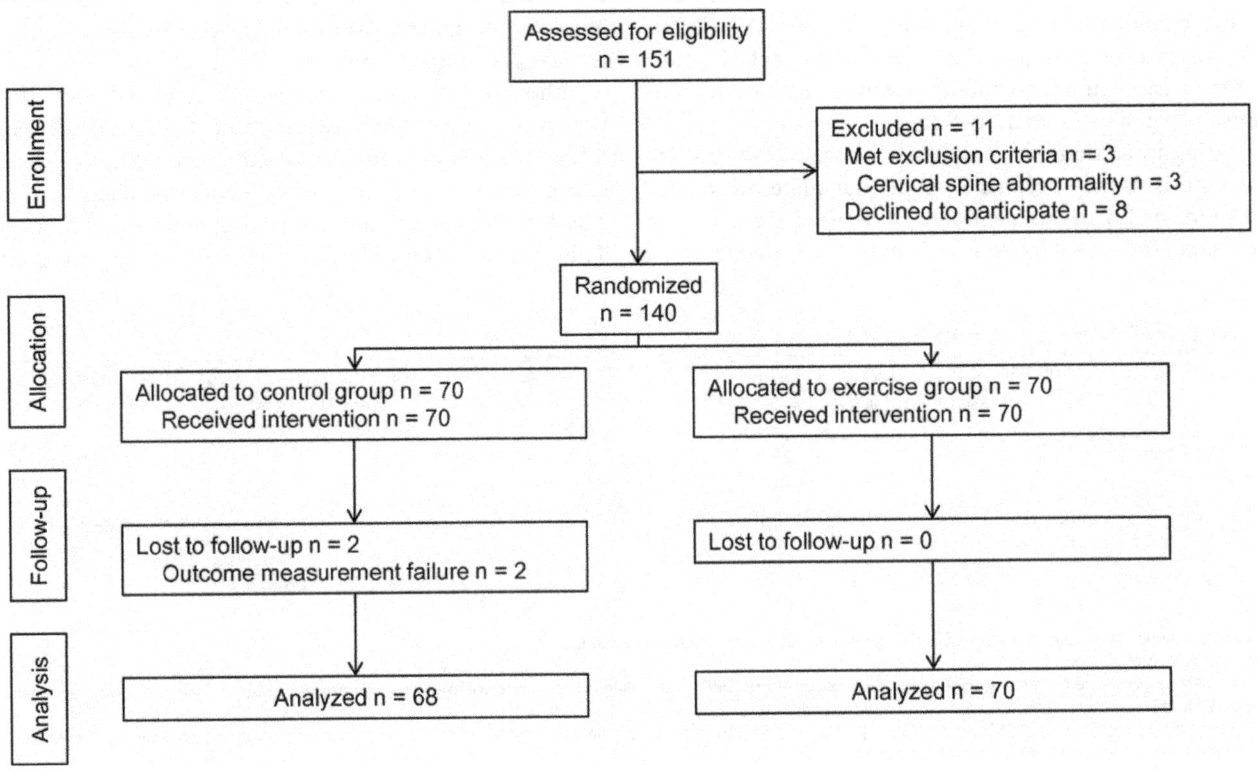

Fig. 3 CONSORT diagram

Table 1 Patients' characteristics, anesthesia, and operational data

	Control ($n = 68$)	Exercise ($n = 70$)
Age (years)	49.5 ± 11.6	50.6 ± 10.6
Male sex	32 (47.1%)	32 (45.7%)
Height (cm)	165.1 ± 9.1	163.9 ± 9.0
Weight (kg)	65.2 ± 11.8	68.0 ± 11.4
ASA class (I/II)	27 (39.7%) / 41 (60.3%)	23 (32.9%) / 47 (67.1%)
Thyromental distance (mm)	91.1 ± 9.8	91.8 ± 10.2
Buck teeth	1 (1.5%)	3 (4.3%)
Induction dose (propofol, mg)	112.6 ± 13.2	114.9 ± 10.5
Anesthetic time (min)	123.6 ± 74.7	139.9 ± 82.4
Operation Position (supine/prone/lateral decubitus)	66/2/0	69/0/1
Nasal surgery	4 (5.9%)	9 (12.9%)

Continuous values are shown as mean ± SD. Categorical variables are expressed as patient numbers (%) or numbers
ASA American society of anesthesiologists

osteoarthritis and rheumatoid arthritis [11, 25–28]. The exercise regimen of our study protocol included active and passive stretching of jaw and neck muscles. A brief stretching session potentially enhances joint flexibility and alleviates muscle stiffness [12, 13, 18]. In a previous study of knee joint exercise, 4 sets of stretching for 20 s each produced a decrease in passive hamstring stiffness, and improved joint range of motion [12]. Massage has been also reported to reduce muscle stiffness [15, 16]. In our protocol, the patients in the exercise group performed masseter muscle massage at the beginning and at the end of the exercise therapy. To our knowledge, this study is the first quantification of the effect of a simple exercise regimen on mouth opening and neck extension during anesthetic induction.

During induction of general anesthesia, orotracheal intubation is usually performed under adequate muscle relaxation that can be achieved by administration of a neuromuscular blocking agent. However, a neuromuscular blocking agent exerts its effects at the neuromuscular junction. It does not modulate the mechanical properties of joints but rather interferes with neural drive to muscle, thereby blocking contraction [29]. Joint flexibility or stiffness is dependent not only upon the contraction of joint muscles, but also on the properties of connective tissue and ligaments [30–33]. Therefore, the enhancement of mouth opening and neck mobility by pre-anesthetic exercise could be maintained even after neuromuscular blocking agent injection. Furthermore, it was reported that general anesthesia employing muscle relaxants did not necessarily increase the passive range of motion of joints [30].

Although SMD examined just before anesthetic induction was comparable between the two groups, the clear differences before and after the regimen within the exercise group showed the definite beneficial effects of our exercise therapy on mouth opening and neck extension. The exercise group showed larger mouth opening and

Table 2 Mouth aperture size, SMD, and Mallampati score

	Control ($n = 68$)		Exercise ($n = 70$)		P_1[a]	P_2[b]	Estimated difference[b] (95% CI)	P_3[c]	Odds ratio[c] (95% CI)	P_4[d]	Estimated difference[d] (95% CI)
	Before	After	Before	After							
Mouth aperture size (mm)	49.3 ± 6.4	49.0 ± 7.5	48.9 ± 5.0	51.3 ± 6.4	0.675	0.042	−2.4(−4.8 to − 0.1)			< 0.001	−2.5(−3.7 to −1.2)
SMD (mm)	183.6 ± 16.0	183.6 ± 16.0	181.8 ± 16.0	187.3 ± 15.8	0.505	0.175	−3.7(− 9.0 to 1.7)			< 0.001	−5.5(− 6.4 to − 4.6)
Mallampati score (I/II/III/IV)	18/22/14/14	18/23/14/13	21/19/8/22	30/19/15/6	0.647	0.039		0.043	2.1 (1.0 to 4.3)		

Continuous values are shown as mean ± SD. Categorical variables are expressed as numbers
SMD Sternomental distance
[a]Comparisons of baseline (before the intervention) mouth aperture, SMD, and Mallampati score between the two groups using Student's t-test (mouth aperture and SMD) and linear-by-linear association (Mallampati score)
[b]Comparisons of mouth aperture, SMD, and Mallampati score after the intervention, between the two groups using Student's t-test (mouth aperture and SMD) and linear-by-linear association (Mallampati score)
[c]Comparison of the incidence of Mallampati score 1 after intervention between the two groups using chi-square test
[d]Comparisons of mouth aperture and SMD between before and after the intervention within the exercise group using paired t-test

Table 3 Intubation difficulty, intubation time, and soft tissue injury

	Control(n = 68)	Exercise(n = 70)	P [a]	Estimated difference (95% CI)	Odds ratio(95% CI)
Number of attempts	1.1 ± 0.4	1.1 ± 0.2	0.253	0.1(− 0.0 to 0.2)	
Additional operator	0 (0%)	0 (0%)			
Alternative techniques required	8 (11.8%)	4 (5.7%)	0.207		0.5 (0.1 to 1.6)
Cormack-Lehane grade (I/II/IIIa/IIIb)	42/20/2/4	45/19/3/3	0.746		
Increased lifting force	28 (41.2%)	17 (24.3%)	0.034		0.5 (0.2 to 1.0)
Laryngeal pressure required	24 (35.3%)	13 (18.6%)	0.027		0.4 (0.2 to 0.9)
Vocal cord mobility (adduction)	2 (2.9%)	0 (0%)	0.241		
IDS	1.6 ± 2.1	1.0 ± 1.7	0.086	0.6(−0.1 to 1.2)	
IDS group (easy/slight difficulty/moderate to major difficulty)	31/31/6	44/23/3	0.112		
Intubation time (s)	18.8 ± 23.1	12.5 ± 5.4	0.032	6.3 (0.5 to 12.0)	
Soft tissue injury	14 (20.6%)	4 (5.7%)	0.009		0.2 (0.1 to 0.8)

Continuous values are shown as mean ± SD. Categorical variables are expressed as patient numbers (%) or numbers
IDS Intubation difficulty scale
[a]Comparisons between the two groups using Student's t-test (continuous variables), chi-square or Fisher's exact test (categorical variables), and linear-by-linear association (Cormack-Lehane grade)

enhanced Mallampati scores, as we had anticipated (Table 2). Strictly speaking, the mouth opening and SMD evaluated in our study are induced by active muscle contraction, and therefore, are different from the passive processes during the orotracheal intubation using direct laryngoscopy. However, improvement of joint flexibility and muscle stiffness by the exercise therapy led to a substantial treatment effect on the measured values (Table 2). The objective increase of mouth opening and neck extension seems to have influenced the clinical differences between the two groups (Table 3).

The IDS comprehensively scores intubation difficulty, because it combines 7 measurable variables (Fig. 2) [2, 22, 34]. In our study, the incidences of increased lifting force and laryngeal compression were lower in the exercise group than in the control group (Table 3). The enhanced joint range of motion and reduced muscle stiffness seem to induce the discrepancies. Conversely, the Cormack-Lehane grade did not differ between the two study groups. This suggests that comparable visualization could be obtained by increasing lifting force or laryngeal compression in the control group. The total IDS scores were also indistinguishable between the two groups (Table 3). However, the additional force and pressure necessary for patients in the control group increased intubation time and caused more frequent oropharyngeal soft tissue injury (Table 3). For the patients with a baseline Mallampati score III or IV, the pre-anesthetic intervention was associated with less intubation difficulty during anesthetic induction, which highlighted the value of the brief regimen (Table 4). The exercise intervention in our protocol was intended to increase the range of motion in jaw and neck joints by enhancing joint flexibility and reducing muscle stiffness, which seemed to be more effective for improving intubation conditions in the patients who had a relatively small mouth aperture size.

In this study, we excluded patients with temporomandibular joint disorders or cervical spine diseases. Unless active movement is impossible or would induce neurologic symptoms, patients at high risk for intubation difficulties should be able to manage the exercise and might benefit from this therapy, which would be clinically valuable. However, since this study was the first clinical trial demonstrating the effect of pre-anesthetic exercise, we excluded those patients to avoid conditions where proper stretching was not possible due to joint pain, and to maintain uniformity in the 5 min intervention. Long-time and steady exercise program might be more helpful

Table 4 Intubation difficulty among the patients with baseline Mallampati score III or IV

	Control (n = 28)	Exercise (n = 30)	P [a]
Cormack-Lehane grade (I/II/IIIa/IIIb)	11/12/2/3	19/9/0/2	0.098
IDS group (easy/slight difficulty/moderate to major difficulty)	8/15/5	19/9/2	0.029

Categorical variables are expressed as patient numbers
IDS Intubation difficulty scale
[a]Comparisons between the two groups using linear-by-linear association (Cormack-Lehane grade) and chi-square test (IDS group)

for this cohort. Further studies would be necessary to identify the effect of preoperative exercise regimen on intubation conditions in patients with an increased risk for difficult intubation.

Some limitations of this study should be mentioned. First, the IDS incorporates some subjective parameters: the perception of lifting force and the application of alternative techniques or laryngeal compression may vary among anesthesiologists. It was also proposed that the intubation difficulty should be evaluated with simple and objective parameters such as Cormack-Lehane grade and intubation time, rather than IDS [35]. However, in our protocol, the orotracheal intubation was performed by a single blinded anesthesiologist in each hospital to exclude any possible inter-assessor bias and increase the reliability of the IDS scoring. Furthermore, there was a significant difference in the intubation time between the control group and the exercise group. However, inter-rater variability still existed between the two hospitals. To minimize the bias, each investigator tried to perform every measurement or intervention uniformly and strictly according to the study protocol standardized in advance. Second, the duration from the end of exercise regimen to the anesthetic induction was not controlled uniformly. In order to maintain the blindness, the intervention was performed at the reception, not in the OR. The time for transportation to the operating room and preparation for general anesthesia was not strictly constant. However, the delay did not extend beyond 5 min in both hospitals, and the exercise significantly improved mouth opening and neck extension during anesthetic induction. In a previous report, simple stretching for less than 2 min alleviated passive hamstring stiffness for 20 min [12]. Third, Mallampati score, the primary outcome of the study, has been criticized for its low predictive value for difficult intubation [36–38]. However, we did not hypothesize that the pre-anesthetic regimen would reduce intubation difficulty, rather, we anticipated that the exercise therapy we describe would increase range of motions of mouth opening and neck mobility during the anesthetic induction, thereby possibly reducing intubation time and tissue injuries associated with intubation (Table 3). We utilized the Mallampati score to assess the clinical effects of the exercises over other simple lengths. Fourth, penlight examination might miss injuries in the deep hypopharyngeal or laryngeal structures. Although the appearance of bloody secretions in the oropharyngeal suction could help identify the injuries, this was also not an objective and accurate measurement. To reduce inter-rater variability and to maintain consistency of the test, a single blinded anesthesiologist in each hospital performed the examinations. Fifth, patients in our study showed a higher proportion of Mallampati score IV, compared to previous studies [39, 40]. No phonation during the measurement and the relatively small number of patients might have influenced the distribution of our findings. However, in previous research, the distribution of Mallampti scores also varied according to the patients' characteristics [41]; the most important outcome of this study was that the exercise regimen significantly changed it.

Conclusion

A 5 min pre-anesthetic exercise session facilitated mouth opening and neck extension during orotracheal intubation, improving intubation conditions and enabling faster intubation with less injury to oropharyngeal soft tissue. The clinical effect of the brief regimen seemed to be more significant in patients with higher Mallampati scores. Our results suggest that incorporation of such therapy into pre-operative procedures may be beneficial for patients. Patients undergoing general anesthesia can easily perform the simple exercise during the waiting time before anesthetic induction.

Abbreviations

ASA: American Society of Anesthesiologists; ISD: Intubation difficulty scale (IDS); SMD: Sternomental distance

Acknowledgements

The authors appreciate Dr. Ji Hun Jo, Pf. Jin-Hee Kim, and Pf. Jung-Hee Ryu of Seoul National University Bundang Hospital for their collecting and analyzing the data. Also, the authors thank Sunkyu Choi, MS, Medical Research Collaborating Center, Seoul National University Bundang Hospital, for his assistance in the statistical analysis.

Authors' contributions

Study design/planning, SYL, JWP; Study conduct, SIB, SHD, JWP; Data analysis, SYL, SIB, JWP; Data interpretation, JTS, JWP; Drafting of manuscript, SYL, SIB; Revising of manuscript: SHD, JTS, JWP. All authors have read and approved the manuscript.

Author details

[1]Department of Anesthesiology and Pain Medicine, ThanQ Seoul Thyroid-Head & Neck Surgery Center, Seoul, South Korea. [2]Department of Anesthesiology and Pain Medicine, Jinju Gyeongsang National University Hospital, Jinju, South Korea. [3]Department of Anesthesiology and Pain Medicine, Seoul National University Bundang Hospital, 82 Gumi-ro, 173 Beon-gil, Bundang-gu, Seongnam, Gyeonggi-do 13620, Republic of Korea. [4]Department of Anesthesiology and Pain Medicine, Seoul National University College of Medicine, Seoul, South Korea. [5]Department of Anesthesiology and Pain Medicine, Gyeongsang National University College of Medicine, Institute of Health Sciences, Gyeongsang National University, Jinju, South Korea.

References

1. Calder I, Picard J, Chapman M, O'Sullivan C, Crockard HA. Mouth opening: a new angle. Anesthesiology. 2003;99(4):799–801.
2. Seo SH, Lee JG, Yu SB, Kim DS, Ryu SJ, Kim KH. Predictors of difficult intubation defined by the intubation difficulty scale (IDS): predictive value of 7 airway assessment factors. Korean J Anesthesiol. 2012;63(6):491–7.
3. Shiga T, Wajima Z, Inoue T, Sakamoto A. Predicting difficult intubation in apparently normal patients: a meta-analysis of bedside screening test performance. Anesthesiology. 2005;103(2):429–37.
4. Carlson JN, Hostler D, Guyette FX, Pinchalk M, Martin-Gill C. Derivation and validation of the Prehospital difficult airway IdentificationTool (PreDAIT): a predictive model for difficult intubation. West J Emerg Med. 2017;18(4):662–72.

5. Eberhart LH, Arndt C, Aust HJ, Kranke P, Zoremba M, Morin A. A simplified risk score to predict difficult intubation: development and prospective evaluation in 3763 patients. Eur J Anaesthesiol. 2010;27(11):935–40.
6. Hirabayashi Y, Seo N. Use of a new videolaryngoscope (airway scope) in the management of difficult airway. J Anesth. 2007;21(3):445–6.
7. Wong DT, Mehta A, Tam AD, Yau B, Wong J. A survey of Canadian anesthesiologists' preferences in difficult intubation and "cannot intubate, cannot ventilate" situations. Can J Anesth. 2014;61(8):717–26.
8. Roth D, Pace NL, Lee A, Hovhannisyan K, Warenits AM, Arrich J, Herkner H. Bedside tests for predicting difficult airways: an abridged Cochrane diagnostic test accuracy systematic review. Anaesthesia. 2019;74(7):915–28.
9. Mourao J, Moreira J, Barbosa J, Carvalho J, Tavares J. Soft tissue injuries after direct laryngoscopy. J Clin Anesth. 2015;27(8):668–71.
10. Ghabash MB, Matta MS, Mehanna CB. Prevention of dental trauma during endotracheal intubation. Anesth Analg. 1997;84(1):230–1.
11. Michelotti A, de Wijer A, Steenks M, Farella M. Home-exercise regimes for the management of non-specific temporomandibular disorders. J Oral Rehabil. 2005;32(11):779–85.
12. Whatman C, Knappstein A, Hume P. Acute changes in passive stiffness and range of motion post-stretching. Phys Ther Sport. 2006;7(4) 195–200.
13. Cronin J, Nash M, Whatman C. The acute effects of hamstring stretching and vibration on dynamic knee joint range of motion and jump performance. Phys Ther Sport. 2008;9(2):89–96.
14. Halbertsma JP, van Bolhuis AI, Goeken LN. Sport stretching: effect on passive muscle stiffness of short hamstrings. Arch Phys Med Rehabil. 1996; 77(7):688–92.
15. Eriksson Crommert M, Lacourpaille L, Heales LJ, Tucker K, Hug F. Massage induces an immediate, albeit short-term, reduction in muscle stiffness. Scand J Med Sci Sports. 2015;25(5):e490–6.
16. Weerapong P, Hume PA, Kolt GS. The mechanisms of massage and effects on performance, muscle recovery and injury prevention. Sports Med. 2005; 35(3):235–56.
17. Wiktorsson-Moller M, Oberg B, Ekstrand J, Gillquist J. Effects of warming up, massage, and stretching on range of motion and muscle strength in the lower extremity. Am J Sports Med. 1983;11(4):249–52.
18. Taniguchi K, Shinohara M, Nozaki S, Katayose M. Acute decrease in the stiffness of resting muscle belly due to static stretching. Scand J Med Sci Spor. 2015;25(1):32–40.
19. Samsoon GL, Young JR. Difficult tracheal intubation: a retrospective study. Anaesthesia. 1987;42(5):487–90.
20. Takahata O, Kubota M, Mamiya K, Akama Y, Nozaka T, Matsumoto H, Ogawa H. The efficacy of the "BURP" maneuver during a difficult laryngoscopy. Anesth Analg. 1997;84(2):419–21.
21. Frerk C, Mitchell VS, McNarry AF, Mendonca C, Bhagrath R, Patel A, O'Sullivan EP, Woodall NM, Ahmad I. Difficult airway society intubation guidelines working g: difficult airway society 2015 guidelines for management of unanticipated difficult intubation in adults. Br J Anaesth. 2015;115(6):827–48.
22. Adnet F, Borron SW, Racine SX, Clemessy JL, Fournier JL, Plaisance P, Lapandry C. The intubation difficulty scale (IDS): proposal and evaluation of a new score characterizing the complexity of endotracheal intubation. Anesthesiology. 1997;87(6):1290–7.
23. Eshraghi Y, Nasr V, Parra-Sanchez I, Van Duren A, Botham M, Santoscoy T, Sessler DI. An evaluation of a zero-heat-flux cutaneous thermometer in cardiac surgical patients. Anesth Analg. 2014;119(3):543–9.
24. Mallampati SR, Gatt SP, Gugino LD, Desai SP, Waraksa B, Freiberger D, Liu PL. A clinical sign to predict difficult tracheal intubation: a prospective study. Can Anaesth Soc J. 1985;32(4):429–34.
25. Aoki O, Tsumura N, Kimura A, Okuyama S, Takikawa S, Hirata S. Home stretching exercise is effective for improving knee range of motion and gait in patients with knee osteoarthritis. J Phys Ther Sci. 2009;21(2):113–9.
26. Bennell KL, Hinman RS. A review of the clinical evidence for exercise in osteoarthritis of the hip and knee. J Sci Med Sport. 2011;14(1):4–9.
27. Minor MA, Hewett JE, Webel RR, Anderson SK, Kay DR. Efficacy of physical conditioning exercise in patients with rheumatoid arthritis and osteoarthritis. Arthritis Rheum. 1989;32(11):1396–405.
28. Leivseth G, Torstensson J, Reikeras O. Effect of passive muscle stretching in osteoarthritis of the hip. Clin Sci. 1989;76(1):113–7.
29. Goyal S, Kothari N, Chaudhary D, Verma S, Bihani P, Rodha MS. Reversal agents: do we need to administer with neuromuscular monitoring - an observational study. Indian J Anaesth. 2018;62(3):219–24.
30. Dompier TP, Denegar CR, Buckley WE, Miller SJ, Hertel J, Sebastianelli WJ. The effect of general anesthesia on passive-knee-extension range of motion. J Sport Rehabil. 2001;10(4):257–66.
31. Alnaqeeb MA, Al Zaid NS, Goldspink G. Connective tissue changes and physical properties of developing and ageing skeletal muscle. J Anat. 1984; 139(Pt 4):677–89.
32. Brandenburg JE, Eby SF, Song P, Zhao H, Brault JS, Chen S, An KN. Ultrasound elastography: the new frontier in direct measurement of muscle stiffness. Arch Phys Med Rehabil. 2014;95(11):2207–19.
33. Witzmann FA, Kim DH, Fitts RH. Hindlimb immobilization: length-tension and contractile properties of skeletal muscle. J Appl Physiol Respir Environ Exerc Physiol. 1982;53(2):335–45.
34. K Nasa V, S Kamath S. Risk factors assessment of the difficult intubation using intubation difficulty scale (IDS). J Clin Diagn Res. 2014;8(7):GC01–3.
35. Sgalambro F. Proposal of a simplified intubation difficulty scale for comparing techniques and devices. BJA: Br J Anaesth. 2016;117(eLetters Supplement). https://doi.org/10.1093/bja/el_13469.
36. Khan ZH, Kashfi A, Ebrahimkhani E. A comparison of the upper lip bite test (a simple new technique) with modified Mallampati classification in predicting difficulty in endotracheal intubation: a prospective blinded study. Anesth Analg. 2003;96(2):595–9 table of contents.
37. Oates JD, Macleod AD, Oates PD, Pearsall FJ, Howie JC, Murray GD. Comparison of two methods for predicting difficult intubation. Br J Anaesth. 1991;66(3):305–9.
38. Adamus M, Fritscherova S, Hrabalek L, Gabrhelik T, Zapletalova J, Janout V. Mallampati test as a predictor of laryngoscopic view. Biomed Pap Med Fac Univ Palacky Olomouc Czech Repub. 2010;154(4):339–43.
39. Pinto J, Cordeiro L, Pereira C, Gama R, Fernandes HL, Assuncao J. Predicting difficult laryngoscopy using ultrasound measurement of distance from skin to epiglottis. J Crit Care. 2016;33:26–31.
40. Ambesh SP, Singh N, Rao PB, Gupta D, Singh PK, Singh U. A combination of the modified Mallampati score, thyromental distance, anatomical abnormality, and cervical mobility (M-TAC) predicts difficult laryngoscopy better than Mallampati classification. Acta Anaesthesiol Taiwanica. 2013; 51(2):58–62.
41. Pilkington S, Carli F, Dakin MJ, Romney M, De Witt KA, Dore CJ, Cormack RS. Increase in Mallampati score during pregnancy. Br J Anaesth. 1995;74(6): 638–42.

Permissions

All chapters in this book were first published by BioMed Central; hereby published with permission under the Creative Commons Attribution License or equivalent. Every chapter published in this book has been scrutinized by our experts. Their significance has been extensively debated. The topics covered herein carry significant findings which will fuel the growth of the discipline. They may even be implemented as practical applications or may be referred to as a beginning point for another development.

The contributors of this book come from diverse backgrounds, making this book a truly international effort. This book will bring forth new frontiers with its revolutionizing research information and detailed analysis of the nascent developments around the world.

We would like to thank all the contributing authors for lending their expertise to make the book truly unique. They have played a crucial role in the development of this book. Without their invaluable contributions this book wouldn't have been possible. They have made vital efforts to compile up to date information on the varied aspects of this subject to make this book a valuable addition to the collection of many professionals and students.

This book was conceptualized with the vision of imparting up-to-date information and advanced data in this field. To ensure the same, a matchless editorial board was set up. Every individual on the board went through rigorous rounds of assessment to prove their worth. After which they invested a large part of their time researching and compiling the most relevant data for our readers.

The editorial board has been involved in producing this book since its inception. They have spent rigorous hours researching and exploring the diverse topics which have resulted in the successful publishing of this book. They have passed on their knowledge of decades through this book. To expedite this challenging task, the publisher supported the team at every step. A small team of assistant editors was also appointed to further simplify the editing procedure and attain best results for the readers.

Apart from the editorial board, the designing team has also invested a significant amount of their time in understanding the subject and creating the most relevant covers. They scrutinized every image to scout for the most suitable representation of the subject and create an appropriate cover for the book.

The publishing team has been an ardent support to the editorial, designing and production team. Their endless efforts to recruit the best for this project, has resulted in the accomplishment of this book. They are a veteran in the field of academics and their pool of knowledge is as vast as their experience in printing. Their expertise and guidance has proved useful at every step. Their uncompromising quality standards have made this book an exceptional effort. Their encouragement from time to time has been an inspiration for everyone.

The publisher and the editorial board hope that this book will prove to be a valuable piece of knowledge for researchers, students, practitioners and scholars across the globe.

List of Contributors

Sanghee Park, Keunbae Yook, Kyung Yeon Yoo, Jeong Il Choi, Hong-Beom Bae and Youngwook You
Department of Anesthesiology and Pain Medicine, Chonnam National University Medical School and Hospital, 42 Jebong-ro, Dong-gu, Gwangju 61469, South Korea

Baoyuan Jin and Seongtae Jeong
Department of Anesthesiology and Pain Medicine, Chonnam National University Medical School and Hospital, 42 Jebong-ro, Dong-gu, Gwangju 61469, South Korea
The Brain Korea 21 Project Center for Biomedical Human Resources, Chonnam National University, Gwangju, South Korea

Amanda S. Deis and Michael P. Schnetz
Department of Anesthesiology & Perioperative Medicine, University of Pittsburgh Medical Center, Pittsburgh, USA

James W. Ibinson
Department of Anesthesiology & Perioperative Medicine, University of Pittsburgh School of Medicine, 3459 Fifth Avenue, UPMC Montefiore, Suite 467, Pittsburgh, PA 15213, USA
Clinical and Translational Science Institute, University of Pittsburgh, Pittsburgh, USA
Department of Anesthesiology, Surgical Service Line, Veterans Affairs Pittsburgh Healthcare System, Pittsburgh, USA

Keith M. Vogt
Department of Anesthesiology & Perioperative Medicine, University of Pittsburgh School of Medicine, 3459 Fifth Avenue, UPMC Montefiore, Suite 467, Pittsburgh, PA 15213, USA
Department of Bioengineering, Swanson School of Engineering, University of Pittsburgh, Pittsburgh, USA
Center for the Neural Basis of Cognition, Pittsburgh, USA

Li-Qin Li, Cong Wang, Mei-Dan Fang, Hong-Yu Xu, Hong-Liu Lu and Hou-Zhong Zhang
Department of Anesthesiology, Jilin University Second Hospital, No. 218 Ziqiang street, Changchun, Jilin 130021, People's Republic of China

Jipeng Song
Graduate School of Peking Union Medical College, Chinese Academy of Medical Sciences, Beijing 100730, People's Republic of China

Ping Yi
Department of Spine Surgery, China-Japan Friendship Hospital, No. 2 Yinghua Dongjie, Hepingli, Chaoyang District, Beijing 100029, People's Republic of China

Zhencheng Xiong and Mingsheng Tan
Graduate School of Peking Union Medical College, Chinese Academy of Medical Sciences, Beijing 100730, People's Republic of China
Department of Spine Surgery, China-Japan Friendship Hospital, No. 2 Yinghua Dongjie, Hepingli, Chaoyang District, Beijing 100029, People's Republic of China

Yun'an Song
Department of Anesthesiology, Shanghai Children's Medical Center, Shanghai Jiao Tong University School of Medicine & National Children's Medical Center (Shanghai), 1678 Dongfang Road, Shanghai 200127, China

Kan Zhang, Lei Wu, Meihua Cai, Mazhong Zhang and Jijian Zheng
Department of Anesthesiology, Shanghai Children's Medical Center, Shanghai Jiao Tong University School of Medicine & National Children's Medical Center (Shanghai), 1678 Dongfang Road, Shanghai 200127, China
Pediatric Clinical Pharmacology Laboratory, Shanghai Children's Medical Center, Shanghai Jiao Tong University School of Medicine & National Children's Medical Center (Shanghai), Shanghai, China

Siyuan Wang
Department of Anesthesiology, 3201 Hospital, Xi'an Jiaotong University Health Science Center, Hanzhong, Shaanxi Province, China

Junko Nakahira, Shoko Nakano and Toshiaki Minami
Department of Anesthesiology, Osaka Medical College, 2-7 Daigaku-machi, Takatsuki, Osaka 569-8686, Japan

Marianna Juhász, Levente Molnár and Csilla Molnár
Faculty of Medicine, Department of Anesthesiology and Intensive Care, University of Debrecen, Nagyerdei krt. 98, Debrecen, Hungary

Dénes Páll
Faculty of Medicine, Department of Medicine, University of Debrecen, Debrecen, Hungary

Béla Fülesdi and Tamás Végh
Faculty of Medicine, Department of Anesthesiology and Intensive Care, University of Debrecen, Nagyerdei krt. 98, Debrecen, Hungary
Hungarian Center, Outcomes Research Consortium, Cleveland, USA

Xiao-Xia Wang, Xiao-Lan Sha, Yu-Lan Li, Chun-Lan Li, Su-Heng Chen and Jing-Jing Wang
Department of Anesthesiology, First Hospital of Lanzhou University, Lanzhou 730000, People's Republic of China

Zhengyuan Xia
Department of Anesthesiology, The University of Hong Kong, Hong Kong 999077, People's Republic of China
Department of Anesthesiology, Affiliated Hospital of Guangdong Medical University, Zhanjiang 524000, People's Republic of China

Zsolt Kovács
Savaria Department of Biology, ELTE Eötvös Loránd University, Savaria University Centre, Szombathely, Hungary

Brigitta Brunner
Savaria Department of Biology, ELTE Eötvös Loránd University, Savaria University Centre, Szombathely, Hungary
Institute of Biology, University of Pécs, Pécs, Hungary

Dominic P. D'Agostino
Department of Molecular Pharmacology and Physiology, Laboratory of Metabolic Medicine, Morsani College of Medicine, University of South Florida, Tampa, FL, USA
Institute for Human and Machine Cognition, Ocala, FL, USA

Csilla Ari
Department of Psychology, Hyperbaric Neuroscience Research Laboratory, University of South Florida, 4202 E. Fowler Ave, PCD 3127, Tampa, FL 33620, USA

Rui Ma and Yu Wei
Department of Anesthesiology, international Peace Maternal and Child Health Hospital, School of Medicine, Shanghai Key Laboratory of Embryo Original Disease, Shanghai Municipal Key Clinical Specialty, Shanghai Jiao Tong University, Huashan Rd. 1961, Shanghai 200030, China

Zifeng Xu
Department of Anesthesiology, international Peace Maternal and Child Health Hospital, School of Medicine, Shanghai Key Laboratory of Embryo Original Disease, Shanghai Municipal Key Clinical Specialty, Shanghai Jiao Tong University, Huashan Rd. 1961, Shanghai 200030, China
Shanghai Key Laboratory of Embryo Original Diseases, Shanghai, China

Wei Yu Yao and Shi Yang Li
Department of Anesthesiology and Perioperative Medicine, Quanzhou Macare Women's Hospital, Quanzhou, Fujian Province, China

Yong Jin Yuan
Department of Anesthesiology, Qinghai University Affiliated Hospital, Xining, Qinghai Province, China

Hon Sen Tan
Department of Women's Anaesthesia, KK Women's and Children's Hospital, 100 Bukit Timah Road, Singapore, Singapore

Nian-Lin R. Han
Division of Clinical Support Services, KK Women's and Children's Hospital, 100 Bukit Timah Road, Singapore, Singapore

Rehena Sultana
Center for Quantitative Medicine, Duke-NUS Medical School, 8 College Road, Singapore, Singapore

Pryseley N. Assam
Singapore Clinical Research Institute, 31 Biopolis Way, Singapore, Singapore

Alex Tiong-Heng Sia and Ban Leong Sng
Department of Women's Anaesthesia, KK Women's and Children's Hospital, 100 Bukit Timah Road, Singapore, Singapore
Anaesthesiology and Perioperative Sciences Academic Clinical Program, Duke-NUS Medical School, 8 College Road, Singapore, Singapore

Jinwei Xie, Jun Ma, Qiang Huang and Fuxing Pei
Department of Orthopaedic Surgery, National Clinical Research Center for Geriatrics, West China Hospital, Sichuan University, No. 37 Guoxue Road, Chengdu, Sichuan Province 610041, People's Republic of China

Yingchun Cai
Department of Orthopaedic Surgery, National Clinical Research Center for Geriatrics, West China Hospital, Sichuan University, No. 37 Guoxue Road, Chengdu, Sichuan Province 610041, People's Republic of China
Department of Orthopaedic Surgery, The First Affiliated Hospital of Zhengzhou University, No. 1 East Jianshe Road, Zhengzhou 450052, People's Republic of China

Chengwei Yang, Sheng Wang, Mingming Han, Song Wang, Fang Kang, Xiang Huang and Juan Li
Department of Anesthesiology, The First Affiliated Hospital of USTC, Division of Life Sciences and Medicine, University of Science and Technology of China, Hefei 230036, China

Yuanyuan Feng
Department of Hematology, The First Affiliated Hospital of USTC, Division of Life Sciences and Medicine, University of Science and Technology of China, Hefei 230031, China

Teng-Fei Wan
Department of First Cadre Ward, the General Hospital of Northern Theater Command, No. 83 Wenhua Street, Shenyang 110016, Liaoning, China

Rui Xu
Department of Neurology, Xinqiao Hospital, the Army Medical University, NO. 183 Xinqiao mian street, Chongqing 400037, China

Zi-Ai Zhao, Yan Lv, Hui-Sheng Chen and Liang Liu
Department of Neurology, the General Hospital of Northern Theater Command , No. 83 Wenhua Street, Shenyang 110016, Liaoning, China

Arpa Chutipongtanate, Sasichol Prukviwat, Nakarin Kamanee and Wichai Ittichaikulthol
Department of Anesthesiology, Faculty of Medicine Ramathibodi Hospital, Mahidol University, Bangkok 10400, Thailand

Nutkridta Pongsakul
Pediatric Translational Research Unit, Department of Pediatrics, Faculty of Medicine Ramathibodi Hospital, Mahidol University, Bangkok 10400, Thailand

Supanart Srisala
Research Center, Faculty of Medicine Ramathibodi Hospital, Mahidol University, Bangkok 10400, Thailand

Nuttapon Arpornsujaritkun and Goragoch Gesprasert
Vascular and Transplantation Unit, Department of Surgery, Faculty of Medicine Ramathibodi Hospital, Mahidol University, Bangkok 10400, Thailand

Nopporn Apiwattanakul
Division of Infectious Disease, Department of Pediatrics, Faculty of Medicine Ramathibodi Hospital, Mahidol University, Bangkok 10400, Thailand

Suradej Hongeng
Division of Hematology and Oncology, Department of Pediatrics, Faculty of Medicine Ramathibodi Hospital, Mahidol University, Bangkok 10400, Thailand

Vasant Sumethkul
Division of Nephrology, Department of Medicine, Faculty of Medicine Ramathibodi Hospital, Mahidol University, Bangkok 10400, Thailand

Somchai Chutipongtanate
Pediatric Translational Research Unit, Department of Pediatrics, Faculty of Medicine Ramathibodi Hospital, Mahidol University, Bangkok 10400, Thailand
Department of Clinical Epidemiology and Biostatistics, Faculty of Medicine Ramathibodi Hospital, Mahidol University, Bangkok 10400, Thailand

Hong Chen, Bin Wang, Qin Li, Juan Zhou, Rui Li and Ye Zhang
Department of Anesthesiology and Perioperative Medicine, The Second Affiliated Hospital of Anhui Medical University, 678# Furong Road, Hefei, Anhui Province, China

Harry Magunia, Anne Jordanow, Marius Keller and Peter Rosenberger
Department of Anaesthesiology and Intensive Care Medicine, University Hospital Tübingen, Eberhard-Karls-University Tübingen, Hoppe-Seyler-Str. 3, 72076 Tübingen, Germany

Martina Nowak-Machen
Department of Anaesthesiology and Intensive Care Medicine, University Hospital Tübingen, Eberhard-Karls-University Tübingen, Hoppe-Seyler-Str. 3, 72076 Tübingen, Germany
Department of Anesthesia and Intensive Care Medicine, Klinikum Ingolstadt, Krumenauerstr. 25, 85049 Ingolstadt, Germany

Xinxun Zheng, Yuming Tan, Yuan Gao and Zhiheng Liu
Department of Anesthesiology, Shenzhen Second People's Hospital, The First Affiliated Hospital of Shenzhen University, Shenzhen 518000, China

Zhen Tian, Bei Hu, Min Miao, Lulu Zhang, Lin Wang and Bin Chen
Department of Anesthesiology, Suqian People's Hospital of Nanjing Drum-tower Hospital Group, Suqian 223800, China
Department of Anesthesiology, The Affiliated Suqian Hospital of Xuzhou Medical University, Suqian 223800, China

Robert G. Hahn
Research Unit, Södertälje Hospital, 152 86 Södertälje, Sweden
Karolinska Institutet at Danderyds Hospital (KIDS), Stockholm, Sweden

Janis Nemme
Department of Anesthesiology and Intensive Care, Riga Stradins University, Riga, Latvia
Paul Stradins Clinical University Hospital, Riga, Latvia

Zemedu Aweke, Fetene Seyoum and Derartu Neme Doba
Department of Anesthesia, College of Medicine and Health Sciences, Dilla University, Dilla, Ethiopia

Tewoderos Shitemaw
Department of Anesthesia, Kotebe Metropolitan University, Menelik II Medical & Health Science College, Addis Ababa, Ethiopia

G. Simpson
Metropolitan Department of Anaesthetics, Critical Care and Pain Management, University of KwaZulu-Natal, 4 Montrose, Hillcrest, Pietermaritzburg, South Africa

R. N. Rodseth
Metropolitan Department of Anaesthetics, Critical Care and Pain Management, University of KwaZulu-Natal, 4 Montrose, Hillcrest, Pietermaritzburg, South Africa
Jones, Bhagwan and Partners, Specialist Anaesthetists, Pietermaritzburg, South Africa

Hye Won Shin, Yoo Kyung Jang, Hae Sun You, Hyub Huh, Seung Uk Choi and Ji Su Hong
Department of Anesthesiology and Pain Medicine, Korea University Anam Hospital, College of Medicine, Korea University, Goryodae-ro 73, Seongbuk-gu, 02841 Seoul, Republic of Korea

Hyun Jung Kim
Department of Anesthesiology and Pain Medicine, Ewha University Magok Hospital, College of Medicine, Ewha University, Seoul, Republic of Korea

Yoon Ji Choi
Department of Anesthesiology and Pain Medicine, Korea University Ansan Hospital, College of Medicine, Korea University, Gyeonggi-do, Republic of Korea

Xiaorong Yin, Xiaoqi Zeng, Ting Wang, Binbin Dong, Menghang Wu and Anna Jia
Department of Anesthesiology, West China Hospital, Sichuan University/ West China School of Nursing, Sichuan University, Chengdu, Sichuan Province 610041, People's Republic of China

Ling Ye
Department of Pain Management, West China Hospital, Sichuan University, Chengdu, Sichuan Province 610041, People's Republic of China

Yinan Li, Hansheng Liang and Yi Feng
Department of Anesthesia, Peking University People's Hospital, Beijing 100044, China

Sue Young Lee
Department of Anesthesiology and Pain Medicine, ThanQ Seoul Thyroid-Head & Neck Surgery Center, Seoul, South Korea

Sung Il Bae
Department of Anesthesiology and Pain Medicine, Jinju Gyeongsang National University Hospital, Jinju, South Korea

Jin-Woo Park
Department of Anesthesiology and PainMedicine, Seoul National University Bundang Hospital, 82 Gumi-ro, 173 Beon-gil, Bundang-gu, Seongnam, Gyeonggi-do 13620, Republic of Korea

Sang-Hwan Do
Department of Anesthesiology and PainMedicine, Seoul National University Bundang Hospital, 82 Gumi-ro, 173 Beon-gil, Bundang-gu, Seongnam, Gyeonggi-do 13620, Republic of Korea
Department of Anesthesiology and Pain Medicine, Seoul National University College of Medicine, Seoul, South Korea

Ju-Tae Sohn
Department of Anesthesiology and Pain Medicine, Jinju Gyeongsang National University Hospital, Jinju, South Korea
Department of Anesthesiology and Pain Medicine, Gyeongsang National University College of Medicine, Institute of Health Sciences, Gyeongsang National University, Jinju, South Korea

Index

www.ingramcontent.com/pod-product-compliance
Lightning Source LLC
LaVergne TN
LVHW060553210926
848485LV00005B/1307